Pathology - From Classics to Innovations

Edited by Ilze Strumfa and Guntis Bahs

Published in London, United Kingdom

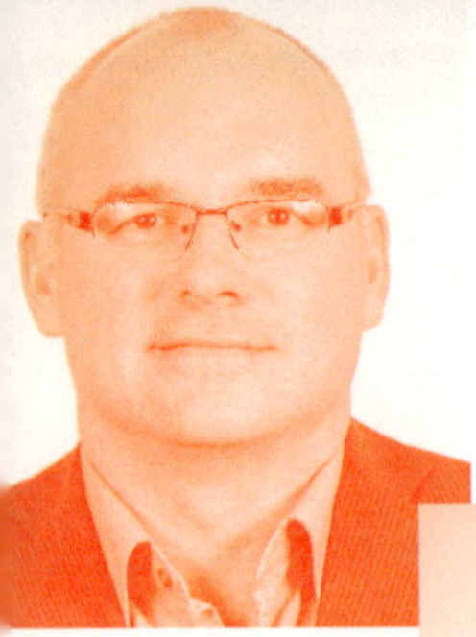
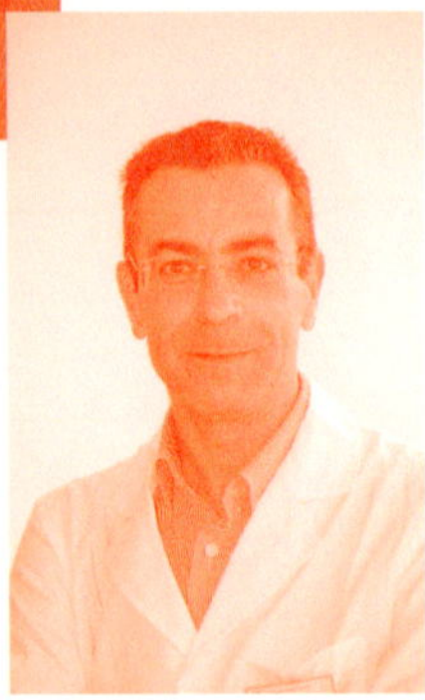
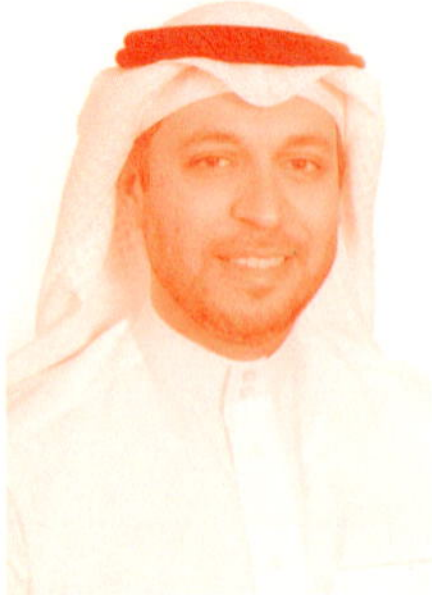
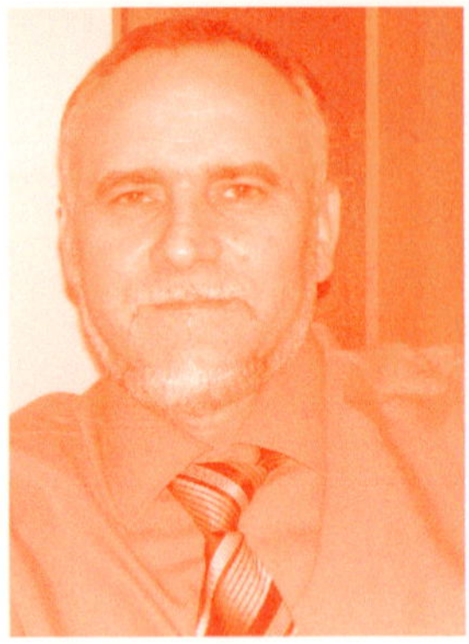
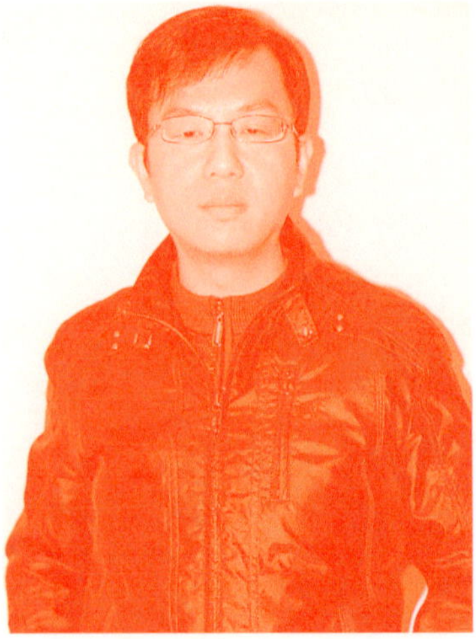
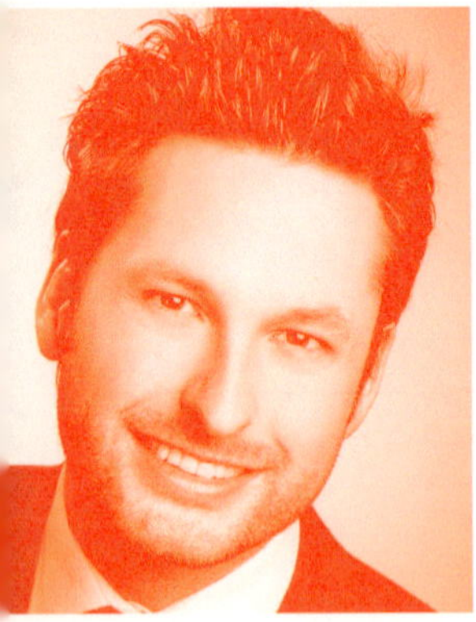
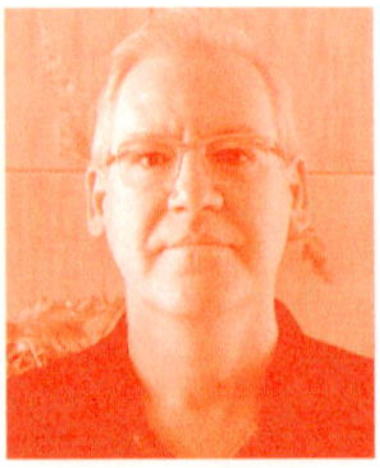

IntechOpen

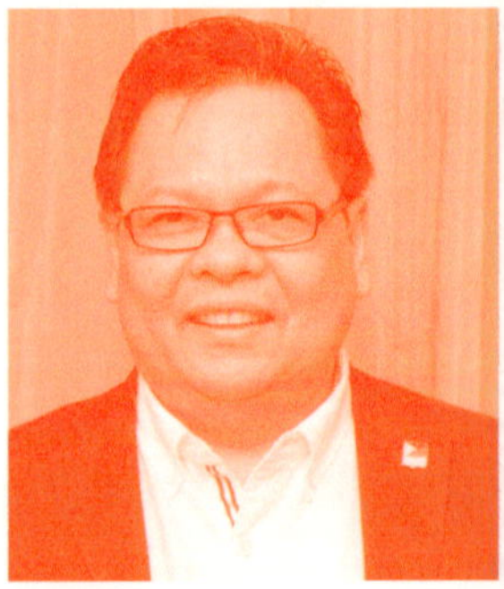
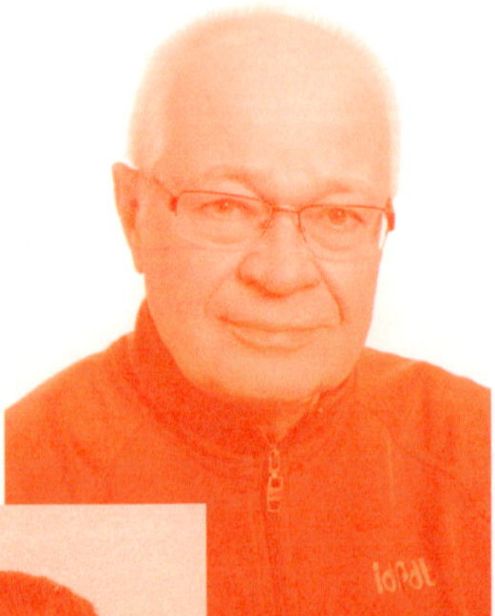
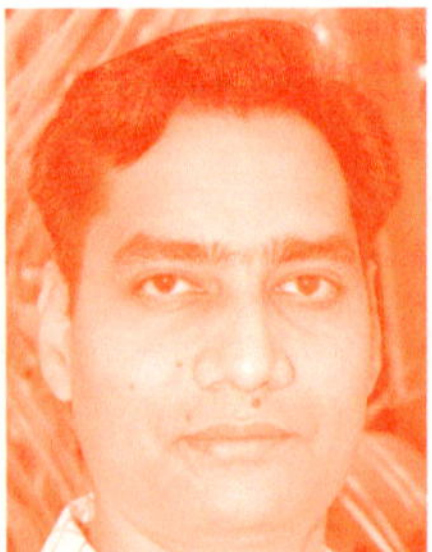
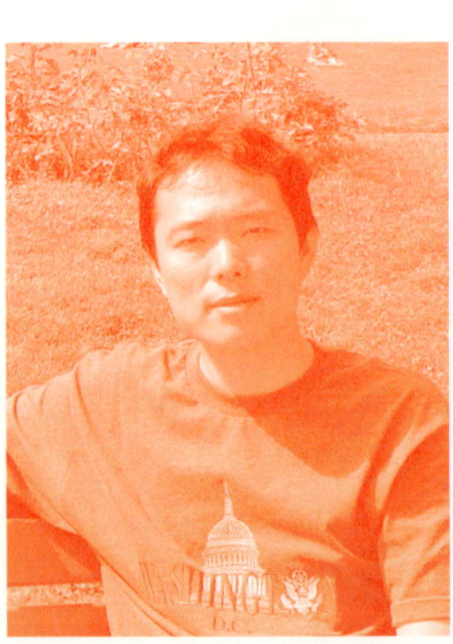
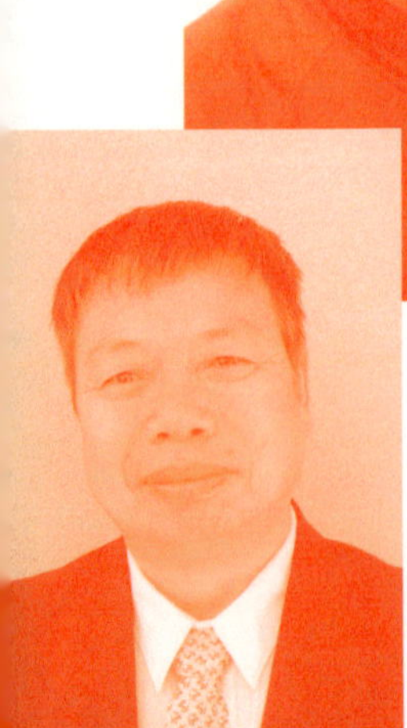
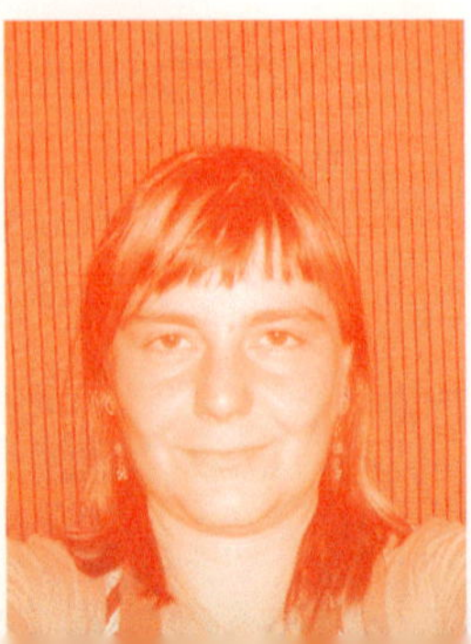

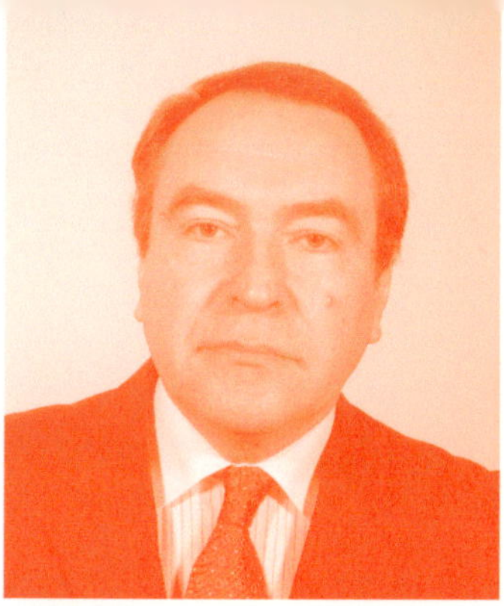
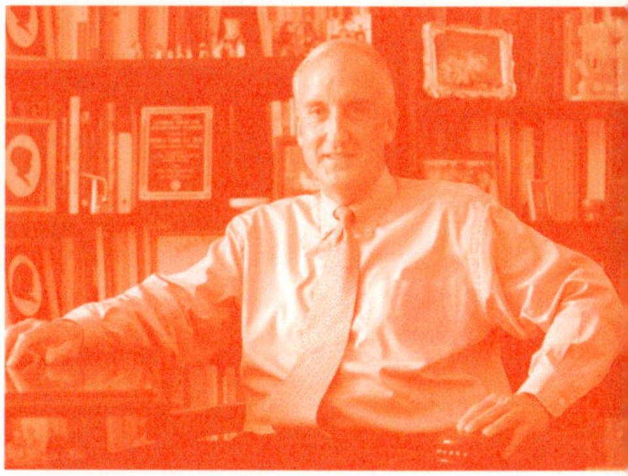
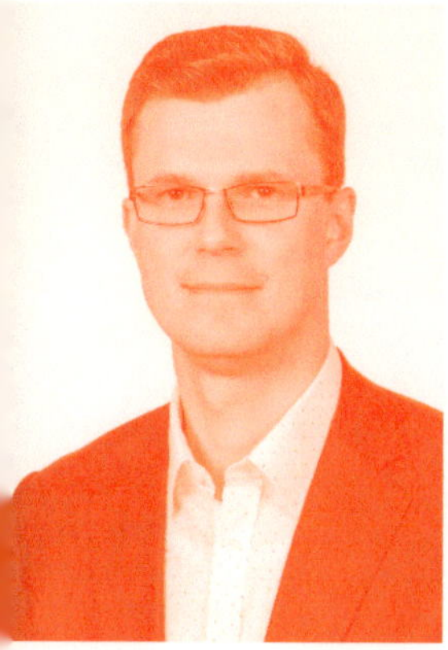
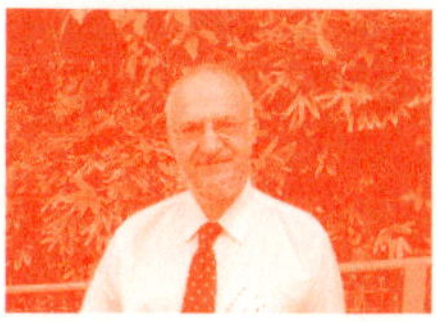
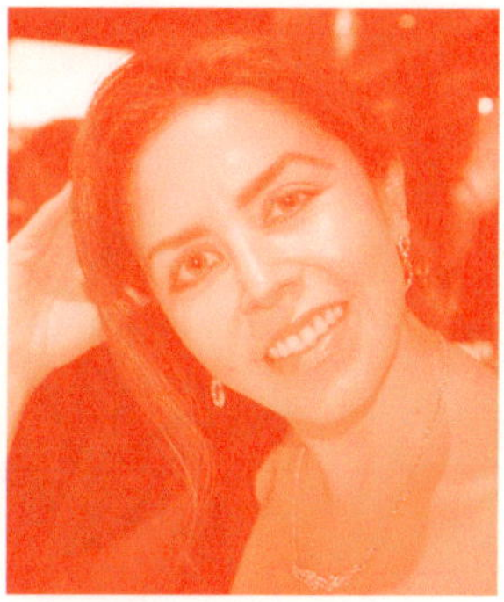

Supporting open minds since 2005

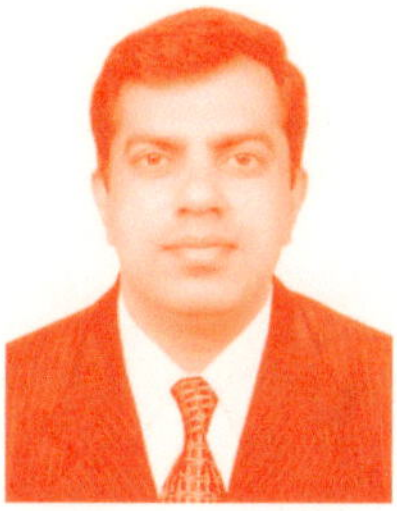
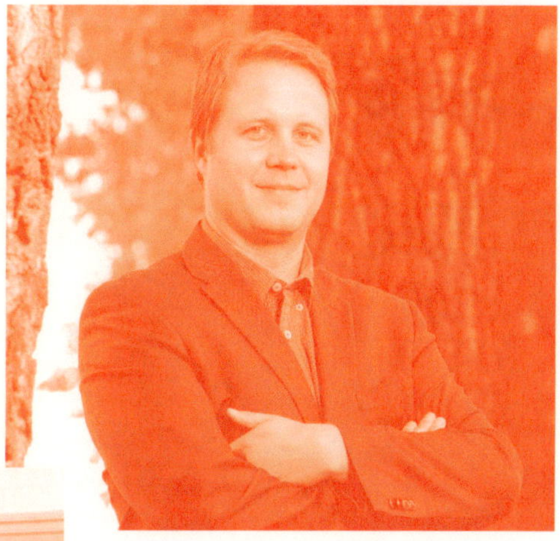
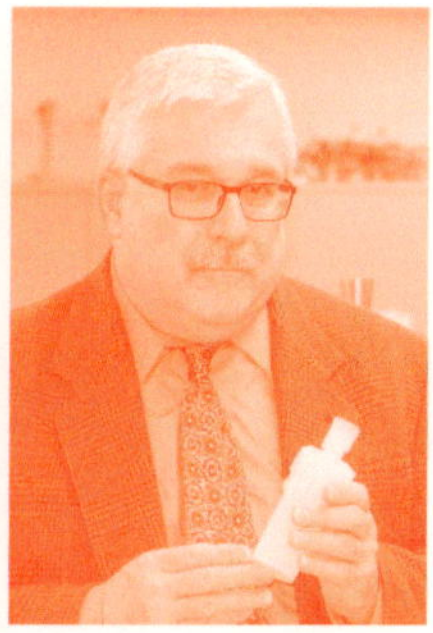
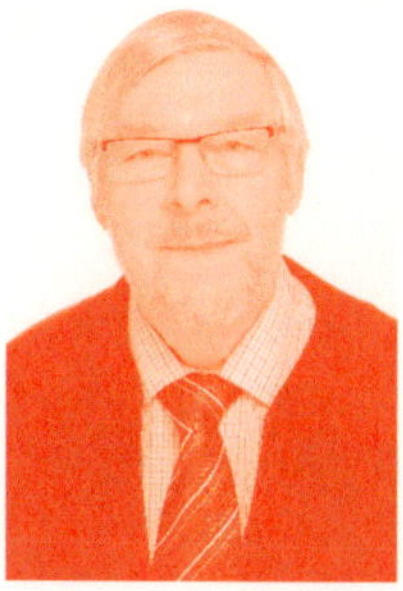
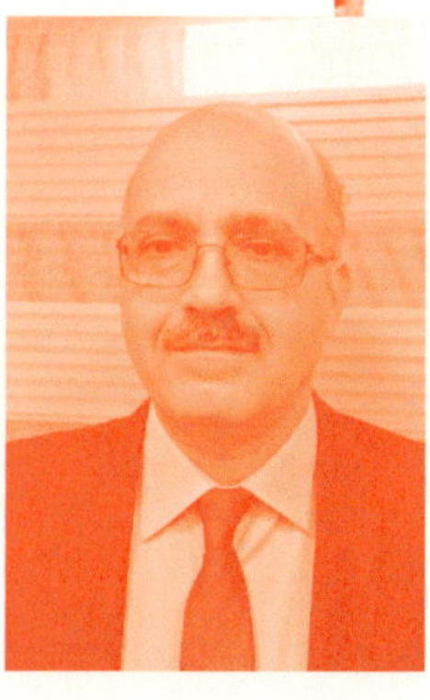
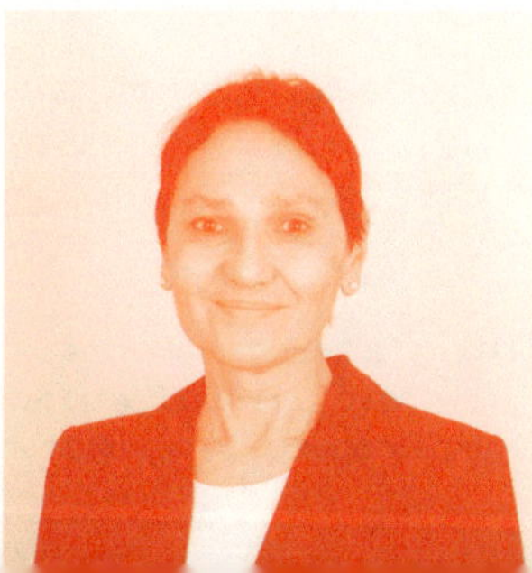
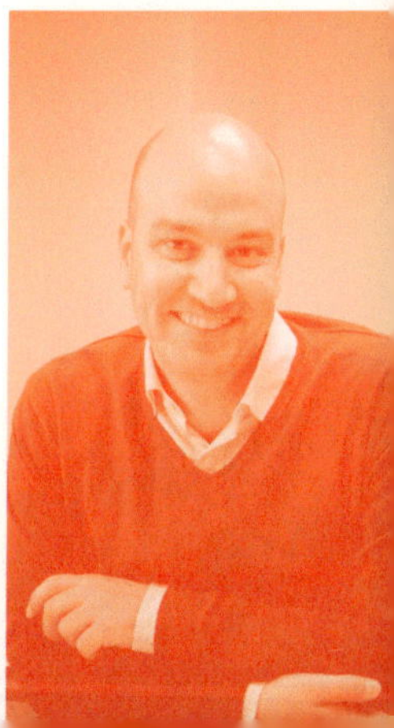

Pathology - From Classics to Innovations
http://dx.doi.org/10.5772/intechopen.87426
Edited by Ilze Strumfa and Guntis Bahs

Contributors
Joe Yeong, Siting Goh, Yue Da Chua, Yiyu Cai, Justina Lee, Meir Warman, Rona Bourla, Elchanan Zloczower, Monica Huszar, Stefania Scarpino, Umberto Malapelle, Rodrigo Vismari de Oliveira, Valeria Cecilia Denninghoff, Ruoyu Li, Junzhou Huang, Mehveş Ece Genç, Emine Nur Özdamar, Ruth L. Katz, Xin Ye, Xiao Zheng Yang, Roberta Carbone, Iris Barschack, Shawn Baldacchino, Rajani Singh

First published in London, United Kingdom, 2021 by IntechOpen
IntechOpen is the global imprint of INTECHOPEN LIMITED, registered in England and Wales, registration number: 11086078, 5 Princes Gate Court, London, SW7 2QJ, United Kingdom
Printed in Croatia

British Library Cataloguing-in-Publication Data
A catalogue record for this book is available from the British Library

Additional hard and PDF copies can be obtained from orders@intechopen.com

Pathology - From Classics to Innovations
Edited by Ilze Strumfa and Guntis Bahs
p. cm.
Print ISBN 978-1-83881-858-6
Online ISBN 978-1-83881-859-3
eBook (PDF) ISBN 978-1-83881-860-9

For EU product safety concerns:
IN TECH d.o.o., Prolaz Marije Krucifikse Kozulić 3, 51000 Rijeka, Croatia,
info@intechopen.com or visit our website at intechopen.com.

Meet the editors

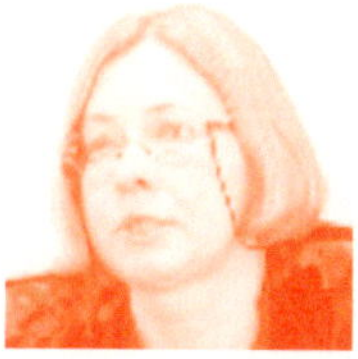

Professor Ilze Strumfa, MD, Ph.D., is an outstanding medical lecturer, actively involved in the research in pathology. She graduated from the Medical Academy of Latvia with distinction in 1998, underwent board certification in pathology in 2001, and received a Ph.D. in 2005. Currently, she is a professor and head of the Department of Pathology, Riga Stradins University (RSU), Latvia. Her twelve years of teaching experience have culminated with the RSU "Lecturer of the Year" Annual Award (2018), given to the most distinguished teachers. As the head of the Department of Pathology, she is leading a skilled, motivated team of teachers and scientists that have won awards such as Best Academic Unit (2011), Best Ph.D. Student (2012), and Best Digital Junior Teacher (2016). Prof. Strumfa is an author/co-author of more than 100 peer-reviewed journal articles and 16 chapters in scientific monographs and medical textbooks. She has been acting as the leading expert in several European and national research projects devoted to the development of diagnostic technologies, neuroendocrine and endocrine tumors, breast cancer, laboratory training in research, and tumor microenvironment. Her main research interests include morphological and molecular diagnostics and prognostic assessment of tumors as well as digital pathology and other innovations in pathology and cytology.

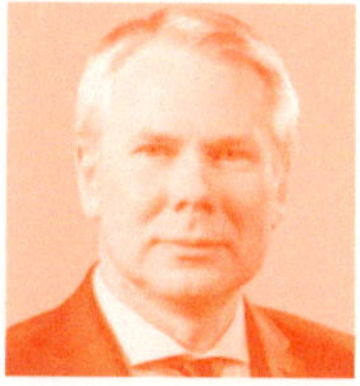

Professor Guntis Bahs, MD, Ph.D., is a dedicated physician who actively translates his excellent clinical experience into research, medical education, and administrative work. He has published numerous peer-reviewed scientific articles and book chapters on biomarkers in the prognosis and pathogenesis of cardiovascular and pulmonary diseases, also addressing adiposity and metabolic and biochemical events in human disease. Prof. Bahs is the head of study courses in pulmonology and cardiovascular diseases, as well as the supervisor of the Medicine and Paediatrics study programs in Riga Stradins University (RSU), Latvia. He has served as the dean of the Medical Faculty and is currently the vice-rector for Health Studies at RSU.

Contents

Preface

Pathology is a diagnostic medical specialty dealing with the evaluation of tissues and body fluids to reach a diagnosis and predict prognosis or response to treatment. A biopsy is a well-known "gold standard" in the diagnostics of most cancers, and its value extends beyond oncology to other subspecialties of medicine. Currently, significant innovations in pathology have pushed the field towards less invasive and more exact diagnostic approaches, going deeper – from the tissues to the molecules. In this journey, microscopes and human minds are being supported by digital pathology and artificial intelligence.

This book is a collection of original peer-reviewed studies and review articles on recent advances in pathology: from classic surgical pathology and application of microscopic tissue evaluation in anatomic studies to immunohistochemistry, molecular pathology, liquid biopsy, and digital pathology.

The book is divided into five sections: "Classic Surgical Pathology and Anatomic Studies," "Molecular Pathology," "Digital Pathology," "Liquid Biopsy," and "Pathophysiology."

The "Classic Surgical Pathology and Anatomic Studies" section includes a brilliant review in Chapter 1 on antrochoanal polyp, a benign unilateral polyp originating from the maxillary sinus and expanding through the accessory or natural ostia into the nasal cavity and choanae. The authors link pathogenesis and histology to clinical features and treatment in a comprehensive and interesting narrative. Regarding anatomic studies, Chapter 2 on tracking cutaneous nerves of the thigh is remarkable not only by its direct findings and meticulous performance but even more so by the ground-breaking technology that can be used in future studies.

Diagnostics of breast cancer represents the brightest, paradigm-setting example of the clinical application of molecular pathology. Therefore, Chapter 3 in the "Molecular Pathology" section reviews advances in the molecular and immunohistochemical assessment of breast cancer. Along with the classic molecular subtypes of breast cancer, the author summarizes current views on the role of germline BRCA gene mutations, cancer stem cells, immunological features of breast cancer and its microenvironment, as well as the molecular events in advanced breast cancer. To further expand the discussion on molecular pathology, Chapter 4 describes the technological prerequisites of molecular testing, including methodological constraints in the work with formalin-fixed, paraffin-embedded tissues. Pre-analytical conditions, such as cold ischemia and tissue fixation, are discussed along with downstream technological steps, for example, tumour microdissection for tumour cell enrichment, PCR assays, and next-generation sequencing.

The "Digital Pathology" section includes two original studies. Chapter 5 presents a computer-based assessment of whole-slide digital pathological images. The authors have targeted the hot topic: how to achieve an objective assessment of very complex images in a reasonable time. They propose a two-stage, superpixel-based approach for the identification of regions of interest, explain the necessity for the innovations in the given point, describe the method, and provide its mathematical basis. Chapter 6 presents an approach to handling multiplex immunohistochemical data by using deep learning-based artificial intelligence methodology.

Liquid biopsy represents a spectrum of technologies for the molecular analysis of blood and other biological liquids (e.g., urine, saliva, tears, or others) to detect cell-free/tumour nucleic acids, exosomes, microRNAs, tumour-educated platelets, and circulating or free-floating tumour or foetal cells, depending on the clinical context. In contrast to classic tumour markers (e.g., prostate-specific antigen (PSA) or carcinoembryonic antigen (CEA)), liquid biopsy is distinguished by high specificity, as it provides genomic, proteomic, and cellular characteristics of the disease. The anticipated outstanding reliability of these tests has been reflected in the term itself: "liquid biopsy" is expected to be at least as informative as tissue biopsy, used as the gold standard in certain diagnostic fields, especially in oncology.

The advantages of liquid biopsy include a non-invasive approach that is patient-friendly, associated with low risk of complications, and technically feasible even in patients who are in serious general condition or affected by tumour or metastases that are not easily accessible by conventional tissue biopsy. The clinically simple application allows the repeated use of liquid biopsy resulting in real-time follow-up for the disease course. Liquid biopsy is also a much-awaited tool to overcome the limitations set by tumour heterogeneity upon conventional tissue biopsy representing only a small part of the whole tumour.

In this book, the "Liquid Biopsy" section (Chapters 7–9) includes extensive in-depth reviews, mainly focusing on circulating tumour DNA and circulating tumour cells; extracellular vesicles are also discussed. The clinical use of liquid biopsies is assessed, highlighting the manifold practical consequences in oncology, from screening and early diagnostics to selection of personalized treatment. The approval status of certain diagnostic tests and indications for their application are described, providing a practically useful general evaluation of the current situation in the field of liquid biopsy. Technological background, the mainstay of any laboratory analysis, is appropriately widely considered. In particular, a fluorescence in situ hybridization approach to detect circulating tumour cells represents an interesting and promising innovation.

In the "Pathophysiology" section, Chapter 10 on dopamine turnover concludes the book, emphasizing that pathology comprises not only morphology but also dynamic understanding of pathophysiological processes in disease.

The book was created by a truly global team of scientists including researchers from Israel, the United Kingdom, Italy, Singapore, Argentina, Brazil, China, the United States, India, and Turkey. We would like to thank sincerely all the authors for their excellent contributions.

We also express our sincere gratitude to the IntechOpen editorial team, especially Mrs. Mia Vulovic and Ms. Ana Simcic for their continuous support and professional help during the editorial process.

"Random discoveries only happen to prepared minds."
Blaise Pascal

Ilze Strumfa, MD, Ph.D. and Guntis Bahs, MD, Ph.D.
Professor,
Riga Stradiņš University,
Latvia

Section 1

Classic Surgical Pathology and Anatomic Studies

Chapter 1

Antrochoanal Polyp: Updated Clinical Approach, Histology Characteristics, Diagnosis and Treatment

Warman Meir, Rona Bourla, Monica Huszar and Elchanan Zloczower

Abstract

Antrochoanal polyp (ACP) is a benign unilateral polyp, originating from the maxillary sinus and expanding through the accessory or natural ostia into the nasal cavity and choanae. It has a 2: 1 male predominance and is more common in children and young adults. The exact pathophysiology is unclear, and it is thought to have less of the inflammatory reactions as opposed to typical bilateral nasal polyps which are commonly seen in diffused chronic rhinosinusitis. The presenting symptoms of ACP are unilateral nasal obstruction and rhinitis. Epistaxis, pain, and foul-smelling secretions are not typically seen and point towards a different etiology. Diagnosis is mainly clinical via endoscopic examination and supported by Computed tomography (CT) imaging. In CT images the three components of the polyp can be identified; an intramaxillary portion, intranasal and choanal components. Treatment is surgical, where Endoscopic sinus surgery (ESS) is the main technique used with other assisting approaches to reach the more challenging anterior and inferior areas of the maxillary sinus. Successful resection depends on complete removal of the intramaxillary component of the polyp to avoid polyp regrowth. The typical histologic characteristics are cyst formation, fibrosis and squamous metaplasia that are significantly more common in ACP than diffused nasal polyps.

Keywords: histoloy, Immunohistochemistry, antrochoanal polyp, nasal polyps

1. Introduction

Antrochoanal polyp (ACP) is a benign, unilateral polyp originating from the maxillary sinus, extending through the natural or accessory ostia into the nasal cavity. This finding is more common in children and young adults [1] with 2:1 male to female ratio. Its etiology is vague and varies from neoplasia to inflammatory polyp or cystic degeneration of intramaxillary retention cyst. The exact anatomic origin of ACP inside the maxillary sinus is not agreed upon in the literature. The medial and posterior walls are the most common origin sites [2, 3], but the polyp may grow from virtually any site inside the maxillary sinus. ACP exits the maxillary sinus through the accessory ostium in at least 70% of cases [4], which may explain why the polyp grows inferiorly and posteriorly into the nasopharynx. Recent publications show evidence that nearly all ACPs extend through the accessory ostium [2, 5]. The most common symptoms of ACP are nasal obstruction and anterior nasal discharge, while epistaxis and pain point towards a different etiology necessitating further workup. The treatment of choice for ACP is surgical resection [1]. While different surgical techniques were described in the past, endoscopic removal of both the intranasal and intramaxillary parts of the polyp is the common practice today. ACP is common in the pediatric population. While it represents only 4–6% of all nasal polyps in adults, up to 35% of nasal polyps in children will eventually be diagnosed as ACP [6]. The common symptoms are the same as with adults, however additional sinus pathologies are rarely seen in children. Oropharyngeal descent is more prevalent in children compared with adults [7]. In addition, children generally present with more advanced disease, probably as a result of delayed diagnosis. The recurrence rate of ACP after endoscopic surgical treatment is not significantly different between children and adults [8]. A meta-analysis conducted by Galluzzi demonstrated a 15% recurrence rate in children with significantly higher rates in patients who underwent endoscopic surgical treatment alone compared with combined approach (i.e. endoscopic and trans-canine sinusoscopy or mini-Caldwell-Luc) [9].

2. Pathophysiology

There are different theories regarding the pathogenesis of ACP; Early studies suggested that ACP grows from an antral mucous retention cyst, a quite common finding in the general population (8–10%) [10]. In their attempt to explain why ACP occurs in only a minority of patients with retention cysts, Frosini et al. hypothesized that increased intra-sinus pressure caused by partial occlusion of the natural ostium due to inflammatory changes and edema is leading an antral cyst to herniate through the accessory ostium [5]. Histologic features of ACP, which include a high rate of inflammatory cells, may support this theory.

The association between ACP and allergy is controversial. While the exact pathogenesis of ACP is unknown, a relationship between ACP and allergic rhinitis or ipsilateral maxillary sinusitis has been shown in pediatric patients [7]. Moreover, increased recurrence rates of ACP after endoscopic surgery were noted in children who were exposed to cigarette smoke (aka 'passive smokers'); Mantilla described a series of 27 cases of recurrent ACP in children in which nearly half of the subjects were considered as passive smokers [11]. While this data may point to a causal correlation between smoking and the development of ACP, such a relationship is not documented elsewhere and more research is needed in this area.

3. Differential diagnosis

The diagnosis of ACP may be challenging, mainly in young children (5–8 years). In this age group, adenoid hypertrophy is a very common finding and the symptoms may resemble those of ACP, like nasal obstruction, chronic rhinorrhea and snoring. Even though the pre-operative management in these cases include nasal endoscopy and/or lateral plain films of the neck, sometimes the diagnosis of ACP may be overlooked. Another unilateral nasal pathology to be ruled out in children is foreign body but it usually manifests with unilateral foul-smelling rhinorrhea. Epistaxis is not a usual clinical feature of ACP. In these cases, vascular lesions (such as juvenile nasopharyngeal angiofibroma, hemangioma or hemangiopericytoma) and neoplasia (inverted papilloma or malignant tumors) should be excluded [12]. The key to

	Adenoiditis / Hypertrophy	Antrochoanal polyp	Allergic rhinitis	Rhinosinusitis
Age	Variable, 4–7 years	7 years <	7 years <	Any age (acute) 12 years < (chronic)
Etiology	Hypertrophy of adenoid tissue	Cystic enlargement of intramaxillary polyp	Inflammatory/ allergic	Infectious (acute) inflammatory (chronic)
Symptoms	Nasal obstruction snoring chronic rhinitis	Nasal obstruction (unilateral progressive to bilateral) rhinorrhea	Rhinorrhea sneezing itching nasal obstruction ocular symptoms	Nasal obstruction rhinorrhea facial pain complications
Signs	Endoscopy: obstructive adnoids X-ray (lateral neck): nasopharynx obstruction	Endoscopy: unilateral nasal polyp	Endoscopy: unilateral nasal polyp	Endoscopy: edema or pus drain from middle meatus
CT	Nasopharynx obstruction	Unilateral maxillary opacification choanal obstruction	Bilateral opacification of sinuses	Bilateral opacification of sinuses complication: (ring enhancement / extrasinus involvement)
Treatment	**Medical:** leukotriene receptor antagonist **Surgical:** adenoidectomy	**Surgical:** resection of antrochoanal polyp	**Medical:** nasal douche, nasal steroid spray, antihistamine, leukotriene receptor antagonist, systemic steroids	**Medical:** nasal douche, antibiotics, nasal steroid **Surgical:** adenoidectomy, endoscopic sinus surgery

Table 1.
Differential diagnosis of pediatric nasal obstruction [14].

differentiate between ACP and other pathologies is a thorough and detailed history along with meticulous physical examination. In cases of limited physical examination, imaging may contribute to the diagnosis. One should keep in mind that adenoid to nasopharynx ratio decreases with age (especially in children >8 years) due to a change in nasopharynx width [13]. Therefore, children older than 8 years must undergo complete nasal flexible endoscopy to rule out nasal polyp (**Table 1**).

4. Clinical manifestations

4.1 History

The most common presenting symptoms of ACP are nasal obstruction and anterior rhinorrhea. Nasal Obstruction may be unilateral or bilateral, depends on the evolution of growth of the polyp. When it emerges from the maxillary sinus ostium to the nasal cavity the patient will complain on unilateral nasal obstruction. However, as the polyp further descends into the choana it may cause bilateral obstruction, as commonly seen in hypertrophic obstructive adenoid tissue. Rhinorrhea is usually unilateral and watery; purulence is rarely seen. Other symptoms may include mouth breathing, snoring and sleep disorders, although ACP does no lead to truly obstructive sleep apnea (OSA). The cystic component is very typical to ACP. Some patients report of a sudden watery or yellow drainage followed by a relief of the nasal obstruction implying to a spontaneous rapture of the cystic part in the ACP.

Very large polyps may descend into the oropharynx and cause a foreign body sensation. As previously noted, the presentation of bilateral nasal obstruction is possible due to expansion of the polyp from one choanae to the other, however true bilateral ACP is extremely rare [15].

5. Imaging

Computed tomography (CT) imaging with nasal endoscopy represent the gold standard in the diagnosis of ACP [5]. All patients must have preoperative sinonasal CT scan, as it is a crucial part of the diagnosis and provides critical information of nasal and sinus bony landmarks prior to surgical intervention.

The classic appearance of ACP in CT is a hypo-attenuating unilateral soft tissue mass that completely occupies the maxillary sinus. It extends through the accessory maxillary ostium into the nasal cavity, medially to the inferior turbinate with progression towards the nasopharynx (**Figure 1**). Less commonly, the polyp

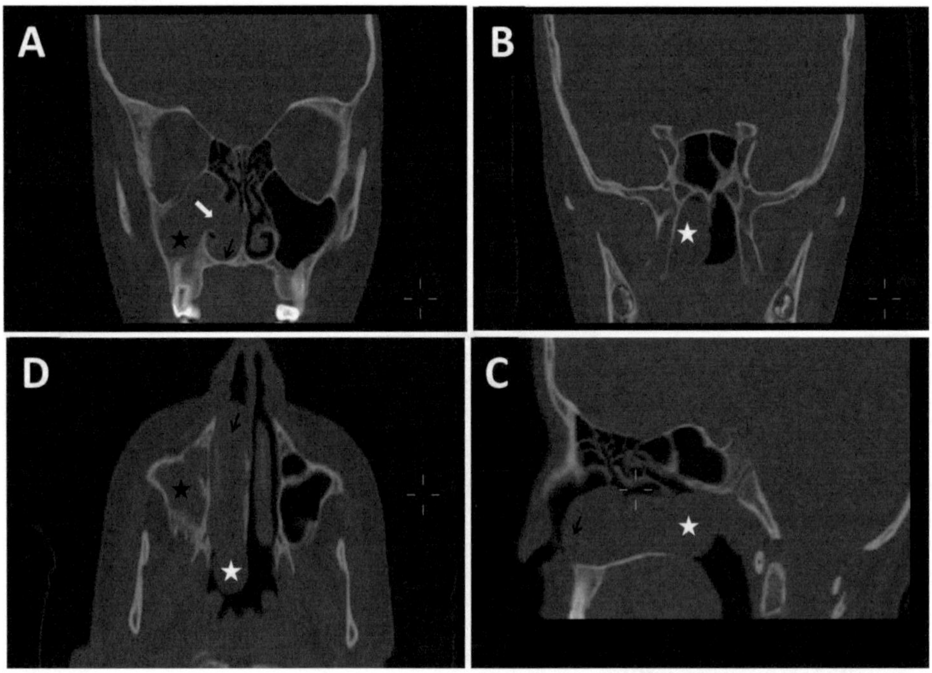

Figure 1.
Computed tomography (CT) imaging of right-sided antrochoanal polyp (ACP). (A) coronal image showing total opacification of the right maxillary sinus and nasal cavity. The antrochoanal polyp has both an intramaxillary component (black asterisk) and an intranasal component (black arrow) this view also demonstrates the enlarged accessory maxillary ostium (white arrow) through which the intramaxillary and intranasal portions are connected via a thin stalk. (B) Coronal view of choanal component of the polyp (white asterisk) obstructing the nasopharynx on the ipsilateral side. (C) and (D) axial and sagittal views demonstrating the different components of the antrochoanal polyp intra-maxillary (black asterisk), intranasal (black arrow) and choanal / nasopharyngeal (white asterisk) potions.

extends anteriorly to the middle turbinate and the anterior inferior turbinate region [16]. Bony changes (bone erosion, destruction or sclerosis) are not typically seen with ACP, although widening of the accessory maxillary ostium may occur, usually due to enlarging cystic portion of the polyp leading to the appearance of expansile maxillary mass (**Figure 1**) [8]. In cases of suspected bone destruction in CT, other pathologies such as malignancy should be considered. However, studies have shown that thinning of alveolar bone in the maxillary sinus may occur secondary to the progressive growing of ACP [2]. Lee classified 3 stages of ACP based on the radiological appearance of the lesion on CT [3, 17]: Stage I (antronasal polyp without extension to the nasopharynx), Stage II (full occlusion of the maxillary sinus ostium with extension to the nasopharynx) and Stage III (partially occlusion of the maxillary sinus ostium with polyp extension to the nasopharynx). In children, advanced CT stages (stage II, III) are more commonly seen due to delayed diagnosis in this population, as previously noted [7]. Magnetic resonance imaging (MRI) shows a hypointense T1 and enhanced T2 signals. With gadolinium administration, the cystic part of the polyp is peripherally enhanced. Although CT is the preferred imaging modality in the diagnosis of any nasal or sinus pathology including ACP, MRI may be considered in children (due to the lack of radiation exposure) and in cases of total unilateral nasal and sinus opacification in CT scans (in order to distinguish between sinus secretions and the mass itself). In nasal endoscopy, ACP appears as a gray-white colored mass with a smooth round surface. Unlike other allergic or inflammatory nasal polyps, ACP has a unique course from the maxillary sinus to the choana and has a bulging expansile behavior due to its cystic component.

6. Histology/histopathology

Macroscopically, ACP is composed of a cystic part filling the maxillary sinus and a solid part emerging through the maxillary ostia and filling the nasal cavity. It has a gross appearance of a "dumbbell" shape with a narrow stalk connecting between the cystic and solid components (**Figure 2**). Microscopically, the antral (or intramaxillary portion) part of ACP demonstrates a central cystic cavity surrounded by a homogeneous edematous stroma with few cells [5]. The intranasal portion of the polyp is covered with a respiratory epithelium similar to the normal mucosa of the sino-nasal tract and the choanal portion occasionally shows squamous metaplasia and reactive fibrosis (**Figure 3**). In comparison to allergic polyp, ACP is characterized by higher inflammatory cell infiltration and edema, lower eosinophilic infiltration and less submucosal glands [18]. These findings indicate that inflammatory changes are the main pathophysiological processes in the pathogenesis of ACP while allergy plays only a minor role. In addition, the paucity of submucosal glands suggests that ACP results from edematous hypertrophy of the respiratory epithelium rather than from distention of the glandular structure, which is the event responsible for the development of ordinary nasal polyps [18]. Angiogenesis is significantly less evident in ACP compared to nasal polyps resulting from chronic rhinosinusitis, with lower expression of angiogenic markers vasculo-endothelial growth factor (VEGF) and CD-34 [12]. These findings further support the idea that ACP is a result of a local inflammatory process and could also explain why ACP has less tendency to bleed compared with other types of polyps, both as a presenting symptom or during endoscopic surgery. ACP is characterized with a significantly high prevalence of intramural cysts [19, 20]. It is speculated that these cysts may have a role in the pathogenesis of ACP, and they contribute to the gross cystic appearance of both its intramaxillary and intranasal components. Moreover, the presence of intramural cysts supports

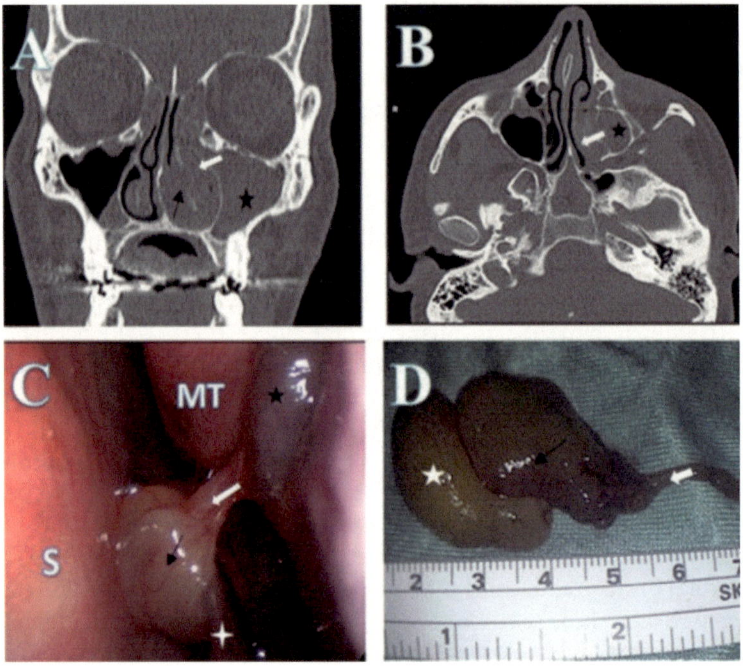

Figure 2.
Combined radiologic and intraoperative views of a left-sided Antrochoanal polyp. (A) & (B). Coronal and axial images showing total opacification of the left maxillary sinus and nasal cavity. The intra-maxillary portion (black asterisk) and the intranasal portion (black arrow) are connected through the enlarged accessory maxillary ostium (white arrow). (C). Endoscopic view of the same patient: The intranasal component of the polyp (black arrow) is medialized with a sinus-seeker (white cross) exposing the stalk (white arrow) that connects it to the intramaxillary component (black asterisk). (D). Gross appearance of the antrochoanal polyp after resection. The intranasal (black arrow) and the choanal (white asterisk) portions are seen clearly, the stalk preserved (white arrow) is seen after separating it from the intra-maxillary portion. MT = middle turbinate. S = nasal septum.

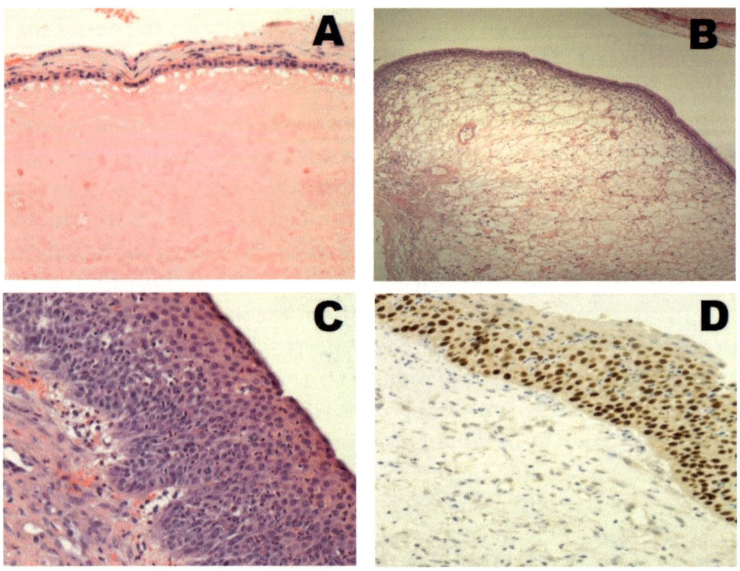

Figure 3.
Typical histologic characteristics of ACP. Image (A) shows a cystic portion of ACP with cuboidal epithelium (H&E original magnification X200). Image (B) demonstrate the intranasal portion of the ACP, edema is seen (H&E X100). Images (C) & (D) demonstrate squamous metaplasia of choanal portion of the ACP (C- H&E X200, (D)- monoclonal P63 antibody stain x200).

Berg's theory [10, 20] that the cystic part of the polyp develops from obstruction in the acinar glands or lymphatic ducts secondary to persistent inflammation. The pressure generated in the process of the polyp's growth through the accessory sinus ostium may be the cause for the substantial edema that is seen.

An explanation of why ACP presents with more cystic changes than diffuse chronic rhinosinusitis with nasal polyps (d-CRS) may be related to their different origins. ACPs develop from the maxillary sinus, characterized by typical respiratory epithelium with thin lamina propria, cyst formation and fewer submucosal glands. On the contrary, nasal polyps in d-CRS typically originate from the ethmoid sinus, which has a thick submucosal layer [21].

When comparing ACP with d-CRS preparations, Warman et al. found that ACP exhibits typical histologic features like cyst formation and edema. ACP demonstrated significantly increased edema when compared to the d-CRS (82.5% vs. 44.4% respectively, $p < 0.001$), and higher cyst formation (40% vs. 6.2% $P = 0.02$). More over ACP preparations demonstrate lower degrees of inflammatory markers than d-CRS [22]. The lack of an inflammatory drive in the pathogenesis of ACP may explain why anti-inflammatory treatment is futile in this population, leading to the common notion that ACP is a rather surgical issue than a medical one.

7. Treatment

Surgery is the standard of care in the treatment for ACP. Since its first description by Killian in 1906, many surgical techniques have been proposed for exposing the maxillary region [4]. Successful ACP resection depends on complete removal of the intramaxillary component of the polyp. The ideal procedure should facilitate excellent approach to all maxillary sinus walls and yet be minimally invasive as possible, especially in children. Currently, various surgical approaches are available: endoscopic sinus surgery (ESS) with polyp removal via either inferior meatus or middle meatus, or a combined inferior and middle meatal naso-antral window. Other options such as ESS with adjuvant canine fossa puncture, or ESS with "mini Caldwel-Luc" procedure aim to facilitate visualization of the anterior and inferior walls of the maxillary sinus [4, 23, 24].

8. Endoscopic inferior meatal antrostomy (EIMA)

Described by Mikulicz in 1887, inferior meatal antrostomy (known as intranasal antrostomy) was a common surgical procedure in the management of maxillary sinus disease. However, the popularity of this technique has declined with the increased use of middle meatal antrostomy due to the growing recognition that an opening in the inferior meatus does not improve sinus drainage, and might even harm the maxillary sinus mucociliary clearance mechanism. Nevertheless, endoscopic approach via inferior meatal antrostomy has the advantage of inferior meatal naso-antral window that avoids violation of the ostiomeatal complex (OMC) and provides better access to anterior-inferior maxillary sinus lesions. Arguments against inferior meatal antrostomy include: persistent sinus disease following surgery, low patency rates, possible injury to the nasolacrimal duct or to developing canine teeth, and technical difficulties associated with the procedure [24, 25]. While these arguments were substantial using anterior rhinoscopy approach, they are not valid with endoscopic approach in EIMA. As the inferior turbinate is carefully medialized, the opening of the nasolacrimal duct (Hasner's valve) is clearly seen and preserved. Then, the maxillary wall is penetrated posterior to that point, and an antrostomy of 8–10 mm is created. Once a satisfactory exposure is achieved, view of the posterior, lateral and anterior portions of the sinus walls is possible with 0- and 45-degree endoscope in respect. The lesion is then removed with straight and curved instruments. At the end of the procedure, the inferior turbinate is lateralized back to its original position [24, 25].

Landsberg and Warman reported 56 patients with multiple maxillary pathologies (45% of them with ACP) in which EIMA was the primary approach for revision surgery. In a follow-up period for at least a year, 93% of patients had no evident sinus disease recurrence. There were no cases of ACP recurrence, and recirculation was not observed during the follow-up period. In addition, no major complications such as nasolacrimal duct injury or bleeding were observed [24].

9. Endoscopic middle meatal antrostomy (EMMA)

Endoscopic sinus antrostomy via the middle meatus (EMMA) is currently considered the gold standard treatment for ACP resection. It is generally recommended that the antral portion should be completely removed together with its stalk to minimize polyp regrowth. As a result, the intranasal and choanal components of the polyp should be resected first (**Figure 2**). Occasionally when the choanal portion is too large, it is easier to push it back to the oropharynx and remove it trans-orally.

Next, the cystic part of the polyp is resected through maxillary antrostomy. The maxillary sinus natural ostium is identified and usually connected with the already enlarged accessory ostium. Resecting the intramaxillary portion includes –45°-70°- endoscopes to better visualize and identify the origin of the polyp. Removal of this intramaxillary portion is extremely important as to minimize post-operative recurrence [4, 26, 27].

Recurrence rate after EMMA is low. Cook et al. observed no recurrence in 33 patients with ACP [28]. Sometimes the intramaxillary portion is tightly adherent to the anterior or antero-inferior walls of the sinus, which makes the dissection a challenging task. In these cases, usage of angled instrumentation is strongly recommended. Nevertheless, the recurrence rate in these cases may increase up to 20% [17, 24, 26, 27].

Ozer et al. reviewed 42 patients who underwent ESS for ACP removal. Transcanine sinoscopy and Caldwell Luc approach were used in addition in 14 and 13 patients respectively. They found recurrence in 3/15 patients after ESS alone (20%), yet there was no recurrence after combined ESS and transcanine sinoscopy or the Caldwell Luc approach [29]. They postulated that the relative high recurrence rate may be due to improper identification of the attachment site of the polyp inside the maxillary sinus (50% of all cases). As a result, they advised considering combined approaches in cases when the attachment site is not clearly recognized. Hong et al. recommended powered instrumentation (Hummer, Stryker Instruments, Kalamazoo, MI) during ESS as an effective technique for removing ACP, especially the antral portion. They found an improvement rate of 96.4% with no significant complications when powered instrumentation was used [29, 30]. Complications following ACP resection are rare.

10. Combining endoscopic middle meatal antrostomy and transcanine sinusocopy

Lee and Huang used the transnasal endoscopic approach for ACPs originated from the inferior and posterior walls of the maxillary sinus, saving the more invasive combined endoscopic and transcanine approach for polyps originated from the lateral wall or in revision surgery. They reported success rate of the transnasal endoscopic approach and the combined endoscopic middle meatal and transcanine approach as 76.9% and 100%, respectively [31].

As mentioned earlier, Ozer et al. found no recurrence after combined ESS and transcanine sinoscopy approach [29].

Transcanine exposure has some complications such as facial swelling pain and rarely injury to the infraorbital nerve. Although rare these complications yet are against using transcanine procedure in ACP resection, especially if the polyp is approachable via EIMA.

11. Combination of ESS and "mini Caldwell-Luc" approach

Kelles et al. retrospectively reviewed 46 patients treated for ACP during a 7-year period. 20 patients underwent endoscopic endonasal surgery (ESS) with mini-Caldwell operation (performing a canine fossa window of 0.5–0.6 cm), while 26 patients underwent ESS alone. The only statistically significant difference between the groups was the recurrence rate, which was higher in the ESS group compared with ESS plus mini-Caldwell group ($P < 0.05$).

In the ESS group, bleeding, synechia, and ostium stenosis were more evident than in the ESS plus mini-Caldwell group, but these differences were not statistically significant. Therefore, Kelles theorized that adding the mini Caldewell-Luc approach allowed better visualization of the maxillary sinus walls and subsequently easier resection of the remnant polyp [23].

Atighechi et al. used a mini-Caldwell approach with ESS in their patients. They reported minimal recurrence and low complication rates, deciding that the technique is useful for the completely removal of ACP [32].

The traditional Caldwell-Luc approach offers good exposure and ensures complete removal of the polyp with the associated antral mucosa. Nevertheless, this approach has been largely abandoned in the treatment of maxillary sinus pathologies, because it does not address the natural ostium of the maxillary hence considered non-functional. Complications include: cheek anesthesia, sensory deficits, cheek swelling and risks for normal teeth development in children [4, 23, 29, 33, 34].

12. Special consideration in ACP resection; ESS in children

As previously noted, the incidence of ACP is higher in children and young adults. Although no difference in the pathophysiology or histology were seen between children and adults, children are at higher risk for recurrence. It is reasonable to believe that the anatomically narrow sinuses, the not-yet erupted teeth, and concern of maxillary growth may affect the surgeon's decision regarding the surgical approach, leading to higher failure rate [17, 31, 35].

In his review of 200 patients with ACP, Forsini described recurrence in 4 patients (2%) all of which were children <7 years of age, in whom only polypectomy was performed. Eventually, in all cases of recurrence ESS was performed without evidence of recurrence [4].

13. Recurrence and follow up

As evident by various published series, recurrence rates range from 0% reported by Tsukidate to 64% reported by Saito and collaborators. Recurrence rates vary between different surgical approaches, patient's age and other factors such as accompanying sinus pathologies [36, 37]. This raises the question – how long should we follow patients ACP resection?

Lee and Huang determined that 65% of their pediatric patients with ACPs had associated chronic sinusitis. Similarly, some authors have also identified association of ACPs with allergic disease. The main hypothesis is the challenge of removing the entire sick mucosa with the origin of the polyp once there is chronic inflammation [31]. Natasha Choudhury reported 29 patients after EMMA surgery for ACP. They described no polyp recurrence, with a mean follow-up period of 14.7 months [8]. Galluzzi reviewed 13 studies and found that recurrence in children is higher than in adults, mostly because of reasons described earlier. The review showed that combined approach had the lowest recurrence rate, with a range of follow-up between 6 to 120 months. Most recurrences were noted between 5 months to 3 years after initial surgery [17]. Some authors claim that different anatomic variations in the nasal cavity such as septal deviation, conchal hypertrophy, and concha bullosa may increase the intramaxillary pressure, hence predisposing for the development of ACP. While these variations were documented in up to 80% of patients with ACP, none of them were linked to increased rates of recurrence [4, 17, 23, 24, 30]. In most relevant studies, the time of recurrence was 1.2 ± 0.6 years. Therefore, it is advised to monitor ACP patients for at least 2 years after surgery in order to detect 95% of recurrent cases [35].

14. Conclusion

ACP originates in the maxillary sinus of children and young adults. Its etiology is speculative, currently considered a benign cystic polyp with limited inflammatory characteristics. It has a consistent three component structure intramaxillary, intranasal and choanal portions. ACP has a typical imaging characteristic and the gold standard of treatment is complete surgical resection. Special attention should be given to identify and resect the intramaxillary portion to prevent recurrence. Long term follow-up is needed to rule out polyp regrowth.

Author details

Warman Meir[1,3]*, Rona Bourla[1], Monica Huszar[2] and Elchanan Zloczower[1]

1 Department of Otorhinolaryngology, Head and Neck Surgery, Kaplan Medical Center, Rehovot, Israel

2 Department of Pathology, Kaplan Medical Center, Rehovot, Israel

3 Hebrew University, Hadassah Medical School, Jerusalem, Israel

*Address all correspondence to: meirwarma@gmail.com

References

[1] Lee TJ, Huang SF, et al. Endoscopic sinus surgery for antrochoanal polyps in children. *Otolaryngol Head Neck Surg.* 2006; 135(5):688-692.

[2] Bidkar VG, Sajjanar AB, et al. Role of computed tomography findings in the quest of understanding origin of antrochoanal polyp. *Indian J Otolaryngol. Head Neck Surg*. 2019; 71(3):1800-1804.

[3] Lee DH, Yoon TM, et al. Difference of antrochoanal polyp between children and adults. *Int J Pediatr Otolaryngolol.* 2016; 84:143-146.

[4] Frosini P, Picarella G, et al. Antrochoanal polyp: analysis of 200 cases. *Acta Otolaryngology Ital*. 2009; 29 (1):21-26.

[5] Yaman H, Yilmaz S, et al. Evaluation and management of antrochoanal polyps. *Clin Exp Otorhinolaryngol* 2010; 3: 110-114.

[6] Larsen K, Tos M, et al. The estimated incidence of symptomatic nasal polyps. *Acta Otolaryngol*. 2002; 122: 179-182.

[7] Balikci HH, Ozkul MH, et al. Antrochoanal polyposis: analysis of 34 cases. *Eur Arch Otolaryngology.* 2013; 270 (5):1651-1654.

[8] Choudhury N. Hariri A, et al. Endoscopic management of antrochoanal polyp: a single UK centre's experience. *Eur Arch Otorhinolaryngol.* 2015; 272(9) 2305-2311.

[9] Mantilla E, Villamor P, et al. Combined approach for paediatric recurrent antrochoanal polyp: a single-centre case series of 27 children. *J Laryngo Otol.* 2019; 133(7): 627-631.

[10] Min YG, Chung J, et al. Histologic Structure of Antrochoanal Polyps, *Acta Oto-Laryngologica.* 1995; 115:4, 543-547.

[11] Gendeh BS, Long YT, et al. Antrochoanal Polyps: clinical presentation and the role of powered endoscopic polypectomy. *Asian J Surg*. 2004; 27(1):22-25.

[12] Hirshoren N, Neuman T, et al. Angiogenesis in chronic rhinosinusitis with nasal polyps and antrochoanal polyps. *Inflamm Res.* 2011; 60 (4):321-327.

[13] Cohen O, Betito HR, et al. Development of the nasopharynx: A radiological study of children. *Clin Anat.* 2020 Oct;33(7):1019-1024.

[14] Flint P.W (2020) Cummings Otolaryngology - Head and Neck Surgery (7th Ed.) chapter 200; Pediatric Chronic Rhinosinusitis 2970-2978. Elsevier

[15] Oner F, Sakat M, et al. Bilateral Antrochoanal Polyp. *J Craniofacial Surg*. 2015; 26 (7): 661-662.

[16] Peric A, Vucadinovic T, et al. Choanal polyps in children and adults: 10-year experience from a tertiary hospital. *Eur Arch Otorhinolaryngol.* 2019; 276(1) 107-113.

[17] Galluzzi F, Pignataro L, et al. Recurrences of surgery for antrochoanal polyps in children: A systematic review. *Int J Pediatr Otolaryngol.* 2018; 106:26-30

[18] Stammberger H, Hawke M. Essentials of functional endoscopic sinus surgery. St Louis: Mosby 1993. p. 103-105.

[19] Maldonado M, Martínez A, et al. The antrochoanal polyp. *Rhinology*. 2004;42(4):178—182.

[20] Berg O, Carenfelt C, et al. Origin of the choanal polyp. *Arch Otolaryngol Head Neck Surg* 1988; 114:1270-1271.

[21] Latta JS, Schall RF. LXXVIII The Histology of the Epithelium of the Paranasal sinuses under Various Conditions. *Ann Otol Rhinol Laryngol*. 1934;43(4):945-971. Doi:10.1177/000348943434300401

[22] Warman M, Kamar Matias A, et al. Inflammatory Profile of Antrochoanal polyps in the Caucasian Population – A Histologic Study. *Am J Rhinol Allergy* 2020 Accepted for publication.

[23] Kelles M, Toplu Y, et al. Antrochoanal polyp: clinical presentation and retrospective comparison of endoscopic sinus surgery and endoscopic sinus surgery plus mini-Caldwell surgical procedures. *J Craniofac Surg*. 2014;25(5):1779-1781

[24] Landsberg R, Warman M, et al. The Rationale for Endoscopic Inferior Meatal Antrostomy. *ORL* 2019; 81:41-47.

[25] Yanagisawa E, Christmas DA Jr, et al. Endoscopic view of a long-term inferior meatal antrostomy. *Ear Nose Throat J*. 2007;86(6):318-319.

[26] Pagella F, Emanuelli E, et al. Clinical features and management of antrochoanal polyps in children: Cues from a clinical series of 58 patients. *Int J Pediatr Otorhinolaryngol.* 2018; 114:87-91.

[27] Stammberger H, Posawetz W, et al. Functional endoscopic sinus surgery. Concept, indications and results of the Messerklinger technique. *Eur Arch Otorhinolaryngol*. 1990;247(2):63-76.

[28] Cook PR, Davis WE, et al. Antrochoanal polyposis: a review of 33 cases. *Ear Nose Throat J*. 72:401-410, 1993.

[29] Ozer F, Ozer C, et al. Surgical approaches for antrochoanal polyp: a comparative analysis. *B-ENT*. 2008;4(2):93-99.

[30] Hong SK, Min YG, et al. Endoscopic removal of the antral portion of antrochoanal polyp by powered instrumentation. *Laryngoscope*. 2001;111(10):1774-1778.

[31] Ta-Jen Lee, Shiang-Fu Huang, et al. Endoscopic sinus surgery for antrochoanal polyps in children. Otolaryngol Head Neck Surg 2006; 135:688-692.

[32] Atighechi S, Baradaranfar MH, et al. Antrochoanal polyp: a comparative study of endoscopic endonasal surgery alone and endoscopic endonasal plus mini-Caldwell technique. Eur Arch Otorhinolaryngol 2009; 266:1245-1248

[33] Paul W. Flint. *Cummings Otolaryngology--Head & Neck Surgery*. 5th ed. Elsevier Saunders, 2014. ISBN: 9781455746965

[34] Datta RK, Viswanatha B, et al. Caldwell Luc Surgery: Revisited. *Indian J Otolaryngol Head Neck Surg*. 2016;68(1):90-93.

[35] Chaiyasate S, Roongrotwattanasiri. K, et al. Antrochoanal Polyps: How Long Should Follow-Up Be after Surgery? *Int J Otolaryngol*. 2015; 297417.

[36] Tsukidate T, Haruna S, et al. Long term evaluation after endoscopic sinus surgery for chronic pediatric sinusitis with polyps. *Auris Nasus Larynx* 2012;39(6)583-7.

[37] Saito H, Honda N, et al. Intractable pediatric chronic sinusitis with antrochoanal polyp, *Int. J Pediatr Otorhinolaryngol.* 2000 31;54(2-3):11-6.

Chapter 2

Tracking of Fascicles of Cutaneous Nerves of Thigh: A Histological Study

Rajani Singh

Abstract

Present study uncovers the secrets of internal morphology of femoral nerve branches namely, cutaneous trunk, subcutaneous trunks, saphenous, medial cutaneous and intermedius cutaneous nerves innervating the skin of anteromedial thigh at fascicular level. Therefore, the aim of the study is to track, correlate, interpret and identify the pathways of fascicles through histological slides. The femoral nerve and its branching points were calibrated in distances from inguinal ligament. These trunks and nerves of a cadaver were processed for histological slides staining with haematoxylin and eosin. The fascicles in the histological slides were identified, tracked, correlated and interpreted from cranial most slide to the last terminal slides of these nerves and trunks. The correlation of the pathways of fascicles revealed that these fascicles are continuous, consistent and traceable interrupted by split, fusion and multiplexing. Femoral nerve branches/fascicles/nerve fibres if damaged, impair the sensation of corresponding area of skin of anteromedial thigh creating helm of neurological complications. Hence the injured fascicles can be repaired with the help of identification and correlation of fascicular pathways carried out in this study with least invasion. The findings of present study will be of paramount importance for intraoperative stimulation to diagnose and identify the fascicle for microneurosurgical repair/graft/regenerate/neurotisation in the cutaneous branches of femoral nerve at fascicular level.

Keywords: cutaneous nerves, microanatomy, transformational process, pathways of fascicles

1. Introduction

There are many variations of femoral nerve and these have been classified by Singh et al. [1]. A femoral nerve cropped from a cadaver was type II of classification of Singh et al. [1]. This femoral nerve bifurcated into muscular and cutaneous trunks at one centimetre below the inguinal ligament. The cutaneous trunk further splits into sub-cutaneous trunk of thigh and the saphenous (S) nerve. The subcutaneous trunk, then, bifurcates into intermedius cutaneous (IC) and medial cutaneous (MC) nerves of the thigh. The group of afferent fascicles of S, IC and MC supply skin of anteromedial thigh.

Though the injuries to the IC and MC nerves have hardly been reported yet few cases of pain and paraesthesia over the anterior and medial aspects of thigh, as a result of engagement of IC and MC nerves of the thigh, are described. However, sensory loss on the medial side of the thigh, leg and foot up to the ball of the great toe because of engagement of the saphenous nerve through iatrogenic lapses or otherwise are well reported. The outcome of injuries may not be fatal or produce unbearably serious signs and symptoms so the patients may not be opting for costly neurosurgical diagnosis (MRI) for detection of location and degree of injury and procedures.

The neuro-therapy of neuropathological morbidity requires accurate diagnosis and treatment. There is very limited scope of investigating location and identification of injured fascicle or nerve fibres under current knowledge of internal morphology of nerve. Though Chhabra et al. claims that location and degree of injury can be identified through MR advanced neurography [2] yet it has its own limitations regarding resolution and image defects. Therefore, a micro-anatomic study has been planned to track fascicles in histological slides of subcutaneous trunk, S, IC and MC for improving identification of injured fascicle, its location and degree of injury for diagnosis and imagery interpretation together with non-invasive neurosurgical repair, grafting and regeneration of injured nerve fibres.

2. Tracking and correlation of fascicles

A24 slide was prepared from the femoral nerve just above the inguinal ligament. This femoral nerve just below the inguinal ligament bifurcated into muscular and cutaneous trunks. Cutaneous trunk then bifurcated into saphenous nerve and subcutaneous trunk which further divided into intermedius and medial cutaneous nerves. Saphenous, intermedius and medial cutaneous nerves innervate skin of anteromedial thigh. Histological slides of cutaneous, saphenous nerve, subcutaneous trunk, medial and intermediate cutaneous nerves were prepared and stained with haematoxylin and eosin. The fascicles in these nerves/trunks were identified, tracked, correlated and interpreted.

3. Naming scheme of fascicles

For deciphering the fascicles of individual nerves and to avoid confusing duplicate numbers, the name of the fascicles at the point of transformational processes was changed in sequential order with prefix from CF of composite fascicles in femoral nerve to CCF in cutaneous trunk and SCCFs in subcutaneous trunk extending it to SCF in S nerve, MCCFs and ICCFs in MC and IC respectively.

The composite fascicles (CFs) in slide A24 1 have been identified as CFs {(303, 304); (280, 257, 270, 312, 313): (316, 317, 318)}* of both cutaneous and muscular trunks. CFs 316, 317, 318 corresponds muscular trunk and CFs {(303, 304); (280, 257, 270, 312, 313)} to cutaneous trunk (**Figure 1**).

4. Tracking and correlation of fascicles in cutaneous trunk

The cutaneous trunk was cut into 6 pieces and six blocks C1, C2, C3, C4, C5 and C6 were prepared. From C1, 13 slides were processed. C1 13 was the cranial most slide of C1. Similarly variable number of slides were prepared from C2, C3, C4, C5 and C6.

In C24 1, composite fascicles, {(303, 304); (280, 257, 270, 312, 313)} correspond to cutaneous trunk, but CF313 of A24 1 splits and formed CCF 318 and 319

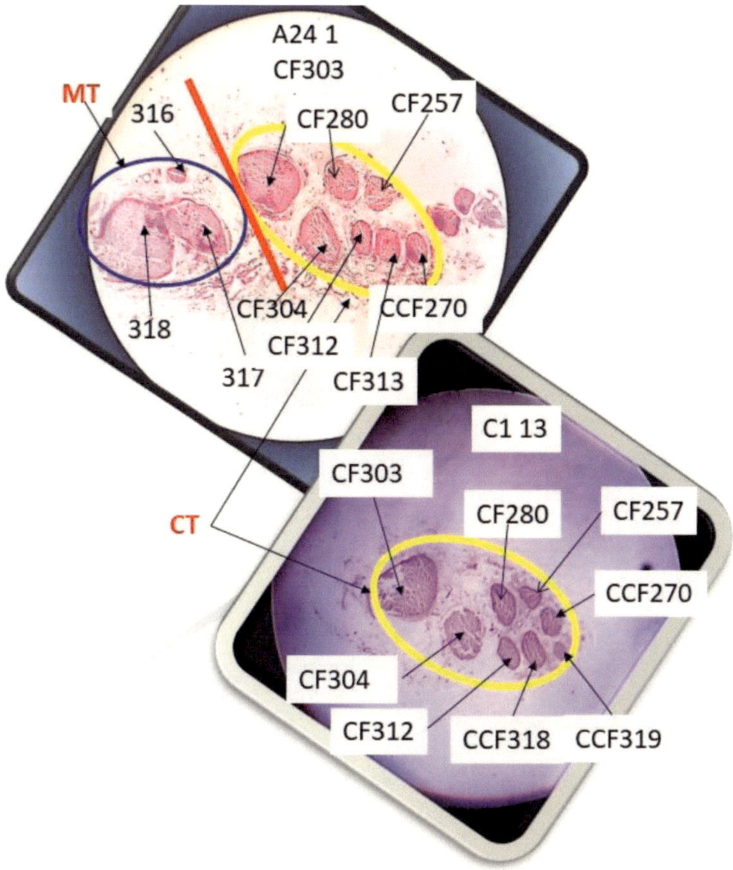

Figure 1.
Correlation between A24 1-C1 13. MT- muscular trunk, CT- cutaneous trunk.

in C1 13. So C1 13 consists of {(303, 304); (280, 257, 270, 312, 318, 319)} (**Figure 1**). These fascicles continuously consistent up to slide C2 16, the cranial most slide of C2 block.

The fascicles in C2 16 were continuous, consistent and correctable up to slide C2 12. In slide C2 12, CF312 and CCF318 fused forming CCF320 and CF280 in slide C2 12 split into CCF321, 322 and 323 in C2 11 (**Figure 2**). C2 11 is traceable to C2 1 meaning that the fascicles which were present in slide C2 11 were continuing up to slide C2 1.

In C2 1 slide CCF321, 322 and 257 fused forming CCF324 in C3 3 (**Figure 3**). So the slide C3 3 consists of CFs 303, 304, CCFs 319, 320, 323, 324 and 270 fascicles. CCF223 changed the shape forming CCF 323. Fascicles of C3 3 were traceable, continuous, and consistent up to slide C3 1.

CCF270 and CCF324 in C3 1 fused forming CCF325 in C4 4 (**Figure 4**). So slide C4 4 consists of CFs 303, 304, CCFs 320, 323, 325 and 319 fascicles. Fascicles of C4 4 were traceable, continuous, and consistent up to slide C4 1.

CCF325 in C4 1 split into CCF326 and 327 in C5 5 (**Figure 5**). So slide C5 5 consists of CFs 303, 304, CCFs 319, 320, 323, 326 and 327 fascicles. C5 5 is traceable, continuous, and consistent up to C6 1.

In C6 1 fascicles CFs 304 and 303 and CCFs 319, 320, 323, 326 and 327 were found to be surrounded by internal epineurium (**Figure 6**) indicating subcutaneous trunk and saphenous nerve are formed and ready to emerge.

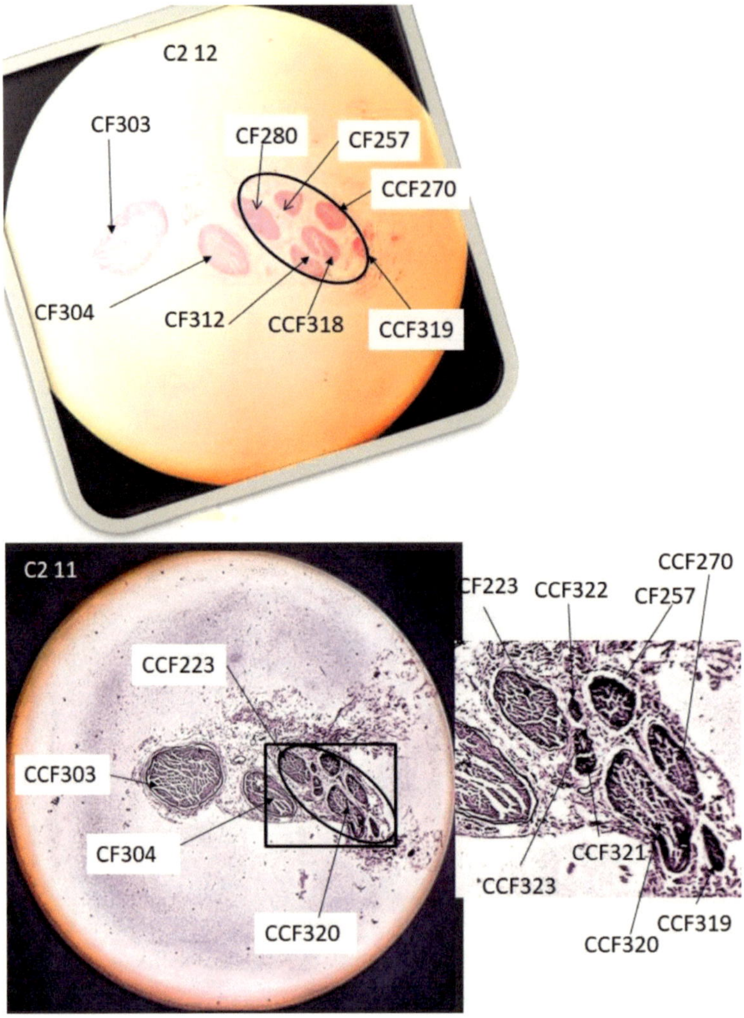

Figure 2.
Correlation between C2 12-C2 11.

After C6 1, cutaneous trunk bifurcated into a) S nerve containing CCFs 319, 320, 323, 326 and 327 as observed in S1 1 of S1 block and b) sub-cutaneous trunk consisting of CFs 304, 305 and 306 in SCT1 1, slide of SCT1 block (**Figure** 7).

5. Tracking and correlation of fascicles in saphenous nerve

S nerve was cut into 6 pieces and six blocks S1, S2, S3, S4, S5 and S6 were prepared. Slides prepared from these six blocks were stained with haematoxylin and eosin and fascicles of S nerve were correlated starting from S1 block to S6 block.

The S nerve having CCFs 319, 320, 323, 326 and 327 in S1 1 emerged out after C6 1 (**Figure** 7). These CCFs were traceable from the slides of block S1 through S2 1 the caudal most slide of S2 block.

The CCFs 319 and 320 in S2 1 fused together forming SCF 328 in S3 13 the cranial most slide of S3 block (**Figure** 8). So, S3 13 slide consists of 323, 326, 327 and 328 fascicles. These fascicles were continuous, consistent and traceable up to slide S3 1.

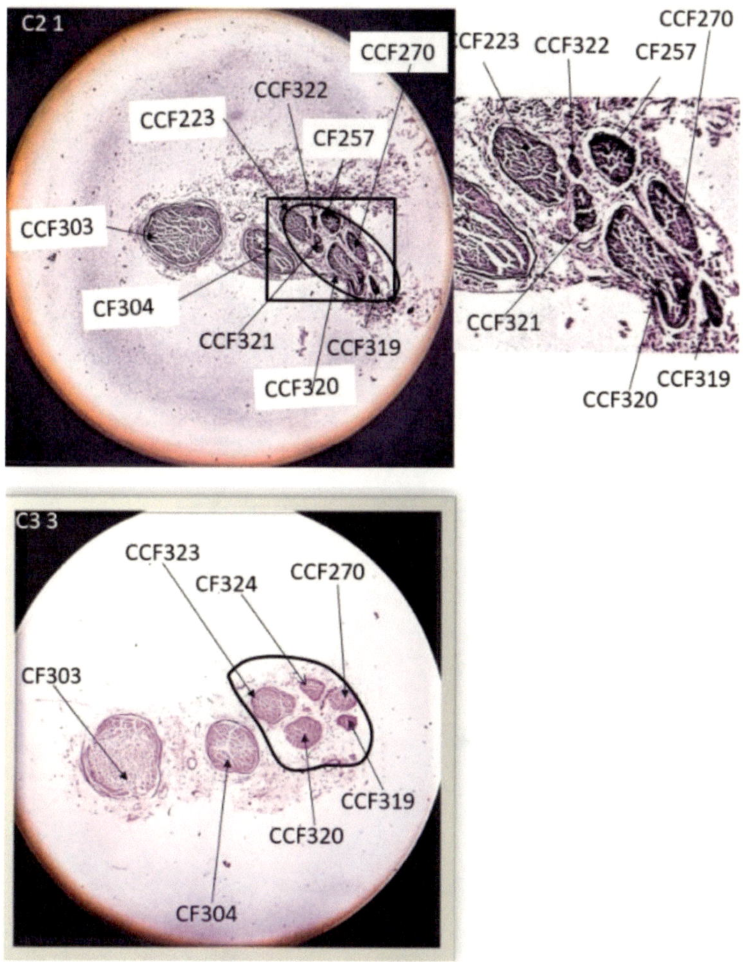

Figure 3.
Correlation of C2 1 with C3 3.

CCF328 in S3 1 slide split into SCFs 329 and 330 in S4 12, the cranial most slide of S4 block (**Figure 9**). So, the slide S4 12 consists of 323, 326, 327, 329 and 330 fascicles. The fascicles of S4 12 slide were continuous, consistent and traceable up to slide S4 1.

CCF330 emerged out as branch of S nerve after S4 1 as this fascicle was not found in next slide. CCFs323 in S4 1 split into SCFs331 and 332 S5 12, CCFs326 in S4 1 into SCF333 and 334 in S5 12, CCF329 in S4 1 into SCF335 and 336 in S5 12. So slide S5 12 consists of 331, 332, 333, 334, 335, 336 and 327 (**Figure 10**). These fascicles in S5 12 were continuous, consistent and traceable up to slide S5 1.

The fascicles from S5 1 reorganise their position through migration and rearrange in S6 11. The fascicles got separated laterally into infrapatellar branch having SCFs (331, 332, 335, 336) and main S nerve having SCFs (327,333, 334) in S6 11 (**Figure 11**) continued caudally.

The fascicles are traceable between S6 11 and S6 7. Again reorganisation of fascicles is taking place from S6 7 to S6 6 (**Figure 12**). These fascicles in S6 6 were continuous, consistent and traceable up to slide S6 1. Infrapatellar branch emanated laterally from S nerve after S6 1.

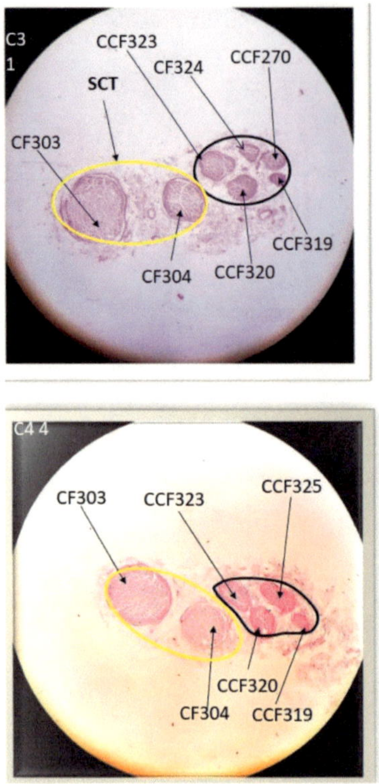

Figure 4.
Correlation of C3 1 and C4 4.

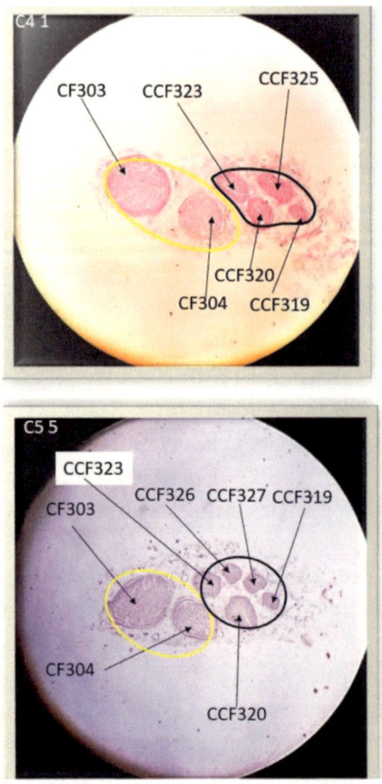

Figure 5.
Correlation of C4 1 and C5 5.

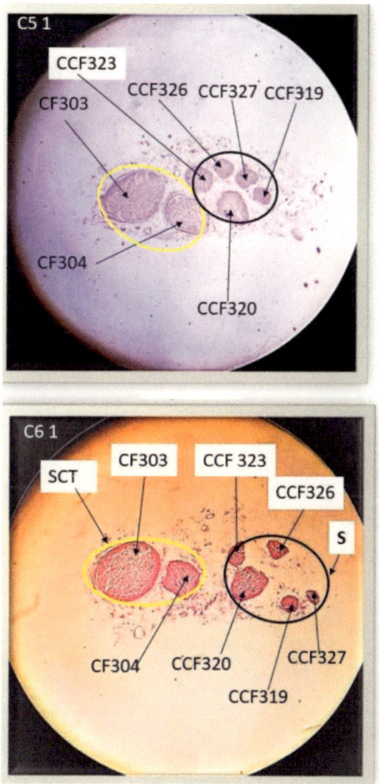

Figure 6.
Correlation of C5 1 and C6 1. SCT- fascicles of subcutaneous trunk, S- fascicles of saphenous nerve.

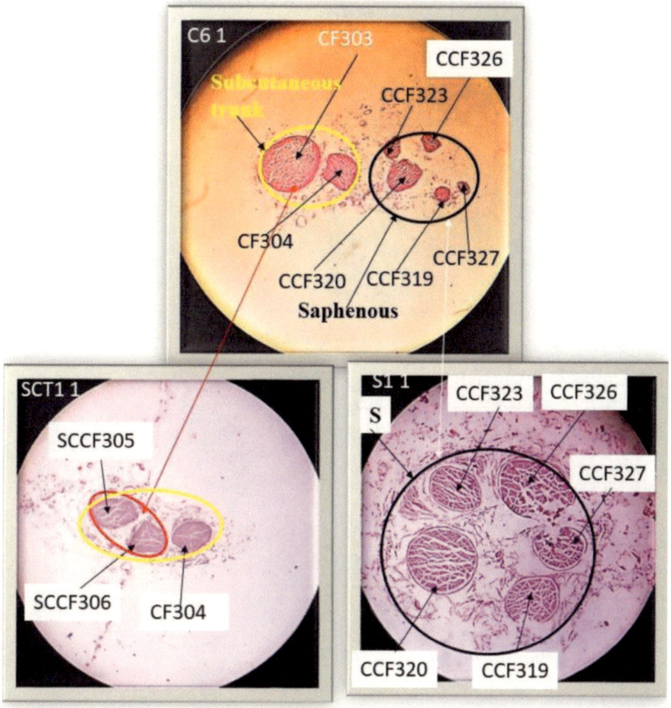

Figure 7.
Correlation of C6 1 and S1 1 and SCT1 1.

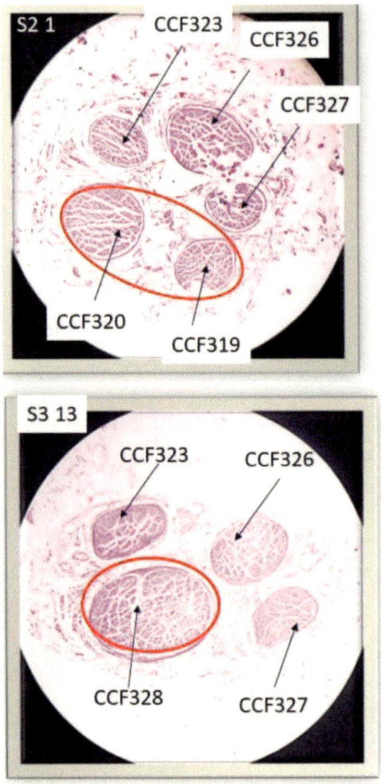

Figure 8.
Correlation of S2 1 and S3 13.

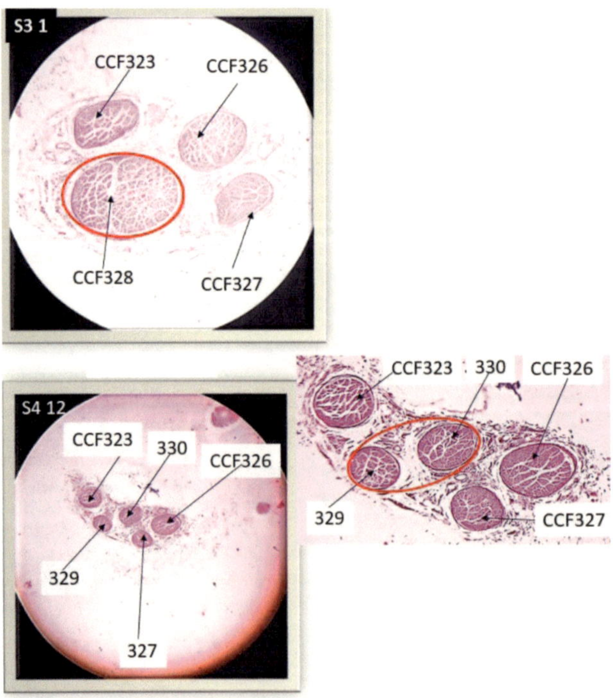

Figure 9.
Correlation of S3 1 and S4 12.

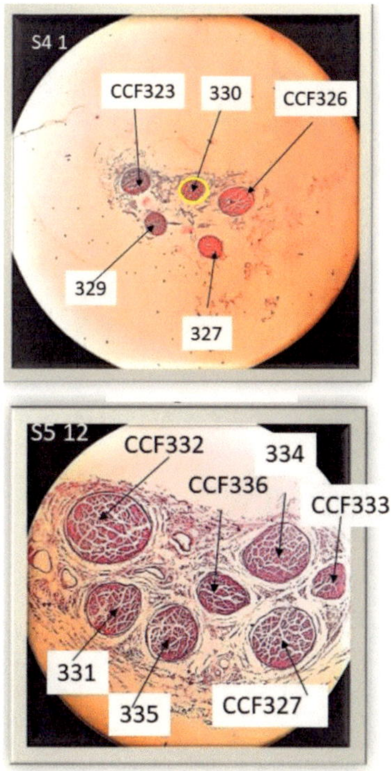

Figure 10.
Correlation of S4 1 and S5 12.

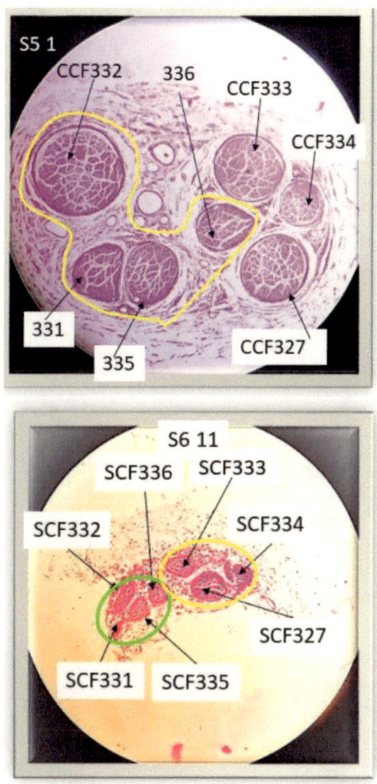

Figure 11.
Correlation of S5 1 and S6 11.

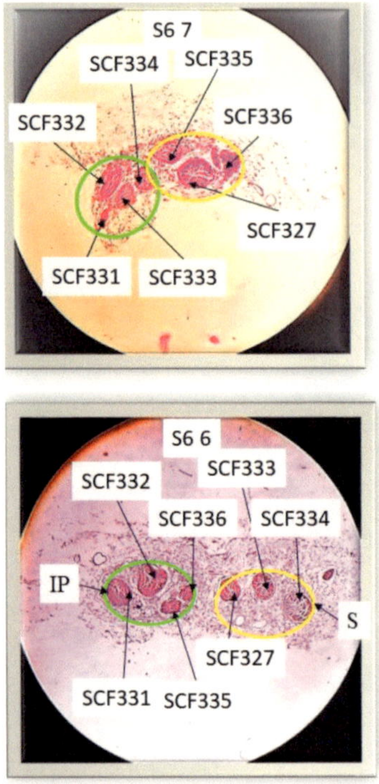

Figure 12.
Correlation of S6 7 and S6 6. IP- infrapatellar branch, S- main saphenous nerve.

6. Tracking and correlation of fascicles in subcutaneous trunk

Subcutaneous trunk was cut into 3 pieces and 3 blocks SCT1, SCT2 and SCT3 were prepared. Subcutaneous trunk bifurcated into MC and IC. One block of

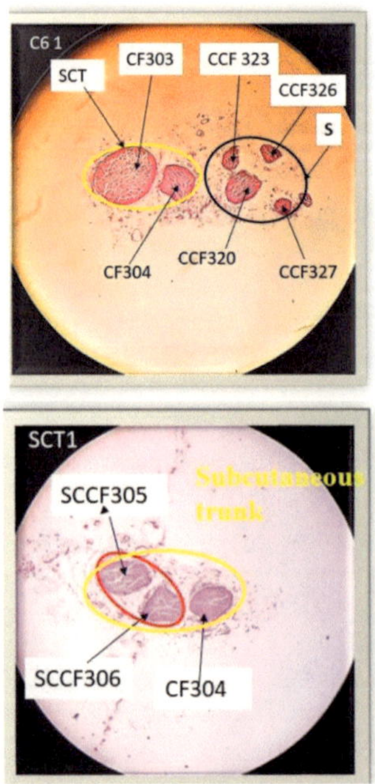

Figure 13.
Correlation of C6 1 with SCT1. SCT- subcutaneous trunk, S- saphenous nerve.

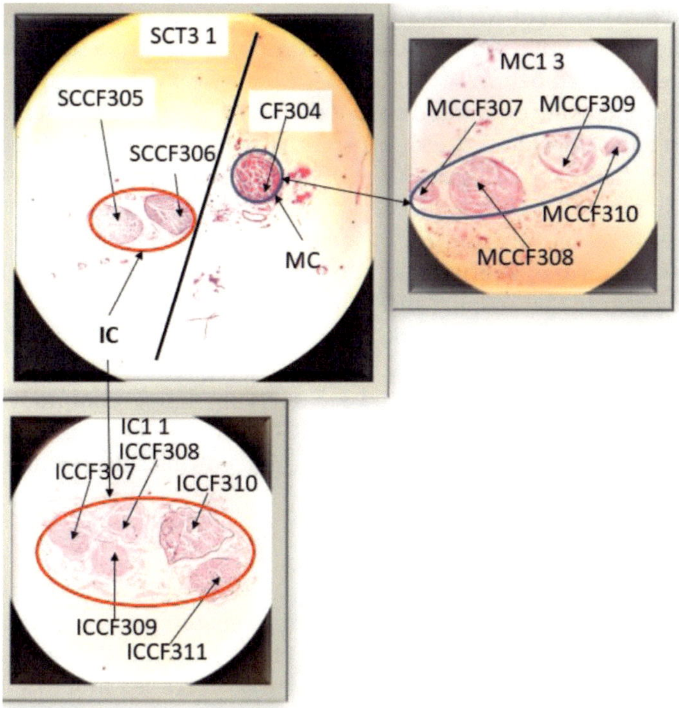

Figure 14.
Correlation of SCT3 1 with IC1 1and MC1 3.

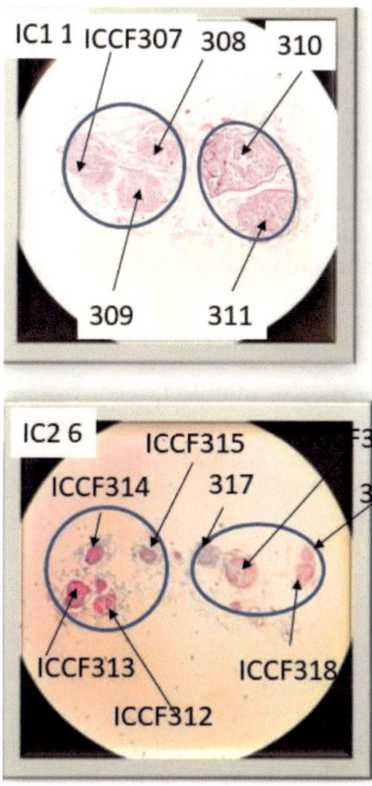

Figure 15.
Correlation between IC1 1 and IC2 6.

MC,MC1 and two blocks of IC, IC1 and IC2 were prepared and slides from aforementioned blocks were stained with haematoxylin and eosin and fascicles were correlated as elaborated below:

The CFs 303 and 304 constituted subcutaneous trunk which was separated laterally from cutaneous trunk after C6 1 (**Figure 6**). Then CF303 split into SCCF 305 and 306 in SCT1 1 slide (**Figure 13**). So the subcutaneous trunk now consists of fascicle CFs 304, SCCFs 305 and 306. After the slide SCT1 1, the CFs 304, SCCFs 305 and 306 were traceable from SCT1 1 up to SCT3 1.

The subcutaneous trunk bifurcated into IC and MC nerves after SCT3 1 slide. The CF304 constitute MC and 305 and 306 IC (**Figure 14**). Then CF304 split into MCCF307, 308, 309, 310 in MC1 3 slide. The SCCF305 split into ICCF307, 308, 309 and SCCF306 into ICCF310, 311 in IC1 1 respectively (**Figure 14**).

ICCF308 IC1 1 split into ICCF314 and 315, ICCF309 IC1 1 split into ICCF312 and 313. ICCF310 split into ICCF316 and 317, ICCF311 split into ICCF318 and 319 (**Figure 15**). These fascicles form fine nervelets innervating skin of thigh.

7. Clinical significance of this study

No such study has been carried out involving sensory nerves of femoral nerve. If the fascicles of S, MC and IC are damaged, the communication of sensory information from the innervated area will be interrupted leading to aggravation of clinical problems. So it is not merely nerve where injury should be investigated rather injured fascicles should be targeted for diagnosis for complications which may occur anywhere in entire fascicular path from origin to point of innervation. The diagnosis of neural insults requires not only the location and degree of injury but also identification, isolation, orientation, directivity, and matching of shape and size of injured nerve CFs for planning surgical repair, grafting and regeneration [3].

The location and degree of injury is investigated by the high resolution MRI advanced neurography [2, 4]. But this has its own limitations of recording and interpretation. This generates uncertainty in diagnosis and thereby in treatment. Thus the radiologists and neurosurgeons face the impediments of pinpointing the probable position of injury and identification of fascicles. Therefore, the imagery coupled with our internal morphological study together can refine the interpretation for identification of injured CF and location of injury. Methodically, it can be done by one to one correlation between images of transverse histological and high resolution MRI advanced neurographic sections at the same position from inguinal ligament. The distance of location of injured fascicle from inguinal ligament may be computed in MRI neurography and then the calibrated histological sections of cutaneous, subcutaneous trunks, S, MC and IC nerves at the same level may be compared and examined for confirmation of identified injured fascicle. After identification of injured fascicle, the idea of shape, size, location and orientation can also be derived from histological slides for matching, alignment and directivity of nerve fibres for repair and grafting.

7.1 Personal communication

The neurosurgery at fascicular level is currently uncommon however, with upcoming science and technology in future, present study will be highly useful for neurosurgeons. The study will help in carrying out less invasive surgery as stimulation of identified injured fascicles will not involve other fascicles which in case of nerve stimulation may be stimulated causing discomfort to the patient.

DOI: http://dx.doi.org/10.5772/intechopen.94461

8. Conclusion

The histological slides of cutaneous, subcutaneous trunks, S, MC and IC nerves brought out correlation of fascicles and grouped fascicles together with their configuration data present the straight, continuous and identified pathways of CFs interrupted by transformational processes calibrated in distance from inguinal ligament. This data will be of utmost importance to imagery guided microneurosurgical interventions more precisely at fascicular level together with the imagery interpretation to radiologists and neurosurgeons to assess injury and its location in an identified fascicular pathway to plan for its repair and surgical access. Fascicular electrode may be designed and developed like nerve cuff electrode [5] to improve neural microsurgery tremendously at fascicular level.

9. Limitation

This study involves variations in the branching pattern of sensory nerves in one individual. Further studies are recommended to encampass variations in other individuals.

Author details

Rajani Singh
Department of Anatomy, UP University of Medical Sciences, Saifai Etawah, UP, India

*Address all correspondence to: nani_sahayal@rediffmail.com

References

[1] Singh R, Tubbs RS, Singla, M. Classification and fascicular analysis of variant branching pattern of femoral nerve for microsurgical intervention. A series of thirteen cadavers. Int J Morphol 2016; 34(2):561-569.

[2] Chhabra Avneesh, Lianxin Zhao, John A Carrino, Eo Trueblood, Saso Koceski, Filip Shteriev et al. 2013. MR Neurography: Advances. Radiology Research and Practice. Volume 2013, 14 pages Article ID 809568.

[3] Payne S Houston. Nerve Repair and Grafting in the Upper Extremity. J South Orthop Assoc 2001; 10(2). https://www.medscape.com/viewarticle/423216_6

[4] Bäumer Philipp, Sabine Heiland, Martin Bendszus, Mirko Pham. MR Neurography - Diagnostic Criteria to Determine Lesions of Peripheral Nerves. Clinical Neurology 2012; page 10-14. Available at Magnetom Flash · 2/2012 www. siemens. com/magnetom-world.

[5] Chandra Naresh, Singh Rajani. Tracking of Fascicles of Sartorius and Pectineus Nerves-A key to Neurosurgery. Journal of Clinical and Diagnostic Research 2019; 13(1):AC01-AC08.

Section 2

Molecular Pathology

Chapter 3

Advances in Molecular and Immunohistochemical Detection of Prognostic and Therapeutic Markers in Breast Cancer

Rodrigo Vismari de Oliveira

Abstract

In the last two decades, new discoveries concerning on breast cancer have contributed to important changes on its classification, from purely morphologic to molecular embased, to establish better correlation with clinicopathologic features. The classification in molecular subtypes, based on hormonal receptor and *HER-2* status, have been remarkable not only for its more accurated clinical correlations, but also for its easy applicability in diagnostic routine, better replication of tumor microenvironment through the selection of paraffinized tumor amounts and cost-effectiveness of the detection method, the immunohistochemistry. Hence, this classification may predict the breast cancer prognosis and became an important target for therapy with hormonal and *HER-2* antagonist drugs. Other study models, like cancer-stem cell hypothesis and immunological aspects of human cancer, have brought new emerging ideas regarding on molecular pathways and accurated prognostic preditions. Putative stem-cell markers and *PD-1/PDL-1*, have highlighted among several emerging molecular markers because of the bad cancer prognosis determinated by stem-cell markers expression and for emerging new drugs with selective action to PD-1/PDL-1, with promising results. The therapy of breast cancer have became diverse, target directed and personalized, in order to take in consideration the clinicopathologic cancer aspects, molecular tumor profile and clinical status of the patient.

Keywords: breast cancer, target therapy, molecular markers, prognostic markers, immunomarkers, cancer stem-cell

1. Introduction

Breast cancer is the one of the three most frequent human neoplastic disease worldwide and is the most common female cancer, remaining with considerable impact on general mortality. Worldwide, in the last 10 years, the incidence is growing up, with approximately 2.1 million of new cases per year and estimated mortality of 15%, at about 300.000 per year [1, 2].

Breast cancer remains as an heterogeneous group of disease from the point of view of biological behavior, therapeutic issues and prognostic features, determining different tracks of overall and free of disease survivals [3, 4]. Thus, the clinicopathologic classification of breast cancer has been challenging over the last years, since the isolated simple morphologic classification of the tumor on histology examination is not necessarily related to the precise biologic behavior of the disease [5, 6].

In this way, especially over the last two decades, important researches revealing novel molecular markers expressed by cancer cells has been published in the literature. The new discoveries have improved the breast cancer classification, which has been progressed from a purely morphologic classification, based on histologic patterns, to a molecular classification, based on expression of oncoproteins and hormonal receptors, detected mainly by immunohistochemical techniques, in paraffin-embedded tumoral specimens [6, 7].

The novel molecular classification of breast cancer seems to exhibit more accurated correlation to the clinicopathological aspects of the tumor, as proliferative index, invasiveness and potential to metastatic spread. Furthermore, some of these molecular markers allowed the development of new drugs with specific actions on populations of cancer cells with specific genes alterations, improving considerably the therapeutic, prognostic and survival issues [7].

Instead of the recent advances on new therapeutic protocols under a new molecular perspective, early breast cancer on clinicopathological classification still remains the single one potencially curative [8]. The management of advanced clinicopathologic stage tumors and some established molecular groups of cancer, especially the 'triple negative' disease, remains with lacks of consensus. Anyway, the molecular markers have just improved the pathophysiology pathways knowledge, with potential future development of promising new drugs for target therapy of breast cancer [8–10].

2. The molecular subtypes of breast cancer of clinicopathologic importance

In the beginning of the 21st century, breast cancer was classified mainly on histologic basis. The WHO current histologic classification of breast cancer is demonstrated in **Table 1**. Photomicrographies of the most frequent histologic subtypes of invasive breast cancer are represented on **Figure 1**. The hormonal status receptors (estrogen and progesterone) expression by the neoplastic cells was just evaluated by immunohistochemistry on paraffin-embedded specimens of tumor (core needle biopsy or the surgical excision specimen) [6, 7].

Breast cancer is known for its heterogeneous behavior [3, 4]. The histologic classification has been satisfactory for malignancy determination [6]. Though, the clinical division based on hormonal status was not enough for accurate prediction of the prognosis and of clinical response to the therapy [5]. Thus, until the last decade of 20th century, the clinical treatment of breast cancer was based on unespecific chemotherapy and hormonal therapy with drugs like tamoxifen, a known hormonal receptor antagonist [12].

The hormone positive breast cancer is more "differentiated" than the negative one, as the cancer cells maintain the epithelial original cell feature of hormonal receptor expression and, therefore, the hormonal antagonist drugs are effective against these tumors [8]. On the other hand, the approaching of hormonal negative cancers were variable, since it was forming a kindly heterogeneous group, with different aggressiveness potentials, imprecise therapeutic response and doubtful prognosis [6, 8, 10].

In the first decade of the current century, it was emerged a promising classification of breast cancer, proposing a division of the disease in 3 molecular subtypes:

WHO classification of epithelial breast tumors (5th edition, 2019)	
Benign epithelial proliferations and precursors • Usual ductal hyperplasia • Columnar cell lesions, including flat epithelial atypia • Atypical ductal hyperplasia **Adenosis and benign sclerosing lesions** • Sclerosing adenoma • Apocrine adenoma • Microglandular adenosis • Radial scar/complex sclerosing lesion **Adenomas** • Tubular adenoma • Lactating adenoma • Duct adenoma **Epithelial-myoepithelial tumors** • Pleomorphic adenoma • Adenomyoepithelioma NOS • Adenomyoepithelioma with carcinoma • Epithelial-myoepithelial carcinoma **Papillary neoplasms** • Intraductal papilloma • Ductal carcinoma *in situ*, papillary • Encapsulated papillary carcinoma • Encapsulated papillary carcinoma with invasion • Solid papillary carcinoma *in situ* • Solid papillary carcinoma with invasion • Intraductal papillary adenocarcinoma with invasion **Non-invasive lobular neoplasia** • Atypical lobular hyperplasia • Lobular carcinoma *in situ* NOS o Classic lobular carcinoma *in situ* o Florid lobular carcinoma *in situ* o Lobular carcinoma in situ, pleomorphic **Ductal carcinoma *in situ* (DCIS)** • Intraductal carcinoma, non-infiltrating, NOS o DCIS of low nuclear grade o DCIS of intermediate nuclear grade o DCIS of high nuclear grade	**Invasive breast carcinoma** • Infiltrating duct carcinoma NOS • Oncocytic carcinoma • Lipid-rich carcinoma • Glycogen-rich carcinoma • Sebaceous carcinoma • Lobular carcinoma NOS • Tubular carcinoma • Cribriform carcinoma NOS • Mucinous adenocarcinoma • Mucinous cystadenocarcinoma NOS • Invasive micropapillary carcinoma of breast • Apocrine adenocarcinoma • Metaplastic carcinoma NOS **Rare and salivary gland-type tumors** • Acinar cell carcinoma • Adenoid cystic carcinoma o Classic adenoid cystic carcinoma o Solid-basaloid adenoid cystic carcinoma o Adenoid cystic carcinoma with high grade transformation • Secretory carcinoma • Mucoepidermoid carcinoma • Polymorphous adenocarcinoma • Tall cell carcinoma with reverse polarity **Neuroendocrine neoplasms** • Neuroendocrine tumor NOS • Neuroendocrine tumor, grade 1 • Neuroendocrine tumor, grade 2 • Neuroendocrine carcinoma NOS • Neuroendocrine carcinoma small cell • Neuroendocrine carcinoma large cell

Table 1.
Current histologic (morphologic) classification of epithelial breast tumors (WHO, 2019, 5th edition). This classification considers the tumors histologic patterns of tumors. The most common histologic breast cancer subtype is the infiltrating duct carcinoma NOS (or invasive ductal carcinoma non-special type), accounting for 65–80% of all breast cancers. Invasive lobular carcinoma corresponds to around 5% of all breast malignancies.

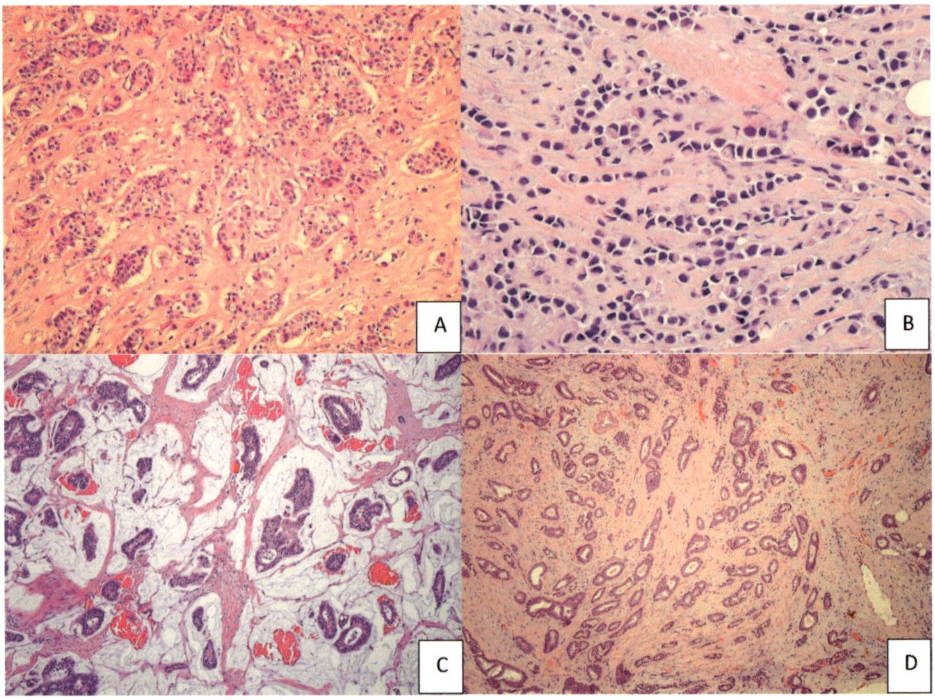

Figure 1.
Photomicrographies of hematoxylin & eosin (H&E) slides illustrating the most frequent histologic subtypes of infiltrating (invasive) breast cancer. (A) Infiltrating duct carcinoma (Invasive ductal carcinoma NOS) is the most frequent histologic subtype of breast cancer (nearly 75–80% of all invasive breast cancer), constituted of cohesive cancer cells forming infiltrative ductal and ribbons structures (4×); (B) Lobular invasive carcinoma is the second most frequent invasive breast cancer (5–15% of all invasive breast cancer), composed of infiltrating cancer cells with diffuse single-file pattern (10×). In this subtype, the cancer cells lose the cohesion (e-cadherin, an immunomarker important for cell adhesion evaluation, is negative on immunohistochemistry); (C) Mucinous carcinoma represents approximately 2% of breast invasive cancer, composed of groups of cancer cells outling ductal structures, immersed in mucin pools, with delicate fibrous strands containing capilaries (10×); (D) Tubular carcinoma represents around 2% of invasive breast cancer, composed of haphazard arrangement of small well-differentiated duct structures, forming tubules (4×). The other listed invasive breast cancers are uncommon, with each one histologic subtype representing 1% or less (figures extracted from [11]).

luminal, *HER-2* overexpressed and "triple negative" (**Table 2**). This new classification has demonstrated better correlation with the breast cancer behavior. Thus, it was adopted on diagnostic routine of breast cancer. Since this study was published, besides of evaluate the histologic patterns and report the pathologic tumor stage, the pathologist has been required to determine the molecular cancer profile, which has became indispensable to therapy planning [12, 13].

The luminal subtype cancer is the hormonal positive tumors. This kind of cancer is frequently well or moderately differentiated on histology, formed by lower grades of cells, with lower proliferative index, which is evaluated by antibody *Ki-67/MIB-1* on immunohistochemistry. The majority of breast cancers are classified as this subtype (**Figure 2**). Eventually, luminal cancer can overexpress or amplify at the same time the protein called human epithelial growth factor receptor 2 (*HER-2*), codified by the oncogen *ERBB2* [14, 15].

ERBB2 is a oncogen localized in chromosome 17, which codifies the *HER-2* protein, a type I transmembrane protein with an extracellular and an intracellular domains, activating signaling pathways from extracellular signals. In last instance, the overexpression/amplification of *HER-2* overactivates the intracellular protein kinases, dysregulating the cell cycle, disrupting the cell adhesion and cell polarity and promoting the invasive phenotype [16].

Molecular subtype	Biomarkers profile	Incidence
Luminal	Hormone receptors positive (ER+ and/or PR+)	50–70%
• Luminal A	• with Ki-67 ≤ 14% of cancer cells	35–50%
• Luminal B	• with Ki-67 > 14% of cancer cells	5–15%
○ Luminal B1	○ HER-2 negative	
○ Luminal B2	○ HER-2 positive	
HER-2 overexpressed	Hormone receptors negative (ER and PR negative) and HER-2 positive	10–20%
"Triple negative"	Hormone receptors negative (ER and PR negative) and HER-2 negative	15–30%

Table 2.
Molecular subtypes of breast carcinoma. The reported absolute incidences of each molecular subtype of breast carcinoma are variable among several studies.

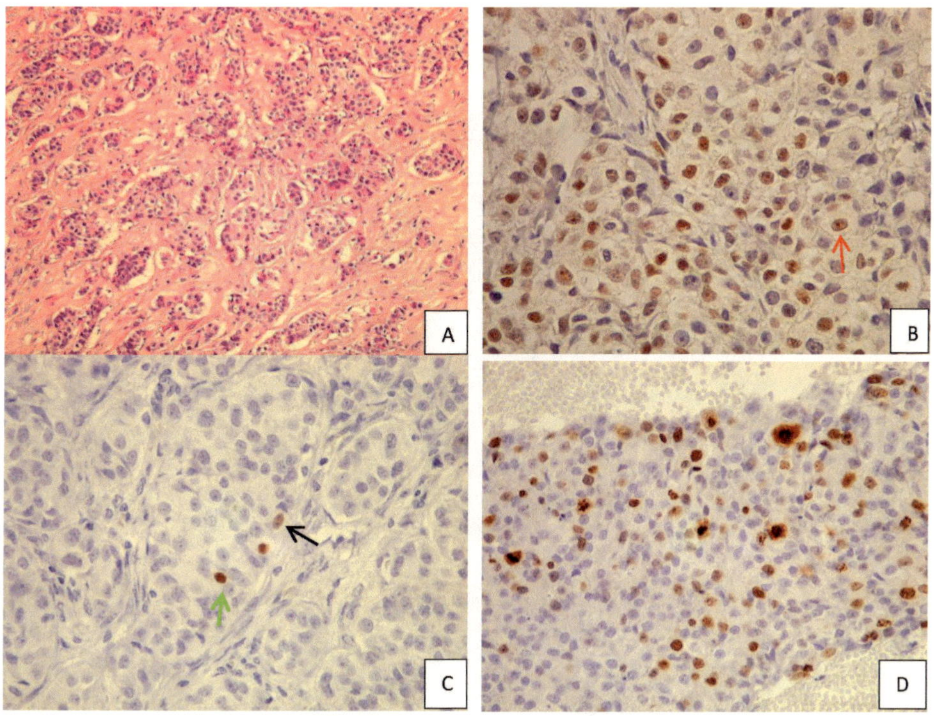

Figure 2.
Photomicrographies of immunohistochemical assessment of invasive breast cancer hormonal expression, in an example of infiltrating duct carcinoma (Invasive ductal carcinoma NOS, WHO 2019), which is the most frequent histologic subtype of breast cancer, constituted by ductal and ribbons structures of cancer cells infiltrating the breast stroma (A). Any kind of nuclear positivity of estrogen receptor (B) and progesterone receptor (C) allows to consider the tumor as positive to hormonal receptor on immunohistochemistry, even when rare cells are positive (C). The hormonal receptors positivities on immunohistochemistry are evaluated for intensity (mild, moderate or strong) and percentages of positive cells (0–100%). Examples of mild positivity (black arrow, C), moderate positivity (red arrow, B) and strong positivity (green arrow, C). Ki-67/ MIB-1 assesses the tumor proliferative index (D), its positivity is nuclear and is expressed in percentages of positive cells (0–100%).

The breast cancer classified as *HER-2* subtype is necessarily negative for hormonal receptors and is featured by overexpression or amplification of *HER-2*. This subtype is frequently less differentiated than the luminal ones on histology, constituted by high grades of cancer cells, with high proliferative index. The presence of elevated concentration of intratumoral lymphocytes (TIL) is not an uncommon finding in these tumors [17].

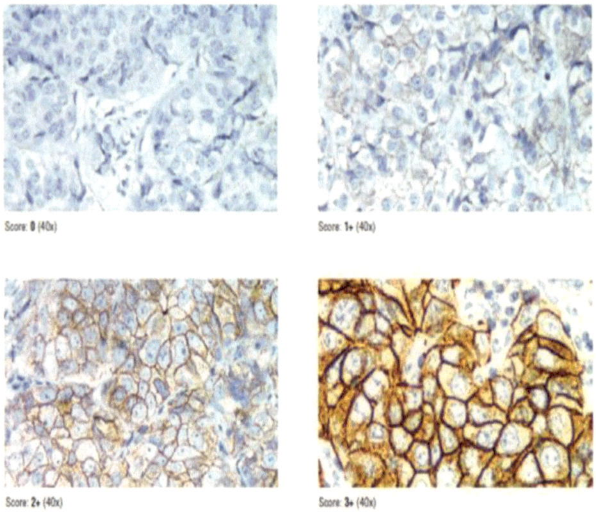

(a)

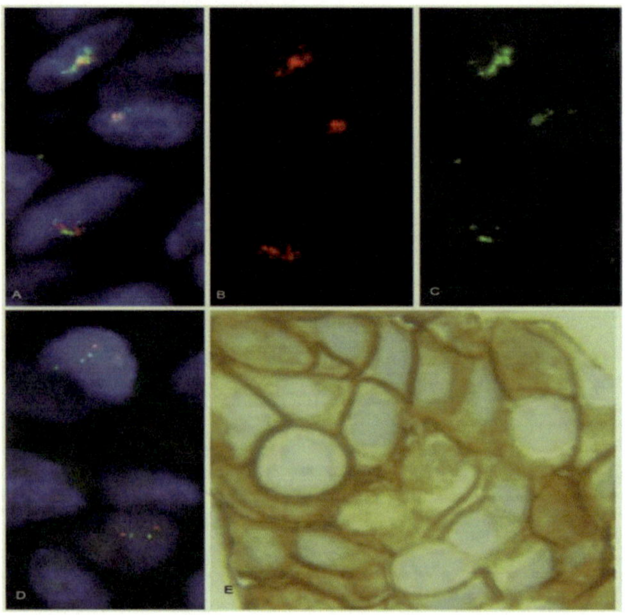

(b)

Figure 3.
(a) Photomicrographies of immunohistochemical assessment of HER-2 expression status by tumoral cells in histologic paraffinized specimen of breast cancer. Score 0 (negative): none tumoral cell is labeled. Score 1+ (negative): incomplete positivity with low intensity in part of tumoral cells. Score 2+ (equivocal): complete positivity with low intensity in majority of tumoral cells. Score 3+ (positive): complete positivity with strong intensity in majority of tumoral cells. (b) Photomicrographies of amplification of HER-2 gene performed through fluorescence in situ hibridization (FISH) in a HER-2-overexpressed breast carcinoma on immunohistochemistry (Score 3+, E). HER-2 gene copies are the orange signals (B) and chromosome 17 centromeres (CEP17) are the green signals (C). The signals of HER-2 gene and CEP17 are present in tumoral cell nuclei (blue, A and D). CEP17 is an internal control on the same chromosome to compare with HER-2 signals in tumoral cell nucleus. According to American Society of Clinical Oncology/College of American Pathologists (ASCO-CAP) guidelines, a HER-2/CEP17 ratio ≥ 2.0 defines a positive result for amplification of HER-2 gene. If HER-2/CEP17 ratio is < 2.0, an average HER-2 copy number ≥ 6.0 signals/cell defines a positive result for amplification of HER-2 gene, an average HER-2 copy number < 4.0 signals/cell defines a negative result for amplification of HER-2 gene and an average HER-2 copy number ≥ 4.0 and < 6.0 signals/cell defines an equivocal result for amplification of HER-2 gene (extracted from [20]).

This new receptor was one of the pioneers for target therapy in molecular era of breast cancer approaching, as it was developed a new class of drug, called trastuzumab, with selective action against the cancer cells overexpressing/amplifying *HER-2*. Besides the *HER-2* subtype tumors, this drug is also recommended for the luminal ones with positive status for *HER-2* [18, 19].

The status of *HER-2* expression is analyzed through immunohistochemistry of paraffin-embedded specimens of the breast cancer (**Figure 3a**). The tumor is considered negative for *HER-2* if it is not labeled (score zero) or the cell membrane is partially labelled for the *HER-2* antibody (score 1+). The tumor is positive for *HER-2* if all the cell membranes outlines are strongly labeled for this antibody (score 3+). Finally, in part of the cases, the *HER-2* antibody can label totally the cancer cell membrane, but with low intensity or can label partially the cell membrane with high intensity. In these situations, the *HER-2* status is considered equivocal (score 2+). The confirmation of overexpression/amplification must be evaluated through fluorescence "in situ" hybridization (FISH) (**Figure 3b**) [21, 22].

The "triple negative" breast cancer is negative for hormonal receptors and *HER-2*. It is the less differentiated tumor subtype on histology, formed by highest grades cancer cells, with highest proliferative index, presenting the worst prognosis among the 3 molecular subtypes. This tumor still does not present an specific therapy, which is chosen depending on the clinicopathological stage. In metastatic disease, the treatment focuses on quality of life and palliation. In "triple negative" tumors, the evaluation of *BRCA* status is mandatory [8, 21].

3. Germline mutations of *BRCA-1/BRCA-2* genes: increased risk of breast cancer development during the life

Identified in 1994, *BRCA-1/BRCA-2* are tumoral suppressor genes, respectively located in chromosome 17 and 13. Mutations of these genes are related to hereditary breast cancer, estimated in 5–10% of all breast malignancies. *BRCA-1/BRCA-2* play a central role in DNA repair [23, 24]. Mutations of these genes increase the susceptibility for DNA damages. "Triple negative" subtypes carry more frequently mutations of *BRCA-1* and mutations of *BRCA-2* increase the risk for luminal subtypes of breast cancer. *HER-2* overexpression is inversely correlated to *BRCA* mutations [24, 25].

It was observed in some studies that "triple negative" breast cancers with *BRCA* mutations present more chemosensitivity than the ones without *BRCA* mutations. Chemotherapy with DNA-damaging drugs, like the alkylating agents and anthracycline, can prolong the free of disease survival for tumors of triple negative phenotypes. This found is expected, since *BRCA* mutation prejudices the DNA repair and, consequently, increase the sensibility to DNA damages of cancer cells by these drugs. Neither therapeutic response nor free of disease survival of luminal subtypes of breast cancer seems to be influenced by *BRCA* mutations [8, 24, 26].

Regarding on prognosis, multiples studies present conflicting results. The prognosis depends on tumor features, especially the molecular subtypes and the clinicopathologic stage. The predictive value depends on the administrated therapy. Thus, *BRCA-1* mutated breast cancer probably present worse prognosis than the *BRCA-2* mutated ones, since *BRCA-1* mutated tumors are mainly of "triple negative" phenotype, therefore intrinsically more aggressive than the luminal subtypes harboring *BRCA-2* mutations [24, 27].

The tumoral suppressor proteins codified by *BRCA-1/BRCA-2* act on homologous recombination repair of double stranded DNA breaks. Homologous recombination mechanism protect the integrity of genome in proliferating cells. *BRCA-1* recognize DNA damage and recruit DNA repair proteins. *BRCA-2* mediates the recruitment of another protein, called *RAD51*, to double stranded DNA breaks, allowing for homologous recombination repair [24, 28].

In *BRCA*-mutant breast tumors, the base excision repair pathway is important for cancer cell survival, in response to single stranded DNA breaks. Polyadenosine diphosphate-ribose (*PARP*) is a family of DNA repair enzymes, playing a key role in base excision repair mechanism. These enzymes are recruited to the site of DNA damage and add ADP-ribose to target nuclear proteins, causing post-translational modifications and restarting stalled DNA replication. *BRCA*-mutant breast cancer presents deficiency of homologous recombination repair, with overactivated *PARP*, leading the cancer cell to avoid apoptosis [24, 26, 28].

The inhibition of *PARP* cause persistance of single stranded break, resulting in stalled replication and double strand breaks. This mechanism leads to accumulation of DNA damage, causing cell cycle arrest and apoptosis. The *PARP* inhibitors form an emerging class of drugs, which have been recommended to chemotherapy for *BRCA*-mutant breast cancer and empirically for metastatic breast cancer, with promising results [24, 25, 28].

4. Cancer stem-cell hypothesis: impact in breast cancer prognosis

In the last two decades, experimental evidences in several studies of neoplastic tissues have revealed a population of cancer cell with properties of self-renewal, differentiation to multiple lineages ability and low proliferative index. These properties have been considered cancer stem-cell like features and attributed to a possible cancer stem-cell lineage present in the tumor bulk [29, 30].

Cancer stem-cell has awaked interest in the context of breast cancer because of its characteristic heterogeneity of biological behavior and therapeutic response. It has been hypothesized that cancer stem-cell might be one of the causes of the high variability of biological and prognostic spectrum of breast cancer. Cancer-stem cells might play an important role on therapeutic resistance and progression of disease, affecting the overall and free of disease survival [31, 32].

Thus, an important feature which allows possible cancer stem-cell resistance to chemotherapy is its low expression of surface proteins. Because of its self-renewal properties, cancer stem-cell does not depends on signaling from other cells to proceed its functions in tumoral tissues. Furthermore, for its low antigenicity and low proliferation index, there are few alternatives for drug interactions. DNA damage agents are poor effective against these cells possibly for a lack of proliferation, as well new classes of drugs, like *PARP* inhibitors, which better act on cells in proliferative phase [31, 33].

One of possible pathways for breast cancer therapeutic resistance acquired along the time might be explained by populations of cancer stem-cells not eliminated, selected by multiple chemotherapy cycles. Tumoral cells in active proliferation phase are more hitten, increasing the proportion of indolent cells with stem-like features in cancer cell population. Through the capacity of multilineage differentiation, cancer stem cells might generate new daughter cells with more aggressiveness and chemoresistance [32, 34].

The identification of cancer stem-cells is challenging. First, because of its irregular distribution in selected tumor amounts. Second, for definition, these cells are frequently scarces in tumor bulk. In this way, these cells are better identified through "in vitro" methods, like cellular cultures. However, the mainly disadvantage of this technique is the fact of stem cells behave in a different fashion in artificial environment, since the cell phenotype expression depends on their interactions [32, 35].

Thus, several studies with cancer stem-cells in different neoplastic tissues have been accomplished with conflicting results. An interesting method to identify these cells in their original environment is the immunohistochemistry performed on amounts of paraffin-embedded neoplastic tissues, with the advantages to allow the evaluation of phenotype expression next to the reality and to be easily performed and cost-effectiveness in diagnostic routine [35].

In the last years, some putative stem-cell markers detected by immunohistochemistry have been tested in paraffinized tissues of breast cancer. Multiple studies have demonstrated that expression of putative stem-cell markers by tumoral cells seems to worse the prognosis and survival in breast cancer. The most frequent studied stem-cell markers are *CD24*, *CD44*, *CD133* and *EPCAM*, with two identified putative stem-cell phenotypes: *CD24* low/*CD44* enriched and co-expression of *CD133* and *EPCAM* (**Figure 4**). Besides of the scarcity of stem-cells in neoplastic tissues, the conflictous results of these studies might be explained by a necessity to qualitative analysis of these markers expression, exactly for the rarity of stem-cells [32, 36].

In some studies, identification of a stem-cell like phenotype *CD24* low/*CD44* enriched have prejudiced the free of disease survival, especially in cases of early stages of breast cancer, with more occurrence of distant metastasis and cancer recurrence after surgical and adjuvant treatments. The presence of cancer cells with positivity for cancer stem-cell phenotype *CD133/EPCAM* is has been related to poor overall survival in breast cancer, with more adjuvant therapeutic fail [32].

For the moment, these putative stem-cell phenotypes seems to be independent prognostic factors in breast cancer. "Triple negative" breast cancer and *BRCA-1* mutant breast cancer have been associated to stem-cell like phenotype *CD24* low/*CD44* enriched. These putative stem-cell markers may become possible future targets for new drugs in the future [30, 32].

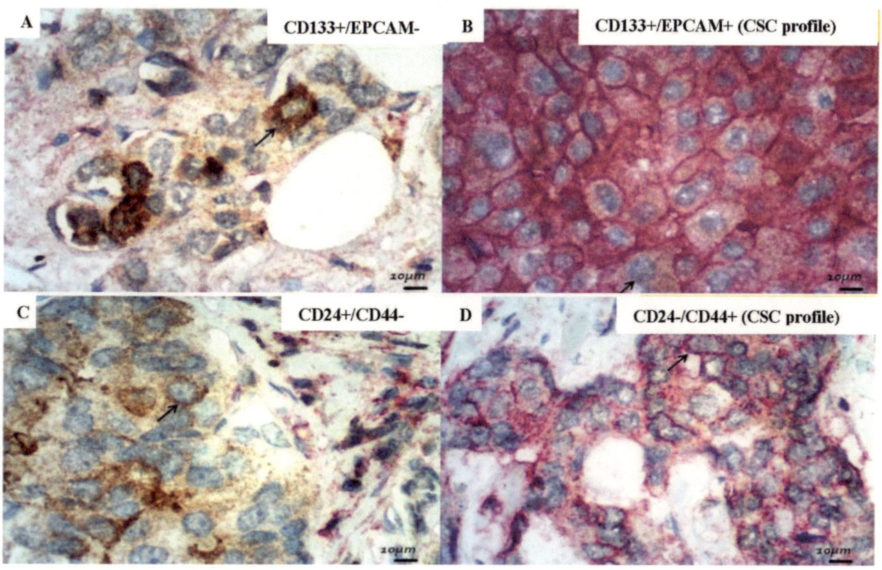

Figure 4.
Photomicrographies of double-labeled simple stained putative CSC antibodies (400×, original magnification, immunoperoxidase and DAB). (A) CD133: cytoplasm positivity (immunoperoxidase); (B) EPCAM: membrane positivity (DAB); (B) CD133+/EPCAM+: CSC profile (black arrow: membrane positivity to DAB and cytoplasm positivity to immunoperoxidase at the same cell); (C) CD24: cytoplasm positivity (immunoperoxidase); (D) CD24−/CD44+: CSC profile (black arrow: membrane positivity only to DAB)

5. Immunologic aspects related to breast cancer

In the context of cancer, the immune system can suppress the tumor growth by the destruction of cancer cells or inhibition of their outgrowth. On the other hand, immune system can play a role on tumor progression by the selection of tumor cells which are adapted to survive in an immunocompetent host or modifying the tumor environment to facilite the tumor outgrowth [37].

Elevated levels of *CD4+* regulatory T lymphocytes (*Tregs*) found in many cancers are associated to poor prognosis. *Tregs* create a favorable immunosuppressive microenvironment to the outgrowth and progression of the tumor. On this way, *FOXP3* is expressed by the *Tregs* and can be detected by immunohistochemistry. *FOXP3* is responsible for induction and maintenance of tolerance to self antigens in normal cells, as well this immunotolerance can be performed by the *Tregs* with cancer cell antigens [37, 38].

Another example of cancer cell escape mechanism from the immune system is *caspase-8* mutations present in "triple negative" breast cancers and other solid malignant tumors. These mutations abolish the death induced by cytotoxic lymphocytes *CD8+* in tumoral cells [37, 39].

The activation of T lymphocytes by foreign antigens occurs by concomitant major histocompatibility complex (*MHC*) antigen presentation and co-expression of T-cell receptor (*TCR*). At the same time, a family of T-cell transmembrane proteins *CD28/B7*, called "immune checkpoints", produces co-inhibitory or co-stimulatory signals. The immune checkpoints regulates the T-cell immunotolerance to protect the tissues from undesirable damages. Cancer cells may produce signals to inhibit T-cell action, through cytotoxic T-lymphocyte associated antigen-4 (*CTLA-4*), programmed cell death-1 (*PD-1*) and its ligands (*PDL-1*) [37, 40].

PD-1 is an inhibitory "immune checkpoint" expressed on the surface of T-cells, B-cells and NK-cells. When T-cells have been activated by their *TCR*, the cells express at the same time *PD-1*, which is a possibility to the attacked cell to escape from the immune reaction (**Figure 5**). Cancer cells express the ligand *PDL-1* on their surfaces, activating *PD-1* of T-cells, escaping from the attack [37, 40].

PD-L1 expression has been associated with large tumor size, high grade, high proliferation, estrogen receptor (*ER*)-negative status, and human epidermal growth factor receptor-2 (*HER2*)-positive status in breast cancer. Survival in breast cancer is inversely related to *PD-1/PDL-1* levels. *PDL-1* expression increases tumor

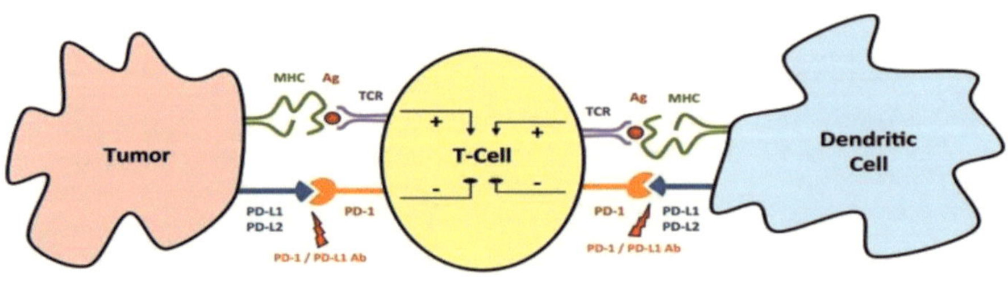

Figure 5.
Simplified schematic illustration of PD-1/PDL-1 interactions in immune responses against cancer cell. Tumoral antigens (Ag) are presented via T-cell by major histocompatibility complex (MHC) of dendritic cells. T-cell recognize tumoral Ag via TCR (T-cell receptor). Interaction Ag-TCR induces an positive immune response against tumoral Ag. Though, there is a scape mechanism of cancer cell from the T-cell attack: interaction of programmed death cell ligands (PDL-1/2) expressed by cancer cell with PD-1 expressed by T-cell inhibit the T-cell action. This scape mechanism of cancer cell mimics the regulation action to avoid immune responses of T-cell against self antigens. The principle of immune therapy is the inhibition of PD-1/PDL-1 (extracted from [40]).

aggressiveness, stimulating tumorigenesis, invasiveness and ability to escape from cytotoxic T *CD8+* lymphocytes attacks [39, 41]. The immunohistochemical evaluation of *PDL-1* is shown in **Figure 6**.

Immune therapies with anti-*CTLA-4* and anti-*PD1*/anti-*PDL-1* agents have been promising for treating several cancers. In breast cancer, some researches reported positive results around 20% of breast tumors on treatment with these agents, mainly the "triple negative" and *HER-2* subtypes, for their higher antigenicity. In general, breast cancer present lower immunogenicity than other cancers and breast cancer cells frequently create an immunosuppressor tumor microenvironment by signaling [37, 43].

The presence of tumor infiltrating lymphocytes (TIL) in some breast cancers has been related to a favorable prognosis, especially in "triple negative" and *HER-2* subtypes. TIL are formed mainly by T-cells *CD3+/CD56* negative, which are either *CD4+* or *CD8+*. A minority component of B-cells *CD20+* and *NK-cells* may be present. The attraction of TIL by cancer cells have been related to their expression of some chemokines, like *CXCL9* and *CXCL13* [37, 44].

In "triple negative" and *HER-2* subtypes of breast cancer, the presence of TIL is related to a better response to neoadjuvant therapy, as well neoadjuvant treatment may modify the tumor microenvironment to attract TIL to tumor site. Furthermore, when the TIL are not attracted instead of neoadjuvance, it is indicative for bad prognosis [44].

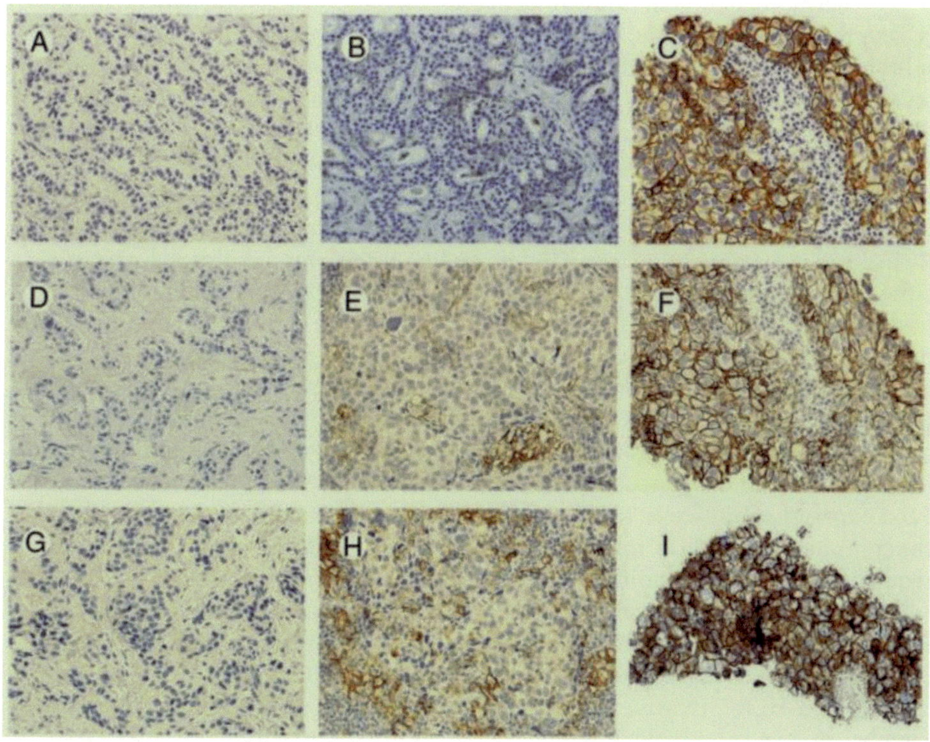

Figure 6.
Examples of PDL-1 expression in breast cancer using 3 different antibodies: Dako 22C3 (D,E and F), Ventana SP263 (G,H and I) and BioCare RbM CAL10 (A, B and C). PDL-1 scoring is divided into 3 groups: zero staining is negative, 1–49% of positive cells are considered "low PDL-1 expression" and 50% of more positive cells are considered "high PDL-1 expression". Examples of negative, low and high PDL-1 expression are represented on A, B and C for BioCare antibody (extracted from [42]).

6. Advanced stage breast cancer: considerations under current approach and futures perspectives

Metastatic breast cancer is considered incurable nowadays with currently therapies. Therapy of metastatic disease aims to guarantee quality of life, palliation of symptoms and prolongation of the patient survival. Advanced stage disease is becoming increasingly chronic, controlled by sequencial therapies, with more personalized approach than the early stage breast cancer [8].

Systemic therapy is frequently the first choice of metastatic disease. Before the new therapeutic decision, it is necessary to consider the previous treatments. If possible, it is recommended to re-evaluate the histologic features and molecular subtype status of the metastatic lesion through a new biopsy, with new immunohistochemical study for hormonal receptor and *HER-2* status. Some studies reported until 40% of discrepances of metastatic lesion histologic features and molecular subtype status *versus* primary tumor histologic and immunohistochemical aspects [45].

The metastatic disease therapeutic choices search for positive targets to hit more effectively the neoplastic cells. Thereby, expression of hormonal receptors by the metastatic lesion is elective for endocrine therapy. Endocrine drugs include tamoxifen, aromatase inhibitors, fulvestrant and progestins. The use of these drugs in metastasis with hormone receptor positive status have demonstrated increase of free of disease survival in several studies [8, 45].

Furthermore, new generation of drugs which inhibit the cyclin dependant kinase (*CDK*) have been successful in prolongation of free of disease survival in luminal subtype *HER-2* negative metastatic disease. *CDK4/6* is a holoenzyme responsible for several extracellular signaling pathways to cell cycle transitions. *CDK4/6* fosforilates and inactivates retinoblastoma tumor supressor protein (*Rb*). Extracellular signals regulate the expression of cyclins and *CDK* inhibitors, like $p16^{\mathrm{INK4a}}$ [46].

In human cancer, this circuit is dysregulated by either overexpression of cyclin D1, loss of $p16^{\mathrm{Ink4a}}$, the mutation of *CDK4* to an *Ink4*-refractory state, or the loss of *Rb* itself. The primary target of *CDK4* is the *Rb* protein, though this holoenzyme either can phosphorylate factors involved in cell differentiation affecting their transcriptional activity, apoptotic factors affecting their activity and other factors that can directly affect mitochondrial function [8, 46, 47].

Therefore, *CDK* inhibitors act in tumor microenvironment, blocking *Rb* phosphorilation and leading to cell cycle exit. Moreover, *CDK* have kinase activity towards *SPOP*, an ubiquitin protein that interacts with *PDL-1*. *CDK* inhibitors lead to inhibition of *SPOP* phosphorilation with blockade of *PDL-1* and stimulus to *PD-1* expression by T-cells, attracting T-cell infiltration to the tumor. In this way, the combined use of *CDK* inhibitors and *PDL-1/PD-1* inhibitors may be promising, requiring more future studies [46–48].

For the moment, hormonal receptors and *HER-2* status are the few validated molecular targets of clinical importance on metastatic breast cancer approaching through chemotherapy and endocrine therapy. For *HER-2* positive metastatic disease, anti-HER-2 treatment with trastuzumab is well established and is recommended as soon as possible. Immune therapy is not standardized for metastatic breast cancer, since metastatic breast disease is highly heterogeneous. Though, it is a promising therapy for the future, as well the target molecular therapies, which become more effective with discovery of novel pathways and mutations by new studies to be developed [8].

A resume of main biomarkers of clinicopathologic importance for breast cancer management is shown in **Table 3** and a proposal of a algorithm for clinicopathologic evaluation of breast cancer is presented in **Table 4**.

Biomarker	Detection technique	Nature	Clinicopathologic importance
Hormonal receptors/ HER2	IHC[1]/FISH	Biomarkers of molecular subtypes of breast cancer	Targets for endocrine and anti-HER2 therapies; prognostic predictors
BRCA1/BRCA2	PCR sequencing	Biomarker of hereditary breast cancer	Target for PARP inhibitors; indication for other malignancies screening
CD24, CD44, CD133, EPCAM	IHC	Putative stem-cell biomarkers	Prediction of poor prognosis, risk of tumor progression and reduction of survival
PD-1/PDL-1	IHC	Biomarker of possible inhibited immune response of T-cell against cancer cell	Target for immune therapy with PD-1/PDL-1 antagonists
TILs[2]	Histologic assessment and IHC	Marker of better cellular mediated immune response against cancer cell	Prediction of better therapeutic responses, mainly of neoadjuvant therapies

[1]*IHC = Immunohistochemistry.*
[2]*TILs = Tumoral infiltrating lymphocytes.*

Table 3.
Resume of main biomarkers of clinicopathologic importance for breast cancer management.

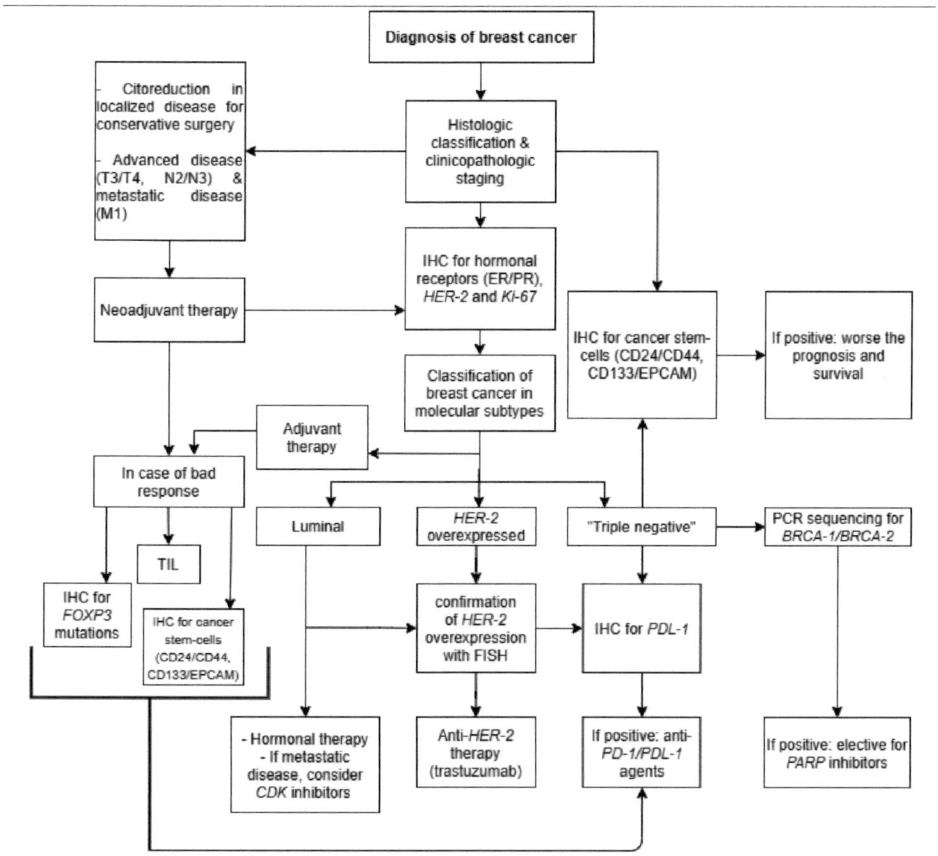

Table 4.
Proposal of an algorithm for clinicopathologic evaluation of breast cancer.

7. Conclusion and final considerations

In the 21st century, breast cancer classification and diagnosis advanced considerably from a purely morphologic/histologic approaching to a immune and molecular basis, with remarkable improvement of the correlation between classification and prediction of biological behavior and prognosis.

The adoption of a clinicopathologic classification based on molecular subtypes of breast cancer in the last decade has modified decisively the management of the disease in the way of molecular era, opening new ways to discovering of multiple targets for novel therapies.

Innovative concepts related to immune reactions related to human cancers, which have been unveiled in the recent years, particularly the immune checkpoints, have offered new treatment tools for several human cancers with promising results, although not still established for breast cancer.

In the molecular era of cancer, the integration of novel knowledges in a direction of more accurated diagnosis and prediction of prognosis to allow personalized therapies is the key to future human cancer management, including the breast cancer.

Author details

Rodrigo Vismari de Oliveira
Rede D'Or São Luiz, São Paulo, Brazil

*Address all correspondence to: rodrigovismari@gmail.com

References

[1] Ahmad, A. (Ed.). (2019). *Breast Cancer Metastasis and Drug Resistance. Advances in Experimental Medicine and Biology.* doi:10.1007/978-3-030-20301-6

[2] Coughlin SS. Epidemiology of Breast Cancer in Women. *Adv Exp Med Biol*. 2019;**1152**:9-29. DOI: 10.1007/978-3-030-20301-6_2

[3] Zardavas D, Irrthum A, Swanton C, Piccart M. Clinical management of breast cancer heterogeneity. *Nat Rev Clin Oncol*. 2015;**12**(7):381-394. DOI: 10.1038/nrclinonc.2015.73

[4] Joseph C, Papadaki A, Althobiti M, Alsaleem M, Aleskandarany MA, Rakha EA. Breast cancer intratumour heterogeneity: current status and clinical implications. *Histopathology*. 2018;**73**(5):717-731. DOI: 10.1111/his.13642

[5] Wesolowski R, Ramaswamy B. Gene expression profiling: changing face of breast cancer classification and management. *Gene Expr*. 2011;**15**(3):105-115. DOI: 10.3727/105221611x13176664479241

[6] Tsang JYS, Tse GM. Molecular Classification of Breast Cancer. *Adv Anat Pathol*. 2020;**27**(1):27-35. DOI: 10.1097/PAP.0000000000000232

[7] Marchio C, Balmativola D, Castiglione R, Annaratone L, Sapino A. Predictive Diagnostic Pathology in the Target Therapy Era in Breast Cancer. *Curr Drug Targets*. 2017;**18**(1):4-12. DOI: 10.2174/1389450116666150203121218

[8] Harbeck N, Penault-Llorca F, Cortes J, et al. Breast cancer. *Nat Rev Dis Primers*. 2019;5(1):66. Published 2019 Sep 23. doi:10.1038/s41572-019-0111-2

[9] Tryfonidis K, Senkus E, Cardoso MJ, Cardoso F. Management of locally advanced breast cancer-perspectives and future directions [published correction appears in Nat Rev Clin Oncol. 2015 Jun;12(6):312]. *Nat Rev Clin Oncol*. 2015;**12**(3):147-162. DOI: 10.1038/nrclinonc.2015.13

[10] Jézéquel P, Kerdraon O, Hondermarck H, et al. Identification of three subtypes of triple-negative breast cancer with potential therapeutic implications. *Breast Cancer Res*. 2019;21(1):65. Published 2019 May 17. doi:10.1186/s13058-019-1148-6

[11] Simpson, Sanders. Differential Diagnosis in Surgical Pathology. Breast: Wolters Kluwer; 2017

[12] Du XL, Key CR, Osborne C. Community-based assessment of adjuvant hormone therapy in women with breast cancer, 1991-1997. *Breast J*. 2004;**10**(5):433-439. DOI: 10.1111/j.1075-122X.2004.21357.x

[13] Prat A, Pineda E, Adamo B, et al. Clinical implications of the intrinsic molecular subtypes of breast cancer. *Breast*. 2015;**24**(Suppl 2):S26-S35. DOI: 10.1016/j.breast.2015.07.008

[14] Bueno GAM. Características clínicas y pronósticas de los subtipos moleculares de cáncer de mama determinados por inmunohistoquímica. Arequipa, Perú [Clinical and prognostic characteristics of the molecular subtypes of breast cancer determined by immunohistochemistry. Arequipa, Peru]. *Rev Peru Med Exp Salud Publica*. 2017;**34**(3):472-477. DOI: 10.17843/rpmesp.2017.343.2530

[15] Irigoyen MA, García FV, Iturriagagoitia AC, Beroiz BI, Martínez MS, Guillén Grima F. Subtipos moleculares del cáncer de mama: implicaciones pronósticas y características clínicas e inmunohistoquímicas [Molecular subtypes of breast cancer: prognostic

implications and clinical and immunohistochemical characteristics]. *An Sist Sanit Navar*. 2011;**34**(2):219-233. DOI: 10.4321/s1137-66272011000200008

[16] Moasser MM. The oncogene HER2: its signaling and transforming functions and its role in human cancer pathogenesis. *Oncogene*. 2007;**26**(45):6469-6487. DOI: 10.1038/sj.onc.1210477

[17] Hida AI, Watanabe T, Sagara Y, et al. Diffuse distribution of tumor-infiltrating lymphocytes is a marker for better prognosis and chemotherapeutic effect in triple-negative breast cancer. *Breast Cancer Res Treat*. 2019;**178**(2):283-294. DOI: 10.1007/s10549-019-05390-x

[18] Ahmed S, Sami A, Xiang J. HER2-directed therapy: current treatment options for HER2-positive breast cancer. *Breast Cancer*. 2015;**22**(2):101-116. DOI: 10.1007/s12282-015-0587-x

[19] Kolarova I, Vanasek J, Odrazka K, et al. Therapeutic significance of hormone receptor positivity in patients with HER-2 positive breast cancer. *Biomed Pap Med Fac Univ Palacky Olomouc Czech Repub*. 2019;**163**(4):285-292. DOI: 10.5507/bp.2019.060

[20] Press MF, Villalobos I, Santiago A, Guzman R, Cervantes M, Gasparyan A, et al. Assessing the New American Society of Clinical Oncology/College of American Pathologists Guidelines for *HER2* Testing by Fluorescence *In Situ* Hybridization: Experience of an Academic Consultation Practice. Arch Pathol Lab Med. 2016 Nov;**140**(11):1250-1258. DOI: 10.5858/arpa.2016-0009-OA Epub 2016 Apr 15. PMID: 27081877

[21] Azizun-Nisa BY, Raza F, Kayani N. Comparison of ER, PR and HER-2/neu (C-erb B 2) reactivity pattern with histologic grade, tumor size and lymph node status in breast cancer. *Asian Pac J Cancer Prev*. 2008;**9**(4):553-556

[22] Ciampa A, Xu B, Ayata G, et al. HER-2 status in breast cancer: correlation of gene amplification by FISH with immunohistochemistry expression using advanced cellular imaging system. *Appl Immunohistochem Mol Morphol*. 2006;**14**(2):132-137. DOI: 10.1097/01.pai.0000150516.75567.13

[23] Talhouet S, Peron J, Vuilleumier A, et al. Clinical outcome of breast cancer in carriers of BRCA1 and BRCA2 mutations according to molecular subtypes. *Sci Rep*. 2020;10(1):7073. Published 2020 Apr 27. doi:10.1038/s41598-020-63759-1

[24] Turk AA, Wisinski KB. PARP inhibitors in breast cancer: Bringing synthetic lethality to the bedside. *Cancer*. 2018;**124**(12):2498-2506. DOI: 10.1002/cncr.31307

[25] Sonnenblick A, de Azambuja E, Azim HA Jr, Piccart M. An update on PARP inhibitors--moving to the adjuvant setting. *Nat Rev Clin Oncol*. 2015;**12**(1):27-41. DOI: 10.1038/nrclinonc.2014.163

[26] Guney Eskiler G, Cecener G, Egeli U, Tunca B. Triple negative breast cancer: new therapeutic approaches and BRCA status. *APMIS*. 2018;**126**(5):371-379. DOI: 10.1111/apm.12836

[27] Baretta Z, Mocellin S, Goldin E, Olopade OI, Huo D. Effect of BRCA germline mutations on breast cancer prognosis: A systematic review and meta-analysis. *Medicine (Baltimore)*. 2016;**95**(40):e4975. DOI: 10.1097/MD.0000000000004975

[28] Tangutoori S, Baldwin P, Sridhar S. PARP inhibitors: A new era of targeted therapy. *Maturitas*. 2015;**81**(1):5-9. DOI: 10.1016/j.maturitas.2015.01.015

[29] Dontu G. Breast cancer stem cell markers - the rocky road to clinical applications. *Breast Cancer Res*. 2008;**10**(5):110. DOI: 10.1186/bcr2130

[30] Honeth G, Bendahl PO, Ringnér M, et al. The CD44+/CD24- phenotype is enriched in basal-like breast tumors. *Breast Cancer Res*. 2008;**10**(3):R53. DOI: 10.1186/bcr2108

[31] Dawood S, Austin L, Cristofanilli M. Cancer stem cells: implications for cancer therapy. *Oncology (Williston Park)*. 2014;**28**(12):1101-1110

[32] Oliveira RV, Souza VB, Souza PC, et al. Detection of Putative Stem-cell Markers in Invasive Ductal Carcinoma of the Breast by Immunohistochemistry: Does It Improve Prognostic/Predictive Assessments? *Appl Immunohistochem Mol Morphol*. 2018;**26**(10):760-768. DOI: 10.1097/PAI.0000000000000513

[33] Czerwinska P, Kaminska B. Regulation of breast cancer stem cell features. *Contemp Oncol (Pozn)*. 2015;**19**(1A):A7-A15. DOI: 10.5114/wo.2014.47126

[34] Das PK, Rakib MA, Khanam JA, Pillai S, Islam F. Novel Therapeutics Against Breast Cancer Stem Cells by Targeting Surface Markers and Signaling Pathways. *Curr Stem Cell Res Ther*. 2019;**14**(8):669-682. DOI: 10.2174/1574888X14666190628104721

[35] Neumeister V, Agarwal S, Bordeaux J, Camp RL, Rimm DL. In situ identification of putative cancer stem cells by multiplexing ALDH1, CD44, and cytokeratin identifies breast cancer patients with poor prognosis. *Am J Pathol*. 2010;**176**(5):2131-2138. DOI: 10.2353/ajpath.2010.090712

[36] Joseph C, Arshad M, Kurozomi S, et al. Overexpression of the cancer stem cell marker CD133 confers a poor prognosis in invasive breast cancer. *Breast Cancer Res Treat*. 2019;**174**(2):387-399. DOI: 10.1007/s10549-018-05085-9

[37] Bayraktar S, Batoo S, Okuno S, Glück S. Immunotherapy in breast cancer. *J Carcinog*. 2019;18:2. Published 2019 May 23. doi:10.4103/jcar.JCar_2_19

[38] Shou J, Zhang Z, Lai Y, Chen Z, Huang J. Worse outcome in breast cancer with higher tumor-infiltrating FOXP3+ Tregs : a systematic review and meta-analysis. *BMC Cancer*. 2016;16(1):687. Published 2016 Aug 26. doi:10.1186/s12885-016-2732-0

[39] Cano-González A, Mauro-Lizcano M, Iglesias-Serret D, Gil J, López-Rivas A. Involvement of both caspase-8 and Noxa-activated pathways in endoplasmic reticulum stress-induced apoptosis in triple-negative breast tumor cells. *Cell Death Dis*. 2018;9(2):134. Published 2018 Jan 26. doi:10.1038/s41419-017-0164-7

[40] Hartkopf AD, Taran FA, Wallwiener M, et al. PD-1 and PD-L1 Immune Checkpoint Blockade to Treat Breast Cancer. *Breast Care (Basel)*. 2016;**11**(6):385-390. DOI: 10.1159/000453569

[41] Sabatier R, Finetti P, Mamessier E, et al. Prognostic and predictive value of PDL1 expression in breast cancer. *Oncotarget*. 2015;**6**(7):5449-5464. DOI: 10.18632/oncotarget.3216

[42] Karnik T, Kimler BF, Fan F, Tawfik O. PD-L1 in breast cancer: comparative analysis of 3 different antibodies. Hum Pathol. 2018 Feb;**72**:28-34. DOI: 10.1016/j.humpath.2017.08.010 Epub 2017 Aug 31. PMID: 28843709

[43] Chen X, Shao Q, Hao S, et al. CTLA-4 positive breast cancer cells suppress dendritic cells maturation and function. *Oncotarget*. 2017;**8**(8):13703-13715. DOI: 10.18632/oncotarget.14626

[44] Wimberly H, Brown JR, Schalper K, et al. PD-L1 Expression Correlates with Tumor-Infiltrating Lymphocytes and Response to Neoadjuvant Chemotherapy in Breast Cancer. *Cancer Immunol Res*. 2015;**3**(4):326-332. DOI: 10.1158/2326-6066.CIR-14-0133

[45] Li Z, Kang Y. Emerging therapeutic targets in metastatic progression:

A focus on breast cancer. *Pharmacol Ther*. 2016;**161**:79-96. DOI: 10.1016/j.pharmthera.2016.03.003

[46] Klein ME, Kovatcheva M, Davis LE, Tap WD, Koff A. CDK4/6 Inhibitors: The Mechanism of Action May Not Be as Simple as Once Thought. *Cancer Cell*. 2018;**34**(1):9-20. DOI: 10.1016/j.ccell.2018.03.023

[47] Deng J, Wang ES, Jenkins RW, et al. CDK4/6 Inhibition Augments Antitumor Immunity by Enhancing T-cell Activation. *Cancer Discov*. 2018;**8**(2):216-233. DOI: 10.1158/2159-8290.CD-17-0915

[48] Lim S, Kaldis P. Cdks, cyclins and CKIs: roles beyond cell cycle regulation. *Development*. 2013;**140**(15):3079-3093. DOI: 10.1242/dev.091744

Chapter 4

Molecular Pathology in the New Age of Personalized Medicine

Valeria Cecilia Denninghoff

Abstract

Personalized medicine is a new approach that allows the identification of patients that can benefit from targeted therapies because of the molecular characteristics of the tumors they present. The molecular profile of the tumor can be studied at the genomic (DNA), transcriptomic (RNA) or protein (protein) level. The next generation sequencing is a useful tool for the study of molecular profile from DNA/RNA. This tool requires molecular pathologists highly trained in pre-analytic processes, tumor area microdissection for tumor cell enrichment, methodology analysis and results. The in-depth study of molecular alterations in patients allows optimizing molecular diagnosis and selecting candidates for receive novel treatments against specific molecular targets. These patients are expected to benefit from multidisciplinary approach and learning. The aim of this chapter is to show the implications of molecular pathology in personalized medicine with an actual approach from the methodological limitations of formalin-fixed paraffin embedded (FFPE) tissues and their pre-analytical conditions.

Keywords: molecular pathology, personalized medicine, next generation sequencing, NGS, clinical benefit, multidisciplinary approach

1. Introduction

Personalized medicine is a new approach that allows the identification of patients that can benefit from targeted therapies, since the molecular characteristics of their tumors could be identified. Over the last decade, new drugs have been incorporated into the treatment, including the development of immunotherapy and treatment against specific molecular targets [1]. Thus, patients can receive specific treatments according to the biology of their tumor, turning oncology a tool for personalized medicine. In order to do so, the development of new DNA/RNA sequencing technologies was required, as well as the development of specific antibodies identifying mutated or altered proteins, and the design of new in situ hybridization techniques. The latter has enabled the selection via genetic biomarkers of patients, who can benefit from therapies targeted against specific molecular alterations [2]. Based on the detection of these point molecular alterations, with a clear oncogenic role, treatments have been developed to block the activation of mutated, amplified proteins or product of translocations by specific drugs. The identification of patients with therapeutic molecular targets in their tumors is currently a standard of care. Notwithstanding that, the initial morphological diagnosis and the eventual tumor classification by immunohistochemistry (IHC), as well as the acquisition, handling and processing of tumor tissue play a pivotal role.

IntechOpen

In advanced-stage patients, a relatively small amount of tissue obtained at a single procedure must be used most efficiently for all studies [3]. In this sense, consensus exists about making histopathological diagnosis using as little material as possible, which should be kept for molecular studies [4, 5]. The combination of less invasive techniques that provide very small samples to carry out an increasing number of determinations is controversial, since it does not allow to increase the amount of tumor cells. Consequently, more sensitive and specific molecular determinations are required [6].

Although several methods are being developed, such as free tumor DNA detection in peripheral blood, most of these determinations are currently experimental and few are validated for clinical use [7, 8]. Therefore, until more sophisticated techniques for these and other molecular markers are validated, the amount/size of the samples should be considered.

The aim of this chapter is to show the implications of molecular pathology in personalized medicine with an actual approach from the methodological limitations of formalin-fixed paraffin embedded (FFPE) tissues and their pre-analytical conditions.

2. Pre-analytical processes

In molecular pathology, several variables should be considered for optimal results, and pre-analytical conditions are evaluated.

2.1 Cold ischemia

One of the crucial phases in tissue management is the period of time immediately after the sample is extracted from the patient until it is placed in a fixation solution (cold ischemia). In an experimental animal model, significant differences in pH values were found between organs at the same cold-ischemia time, and in the same organ at different times. However, no differences were seen in the RNA quality assessed by its integrity number or absorbance ratios [9]. These results reveal a high pH in tissues undergoing ischemia. Firstly, although RNA integrity number (RIN) is a powerful tool to analyze the ribosomal profile and to further infer RNA quality from fresh and frozen tissues (and to compare samples RIN values given the same organism/tissue/extraction method), it is not enough to predict the integrity of mRNA transcripts or to describe the real biological conditions. Secondly, acidic duodenal pH has been reported to alter gene expression in the pancreas of a cystic fibrosis mouse. Upon correction of duodenal pH, either genetically (breeding CFTR-null with gastrin-null mice) or pharmacologically (proton pump inhibitor omeprazole), expression levels of genes measured by quantitative RT-PCR were significantly normalized [10]. Whether alkalosis is secondary to ischemic cell damage, or it may contribute to ischemic cell damage, is yet unknown. Thus, tissue alkalosis in cold-ischemia time may be an underlying mechanism of gene expression changes. Therefore, tissue-pH regulation after organ removal may minimize biological stress in human tissue samples. To date, no consensus exists about the optimal preservation solution. Further optimization of the composition of preservation solutions is required to prolong organ preservation time, and to maximize the yield of successful transplantations by improving the quality and function of organs [11]. Most laboratories have neither control nor record of how long it takes between tissue removal and immersion in the fixer, and its arrival in the laboratory. In addition, most automatic tissue processor machines include a fixation step that further increases the fixation time, which is not often considered.

2.2 Tissue fixation

Once the tissue has been obtained it should be fixed and 10% Neutral buffered formalin (NBF) fixation is recommended. Pre-fixation in alcohol-based fixative, decalcifying acidic solutions, acidic fixatives (such as Bouin) or those containing metallic salts may alter DNA antigenicity or integrity. Setting a period of more than 6 hours and less than 48 hours is recommended [12]. Short or excessive fixation time may have deleterious effects on DNA and protein antigenic epitopes [13, 14]. The most frequently described effect of formalin in DNA is its fragmentation into small pieces. The use of polymerase chain reaction (PCR) techniques in formalin fixed paraffin embedded (FFPE) tissues is associated with a higher incidence of sequence artifacts and risk of misinterpretation in PCR results, compared with the use of fresh samples [15, 16]. After the inclusion of the tissue in paraffin, the sample remains stable and is preserved against oxidative damage or other degenerative effects. However, in addition to fixation, the type of storage is another documented source that can damage DNA and cause artifacts in the PCR. For a better preservation of DNA, FFEP blocks should be stored below 27°C in humidity-free conditions. Although humidity can affect DNA stability, the acceptable humidity control range is not described. In our experience, up to ten-year-old FFEP blocks have been used. Provided that storage is accurately done and the pre-analytical parameters indicated in this chapter are met, blocks can be preserved up to this time [17]. Since FFPE tissue is currently used for genetic analysis, results should always be carefully interpreted. Mutations detected from FFPE samples by sequencing must be confirmed by independent PCR reaction. Determining the nature and duration of fixation is a great challenge to pathology laboratory, which receives samples from other centers. Therefore, it was suggested that the cold ischemia time, the type and time of tissue fixation should be registered in the pathology report [18].

3. Tumor area microdissection for tumor cell enrichment

For a molecular analysis, the following data are required: type of biopsy (primary tumor or metastasis), type of block, and percentage of tumor cells needed for each method.

3.1 PCR amplicon size

As above mentioned, fixation breaks the genetic material into small fragments, and then PCR of FFPE tissue needs a design of specific-sequences primers that flank targets with molecular weight less than 300 bp. Should the designed primers flank a fragmented-amplicon, they fail to perform the enzyme amplification because they need the continuity of the DNA/RNA mold to generate a strand, thus leading to lower sensitivity or false-negative results. Thus, the input for a PCR reaction performed from FFPE tissue requires mandatory quantification with DNA/RNA calculator spectrophotometer. Thus, each methodology uses a different sample input to obtain the analytical sensitivity (LOD). Every PCR requires a balance between its reaction components, and then the sample input has a direct relationship with the concentration of the primers.

Therefore, somatic mutations, which are generated in tumors and are not present in normal cells, require a minimum percentage for each method.

3.2 Tumor cell enrichment

Based on the premise that somatic mutations occur, for the most part, in one of the alleles present in human genome, knowing that in humans there are two equal alleles on somatic chromosomes, one of maternal and one of paternal origin, we must understand that if we seek a tumor marker, we must enrich our input in this allele (**Figure 1**).

Sequencing of tumors is now routine and guides personalized cancer therapy. Mutant allele fractions (MAFs, or the 'mutation dose') of a driver gene may reveal the genomic structure of tumors and influence response to targeted therapies [19]. Mutation fraction can be defined as the ratio between mutant and wild-type (wt) alleles in a tumor sample. Allelic fraction is generally applied to a single mutation in a tumor, and is therefore distinct from allelic frequency, which examines the frequency of an allele in a population. To date, however, these terminuses are unfortunately exchanged. Dideoxynucleotide sequencing is a routine method for identifying genetic changes. Since both alleles are amplified in this method, enough input of mutant allele (as compared to the input of normal allele) must be detected. However, this detection requires at least 10–20% of allelic presence. Mutations below this threshold due to normal cells high contamination or tumor heterogeneity could not be detected by this method [20]. Low percentages of neoplastic cells are sometimes associated with unreliable results. Therefore, the percentage of tumor cells must be estimated either through microdissection technique or selection of block interest region [5, 21]. The normal tissue and the lymphocyte infiltration areas must be removed from the tissue for analysis since both are nucleated elements that provide normal DNA. Areas of necrosis should be also removed, since the cell causing necrosis cannot be identified and may be normal or neoplastic. As we know, cell/tumor free DNA drained by biological mechanisms such as secretion, apoptosis and necrosis can be amplified by new generation methods that require smaller chain fragments, this allows us to infer that necrotic cell DNA can be amplified too, considering that an amount of intact nucleic acid chains still present in necrotic masses, unknowing the normal/tumor cell origin. In case microdissection is performed, higher sensitivity is obtained and more chance to detect a tumor specific mutation.

Depending on the method of extraction, hematic areas might be removed. However, they fail to provide normal DNA, because they are anucled cells, but hemoglobin is one of the main polymerase inhibitors in PCR [22]. Regarding the use of clots, a DNA purification method is required to extract hemoglobin. In this sense, specific columns for FFPE tissues are of value. In several cases, Fine Needle Aspiration (FNA) is the first (and often the sole) diagnostic technique, given its low invasiveness, with

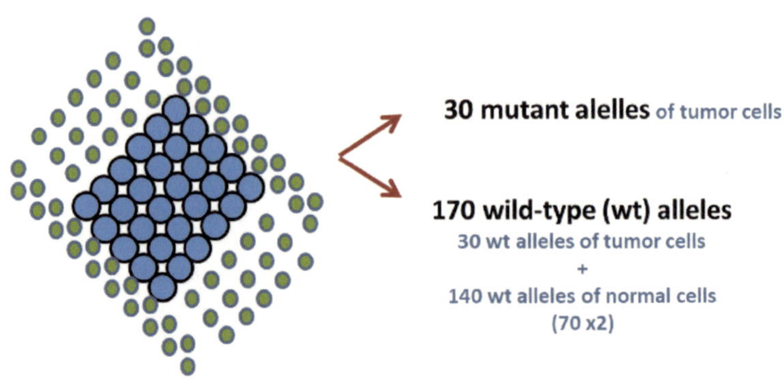

Figure 1.
Mutant allele fractions (MAFs, or the 'mutation dose').

the clot being all the material available for molecular studies. Here formalin fixation is recommended, and although some reports propose 70% ethanol as an alternative, as above mentioned, DNA antigenicity or integrity may be altered by alcohol-based fixatives [5, 6, 23]. To increase the sensitivity of Sanger sequencing, and to discriminate from technical background, at least 70% of tumor cells are required [5]. The chromatogram obtained failed to discriminate specific signal from background. Such chromatogram type may be determined by pre-analytical conditions (pre-fixing, fixative type or fixation time).

As expected, there was a statistically significant difference between large and small samples DNA concentration. However, no significant differences were observed in concentration, fragments number or tumor initial percentage among different small sample types [18]. We can infer that all these types of tissue samples are similarly useful and depend on interdisciplinary medical team (surgeons, radiologists, clinicians, pathologists and oncologists) [6]. Large samples are blocks from surgical specimens, while small samples could be a core biopsy (yielding tissue samples approximately 1 mm in diameter), biopsies from bronchoscopy, nodal biopsies obtained by mediastinoscopy, and fine needle aspiration resulting in cytological specimens and clots. However, no significant differences were observed in concentration, fragments number or tumor initial percentage among different small sample types. **Figure 2** shows that the amount of tissue obtained from small biopsies is often inadequate for a complete evaluation [18].

Over the last decade, genomic research of various solid tumors has suddenly progressed through the discovery of several molecular biomarkers that eventually impact on the prognosis and treatment of most common cancers. Recent technical innovations, such as "next or second generation" sequencing or "massively parallel" sequencing, have the potential to detect many abnormalities in a single assay, and are probably the solution to tissue shortage [24, 25].

This definitely results into multiple activities for surgeons and pathologists, who must obtain and process samples, write a pathology report, choose the material for molecular biology. In furtherance, those molecular biosciences technicians performing studies must draw up guidelines to standardize these practices, and algorithms to cover cyto- and histopathological diagnoses, IHC and molecular studies [4, 5, 23, 24, 26].

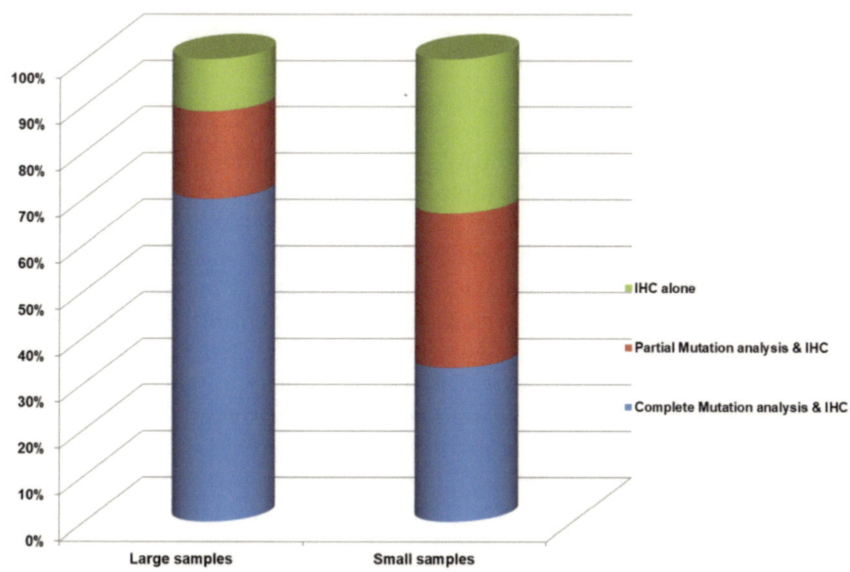

Figure 2.
Performance of IHC and molecular study of large and small biopsies.

4. Methodological analysis and results

Detection of tumor-derived mutations in FFPE is challenging because the tumor DNA is often scarce, fragmented, at a very low concentration and diluted by the presence of a background of non-mutant DNA (both tumor and non-tumor origin). Once the area of tumor cells is selected to be processed, the method of purification of the macromolecules must be chosen. Although manual non-expensive forms (phenol-chloroform-PK) exist, they fail to provide the necessary amount and quality of DNA. There are affinity columns for DNA, RNA or DNA/RNA together, which can be used on a low scale; and finally automated nucleic acid extraction equipment. Some years ago manual extraction was used for FFPE tissue because the columns were developed only for fresh samples. In the last decade the advent of personalized medicine boosted the development of new methodologies for this purpose. Heydt *et al.* used FFPE tissue samples for the comparison of five automated DNA extraction systems, the BioRobot M48, the QIAcube and the QIAsymphony SP all from Qiagen (Hilden, Germany), the Maxwell 16 from Promega (Mannheim, Germany) and the InnuPure C16 from Analytik Jena (Jena, Germany). The results revealed that the Maxwell 16 from Promega seems to be the superior system for DNA extraction from FFPE material. This study also evaluated DNA quantification systems using the three most common techniques, UV spectrophotometry, fluorescent dye-based quantification, and quantitative PCR. The comparison of quantification methods showed inter-method variations, but all methods could be used to estimate the right amount for PCR amplification and for massively parallel sequencing. DNA extracts were quantified as follows: NanoDrop 2000c spectrophotometer (Thermo Fisher Scientific), Quant-iT dsDNA HS Assay on the Qubit 2.0 fluorometer (Life Technologies), QuantiFluor dsDNA Sample Kit on the QuantiFluor-ST fluorometer (Promega) and Quant-iT Pico-Green dsDNA reagent (Life Technologies) on the LightCycler 480 Instrument (Roche). No difference was observed in mutation analysis based on the results of the quantification methods. These findings emphasize that it is particularly important to choose the most reliable and constant DNA extraction system, especially when using small biopsies and low elution volumes [27]. Once DNA/RNA has been obtained and quantified, analysis requires highly sensitive and specific assays. Different techniques with their own advantages and disadvantages can be used to identify and monitor mutations.

4.1 Real-time qPCR assays

A real-time PCR or quantitative PCR (qPCR) amplifies, both quantitatively and semi-quantitatively, a targeted DNA molecule during the PCR process. There exist at least two methods for the detection of PCR products: non-specific fluorescent dyes that bind double-stranded DNA molecules by intercalating between the DNA bases. This method is used in qPCR because the fluorescence can be measured at the end of each amplification cycle to determine, either relatively or absolutely, how much DNA has been amplified. The other method is sequence-specific DNA probes consisting of oligonucleotides that are labeled with a fluorescent reporter, which permits detection only after hybridization of the probe with its complementary sequence (TaqMan).

There is also a revolutionary method that uses PlexZyme™ technology. The revolution in this technology is given by a structure called partzyme (A and B). Each partzyme has 3 different regions: (I) the region that joins the target sequence of DNA, (II) the catalytic constituent region, and (III) the region that joins the probe. Once the primers generate the amplicons, both partzymes join their complementary sequences through the region (I), acquiring a characteristic structure thanks to the region (II) that allows the region (III) to be exposed. The fluorescently labeled reporter probe also binds to the partzymes in the region (III) exposed, and once the active catalytic core is formed, the probe is cleaved, producing a signal that is indicative of successful amplification of the target gene. This technology can produce a robust quintuplex with five target assays into a single reaction tube that contained 10 partzymes (5 A and 5 B), 10 primers (5 forwards and 5 revers), and 5 probes, with a 5 different fluorophores. All consumables required for sample preparation and RT-PCR amplification and detection are provided in a single cartridge loaded into the Idylla™ system. Handling time is less than two minutes per sample, with the liquid-tight, disposable cartridges greatly reducing the risk of contamination (Biocartis NV, Belgium).

4.2 ddPCR assay

In the non-sequencing space, digital PCR (ddPCR), is a highly sensitive and specific technique for the detection of mutations. DNA molecules are split into droplets that form a water oil emulsion. Droplets are like individual test tubes or wells on a plate where a PCR reaction occurs from a DNA template. Each drop is analyzed or read to determine the fraction of positive droplets in the total sample and can accurately and sensitively quantify a mutation. The creation of thousands of drops means that a single sample can generate thousands of data, which are statistically analyzed. For digital PCR the assays are limited to specific single mutations or sets of highly related mutations at the same locus. The analysis of broader genomic regions using ddPCR is not feasible. However, discriminatory multiplex ddPCR assays can be developed, which enable very rapid and cost-effective monitoring for a limited number of mutations in serial plasma samples [28].

4.3 Sanger capillary sequencing

Sanger sequencing is a DNA sequencing method based on the selective incorporation of chain-terminating dideoxynucleotides by DNA polymerase during in vitro DNA replication [29, 30]. This method was first developed by Frederick Sanger and colleagues in 1977, and became the most widely used sequencing method for over 40 years. However, the Sanger method remains widely used for smaller-scale projects and for validation of NGS results.

4.4 Next-generation sequencing (NGS)

In this decade, the treatment of cancer patients has evolved with the addition of new massive sequencing technologies. This contributed to the study of tumor biology with an accurate and highly covered diagnostic method that allows the selection of those patients likely to benefit most from target-specific targeted therapies. NGS, massively parallel or deep sequencing, refers to a DNA sequencing technology that has revolutionized genomic research. NGS can be used to sequence the whole human genome within a single day. In contrast, the previous Sanger sequencing technology used to decipher the human genome took over a decade to deliver the final draft [31]. Over the last years, massively parallel sequencing has rapidly evolved and has now transitioned into molecular pathology routine laboratories. This is an interesting platform for the simultaneous analysis of multiple genes with low input material. Therefore, laboratories working with FFPE material and high sample throughput largely require high-quality DNA obtained from automated DNA extraction systems. The spectrum of DNA variation in a human genome comprises small base changes (substitutions), insertions and deletions of DNA, large genomic deletions of exons or whole genes and rearrangements, such as inversions and translocations. Traditional Sanger sequencing focuses on the discovery of substitutions and small insertions and deletions.

There are a number of different NGS platforms using different sequencing technologies, but all these platforms sequence millions of small fragments of DNA in parallel. The aim of bioinformatics analyses is to piece together these fragments by mapping the individual reads to the human reference genome (pipelines). Each of the three billion bases in the human genome is sequenced several times, in order to provide accurate data and an insight into unexpected DNA variation. NGS can be used to sequence either whole genomes or specific genomic areas of interest, including all 22,000 coding genes, the whole-genome sequencing (WGS), the whole exome sequencing (WES). This is a genomic technique for sequencing all of the protein-coding regions of genes in a genome, known as the exome; or small numbers of individual genes (NGS panels).

Parallel sequencing requires target enrichment, which is a pre-sequencing step that only allows part of a whole-genome be sequenced, or regions of interest, without sequencing the entire genome of a sample. The two most commonly used techniques for NGS target enrichment are capture hybridization and amplicon-based (multiplex PCR). In capture hybridization, genomic DNA is cut to produce small fragments that join sequencer-specific adaptors and indexes to prepare the library, and then the sample is hybridized with biotinylated RNA library primers. Target regions are extracted with magnetic streptavidin beads, amplified and sequenced. Capture hybridization is a screening method for large genetic panels and a large DNA input (more than 1 ug DNA), with a laborious and complex workflow, but a better performance. In amplicon sequencing, custom oligo capture probes are designed to flank DNA specific regions without fragmenting. Extension/ligation takes place between hybridized probes. Finally, the uniquely labeled amplicon library is ready for cluster generation and sequencing. The extension/ligation occurs between hybrid probes which determines a uniquely tagged amplicon library ready for cluster generation and sequencing. Amplification sequencing is used for small gene panels or somatic mutation hotspots (target from kb to Mb), with lower DNA input (100 ng). It has a simple and fast protocol (combining sample preparation and enrichment in one assay), but it is more liable to false positive and negative calls. Considering the WGS method in the same fresh and FFPE samples, hybrid capture sequencing showed higher sensitivity compared to amplicon sequencing, while maintaining 100% specificity using Sanger sequencing as a validation method. Amplicon method has higher target rates. Hybridization capture-based approaches demonstrated that many of them could be false positives or negatives [32]. These results reveal advantages and disadvantages of both methods. Therefore, a greater number of trials must be undertaken to demonstrate both clinical usefulness and socioeconomic benefits. On occasions, an extremely sensitive method is not worth using given its clinical implications.

The basic premise of cancer genomics is that cancer is caused by somatically acquired mutations, and is therefore a disease of the genome. Capillary-based cancer sequencing has been ongoing for over a decade. However, these investigations were restricted to relatively few samples and small numbers of candidate genes. Tumor heterogeneity and the addition of new molecular targets have become a challenge that needs a multidisciplinary approach and learning, with the study of the molecular profile of the tumor at the genomic (DNA), transcriptomic (RNA) or protein (protein) level. NGS technique is a useful and novel tool for the study of molecular profile from DNA/RNA. To do the library using amplicon methods it is only necessary to obtain 10 ng of DNA just from the tumor, and 10 ng of RNA, which is feasible, even from small samples, fixed in formalin and included in paraffin [31].

Thus, three of the major technical drawbacks of the massive analysis required for the approach of multiple specific biomarkers for the treatment are resolved. These drawbacks include the small size of biopsy sample and material scarcity, paraffin fixation of tissues and its effect on DNA/RNA and the impossibility to collect and store fresh material in standard clinical practice. Therefore, this type of studies is necessary to optimize the quality of patient care, avoiding errors and false positives or negatives. Thus, the use of NGS panels with small and overlapping amplicons would solve all these drawbacks, always associated with a bioinformatics algorithm (pipeline) that allows the overlap of the fragments obtained with a reference sequence.

5. In-depth study of molecular alterations

The prevalence of molecular alterations with targeted treatment may vary according to different variables, such as the region of the world, race and gender [33, 34]. About 86% of tumors have molecular alterations that can potentially be treatable with approved or developing drugs, of which approximately 30% have clinically available drugs. The distribution of these alterations in patients with metastatic disease varies compared to those observed in resected tumors at earlier stages [35].

Different analysis options may be combined according to the molecular target to be identified, the type of molecular alteration and the type of sample required. Regarding the KRAS gene, a GTPase which functions as an upstream regulator of the MAPK and PI3K pathways, it is frequently mutated in various cancer types including pancreatic, colorectal and lung cancers [36].

KRAS was one of the first markers to be used as a therapeutic target in colorectal cancer (CRC) in clinical practice since the approval of cetuximad in the second line in 2008. Both the European Medical Agency (EMEA) and the Food and Drug Administration (FDA) in 2008 approved the use of anti-EGFR monoclonal antibodies in patients with tumors with non-mutated KRAS (KRAS-wt). The selection of patients for anti-EGFR treatment based on the mutational status of codons 12 and 13 of the KRAS gene is highly specific to non-responder patients. At that time, the tissue was not macro-dissected, biopsies containing more than 70% of tumor cells were processed by sequencing for the reasons mentioned above, and approximately 30% of cases could not be evaluated since they failed to meet these criteria. Codon 12 and 13 of exon 2 of the KRAS gene were studied and the type of mutation found was irrelevant. For exon 2, 40% of the CRC patients were mutated and 60% were wt (codon 12 and 13). Results showed that 95% of patients with mutated CRC for KRAS did not benefit from anti-EGFR treatment. However, it was not sensitive enough because only half of patients with KRAS-wt tumors responded to treatment [37]. Then, the 59 and 61 codons of exon 3 and the 117 and 146 codons of exon 4 were eventually added. Automated qPCR methods were developed, which covered these hot-spots and dually reported wt or mutated. Nowadays, these binomial methods (wt/mutated) would not serve to identify the G12C amino acid change (c.34G > T p.Gly12Cys). Target therapies like KRAS G12C covalent inhibitors, such as AMG-510, are currently in early phase clinical trials and show promising results for the treatment of KRAS G12 mutant lung cancer patients. However, KRAS G12C colorectal cancer patients have not shown the same response. KRAS mutation testing was carried out using 13 technologies and assays. Limits of detection (LD) of the 13 methods were showed in the following table. Of 13 assays evaluated in this work, 9 showed relatively similar levels of accuracy and reliability in detecting KRAS mutations at low levels with varying sensitivities (50 copies mutant allele frequency by each technology). The best performances were obtained by three assays: Oncomine Focus Assay, Idylla KRAS Mutation Test and UltraSEEK, with high sensitivity and specificity across the entire cell line panel. The worst performances in detection were Illumina Nextera Rapid Capture Custom Lung Panel and Sanger capillary sequencing [38].

	Real-time quantitative PCR			MALDI-TOF		NGS						ddPCR	Sanger
	1	**2**	**3**	**4**	**5**	**6**	**7**	**8**	**9**	**10**	**11**	**12**	**13**
LD	5	5	5	10	0,1	5	5	5	10	5	5	0.001	20

1. **therascreen KRAS RGQ PCR Kit**
2. **cobas KRAS Mutation Test**
3. **Idylla KRAS Mutation Test**
4. **iPLEX Pro**
5. **UltraSEEK**
6. **ThunderBolts**
7. **Oncomine Focus Assay**
8. **Sentosa SQ NSCLC Panel**
9. **Illumina Nextera Rapid Capture Custom Lung Panel**
10. **Ion AmpliSeq Cancer Hotspot Panel v2**
11. **TruSight Tumor 15 panel**
12. **PrimePCR ddPCR Mutation Assays KRAS**
13. **ABI3730 sequencing**

The NGS study may infer biological mechanisms that may explain primary resistance (absence of response to tyrosine kinase inhibitors and disease progression as a better response). This information is required for decision-making of the allelic frequency data for DNA sequence variants, amplified reads for fusions, or the number of copies of amplified genes, since in order to determine that a sequence variant has a clear oncogenic role in the tumor, its representative presence is required. One of the most common false positives with NGS, partly due to its high sensitivity, is the amplification and sequencing of variants from clonal hematopoiesis. Obtaining DNA from FFPE is a methodology used for more than decades, with satisfactory results, since the DNA obtained was degraded by fixation-paraffinization process, as well as its opposite effect which is the deparafinization of tissue. Obtaining RNA from this type of sample is most controversial given its increased lability, and was recently accepted due to the incorporation of new purification strategies. Therefore, obtaining RNA from FFPE was the greatest difficulty of this DNA/RNA NGS method, and required this minimum learning curve to achieve optimal 80% performance (**Figure 3**). The effectiveness of RNA isolation was calculated, taking into account criterion >5000 reads as evaluable sample, for each run/chip. Increased performance was achieved as the long runs occurred. The initial yield was less than 50%, reaching 80% maximum, because the fixation of the tissue as well as the deparanization process are counterproductive effects for obtaining RNA. Pre-analytical pathological processes for NGS take a crucial role.

This has been especially relevant in RNA sequencing from paraffin block. A learning curve is required before using this methodology in the clinical field. The acquisition of macromolecules management is critical. On the other hand, multidisciplinary work is crucial for the correct interpretation of the information provided by these new technologies. Crude data alone, without associated bioinformatics information, should not be used for the treatment of patients. The main pitfall of NGS in the clinical setting is the infrastructure, such as computer capacity and

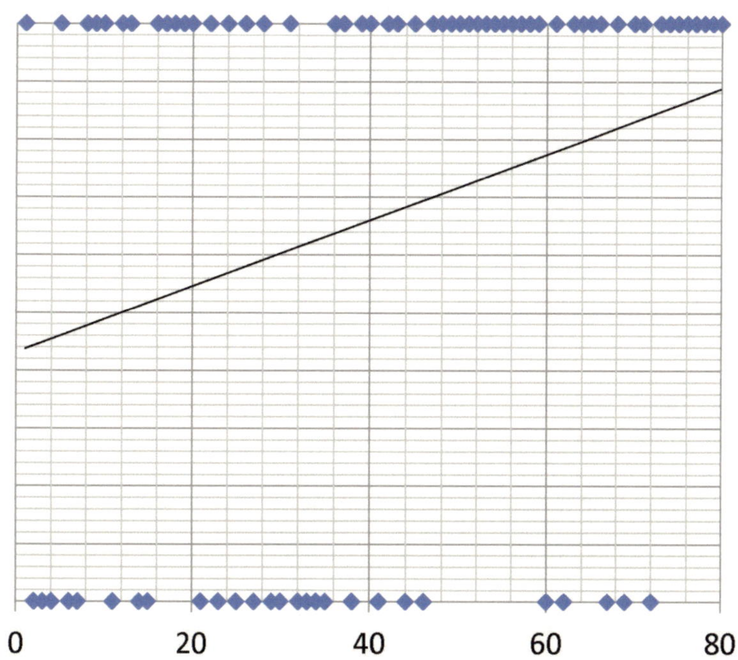

Figure 3.
RNA performance (1= > 5000 reads, 0 < 5000 reads).

storage, and personnel trained in comprehensive analyses and interpretation of the subsequent data. In addition, and in order to obtain clinically relevant information in a clear and robust interface, the volume of data needs to be proficiently managed. However, to make NGS cost effective one would have to run large batches of samples which may require supra-regional centralization. The objective of implementing new technologies is to develop personalized treatment strategies that result in prolongation of survival of patients with a better quality of life.

6. Conclusion

The analysis of the biology of tumors, using NGS, allows to expand the number of molecular alterations to be studied, and allows to detect more patients who can benefit from targeted treatments, modifying the survival in patients with detected and treated molecular alterations. A continuous and inexorable shift in surgical pathology can be observed, with histological diagnosis being just one of its components. The molecular profile is nowadays an essential tool for anatomic pathology practice, which invariably requires highly trained specialists. The in-depth study of molecular alterations in patients allows optimizing molecular diagnosis and selecting patients to receive novel treatments, targeted against specific molecular targets for the clinical benefit of patients, through a multidisciplinary approach and learning.

Acknowledgements

The author thanks Dr. Boris Elsner & Dr. Alejandra Avagnina for their mentorship; Dr. Alejo Garcia† for being an excellent scientific partner; and Valeria Melia for proofreading of the manuscript.

Conflict of interest

The author declares no conflict of interest.

Author details

Valeria Cecilia Denninghoff
CEMIC-CONICET Interacting Units, (CEMIC: Center for Medical Education and Clinical Research "Norberto Quirno" – CONICET: National Scientific and Technical Research Council) and Buenos Aires University (UBA), Ciudad Autónoma de Buenos Aires, Argentina

*Address all correspondence to: vcdennin@gmail.com

References

[1] Carlisle JW, Ramalingam SS: A banner year for immunotherapy and targeted therapy. Nat Rev Clin Oncol 2019;16:79-80. DOI: 10.1038/s41571-018-0138-4

[2] Camidge DR, Doebele RC, Kerr KM: Comparing and contrasting predictive biomarkers for immunotherapy and targeted therapy of NSCLC. Nat Rev Clin Oncol 2019;2016:341-335. DOI: 10.1038/s41571-019-0173-9

[3] TsaoMS, SakuradaA, CutzJC, ZhuCQ, Kamel-Reid S, Squire J, Lorimer I, Tong Zhang, Ni Liu, Daneshmand M, Marrano P, da Cunha Santos G, Lagarde A, Richardson F, Seymour L, Whitehead M, Ding K, Pater J, Shepherd FA: Erlotinib in Lung Cancer - Molecular and Clinical Predictors of Outcome. N Engl J Med 2005;353:133-144. DOI: 10.1056/NEJMoa050736

[4] Pirker R, Herth F, Kerr K, Filipits M, Taron M, Gandara D, Hirsch FR, Grunenwald D, Popper H, Smit E, Dietel M, Marchetti A, Manegold C, Schimacher P, Thomas M, Rosell R, Capuzzo F, Stahel R, European EGFR Workshop Group: Consensus for EGFR Mutation Testing in Non-small Cell Lung Cancer. Results from a European Workshop. J Thorac Oncol 2010;5:1706-1713. DOI: 10.1097/JTO.0b013e3181f1c8de

[5] Lindeman N, Cagle P, Beasley M, Chitale DA, Dacic S, Giaccone G, Jenkins RB, Kwiatowski DJ, Saldivas JS, Squire J, Thunnissen E, Ladanyi M: Molecular testing guideline for selection of lung cancer patients for EGFR and ALK tyrosine kinase inhibitors: guideline from the College of American Pathologists, International Association for the Study of Lung Cancer, and Association for Molecular Pathology. J Thorac Oncol 2013; 8: 823-859. DOI: 10.1097/JTO.0b013e318290868f

[6] EllisP, BlaisN, SoulieresD, IonescuDN, Kashyap M, Liu G, Melosky B, Reiman T, Romeo P, Shepherd FA, Tsao MS, Leigh NB: Systematic Review and Canadian Consensus. Recommendations on the Use of Biomarkers in the Treatment of Non-small Cell Lung Cancer. J Thorac Oncol 2011;6:1379-1391. DOI: 10.1097/JTO.0b013e318220cb8e

[7] Aparicio S, Caldas C: The Implications of Clonal Genome Evolution for Cancer Medicine. N Engl J Med 2013; 368:842-851. DOI: 10.1056/NEJMra1204892

[8] Diaz L, Bardelli A: Liquid Biopsies: Genotyping Circulating Tumor DNA. J Clin Oncol 2014;32:579-586. DOI: 10.1200/JCO.2012.45.2011

[9] Denninghoff V, Olivieri EHR, Fresno C, Uceda A, Mota L, Suenega AP, Carraro DM, Martins VR, Avagnina A, Soarres FA, Fróes Marques Campos AHJ: Tissue alkalosis in cold-ischemia time. Sci Rep 2017;7:10867. DOI: 10.1038/s41598-017-11284-z

[10] Kaur S, Norkina O, Ziemer D, Samuelson LC, De Lisle RC: Acidic duodenal pH alters gene expression in the cystic fibrosis mouse pancreas. AJP Gastrointestinal and Liver Physiology;287:G480-490. DOI: 10.1152/ajpgi.00035.2004

[11] Petrenko A, Carnevale M, Somova A, Osorio J, Rodríguez J, Guibert E, Fuller B, Froghi F: Organ Preservation into the 2020s: The Era of Dynamic Intervention. Transfus Med Hemother 2019;46:151-172. DOI: 10.1159/000499610

[12] Wolff AC, Hammond MEH, Schwartz JN, Hagerty KL, Allred DC, Cote RJ, Dowsett M, Ftzgibbons PL, Hanna WM, Lamger A, McShane LM, Paik S, Pegram MD, Perez EA, Press MF,

Rhodes A, Sturgeon C, Taube SE, Tubbs R, Vance GH, van de Vijver M, Wheeler TM, Hayes DF, American Society of Clinical Oncology/College of American Pathologists: American Society of Clinical Oncology/College of American Pathologists guideline recommendations for human epidermal growth factor receptor 2 testing in breast cancer. Arch Pathol Lab Med 2007; 131:18-43. DOI: 10.1043/1543-2165(2007)131[18:ASOCCO]2.0.CO;2

[13] Eberhard D, Giaccone G, Johnson B, Non-Small-Cell Lung Cancer Working Group: Non-Small-Cell Lung Cancer Working Group. Biomarkers of response to epidermal growth factor receptor inhibitors in Non-Small-Cell Lung Cancer Working Group: standardization for use in the clinical trial setting. J Clin Oncol 2008;26:983-994. DOI: 10.1200/JCO.2007.12.9858

[14] Greer C, Lund J, Manos M: PCR amplification from paraffin embedded tissues: recommendations on fixatives for longterm storage and prospective studies. PCR Methods Appl 1991,1:46-50. DOI: 10.1101/gr.1.1.46

[15] Williams C, Ponten F, Moberg C, Söderkvist P, Uhlén M, Pontén J, Sitbon G, J Lundeberg J: A high frequency of sequence alterations is due to formalin fixation of archival specimens. Am J Pathol 1999,155:1467-1471. DOI: 10.1016/S0002-9440(10)65461-2

[16] Akbari M, Hansen M, Halgunset J, Skorpen F, Krokan HE: Low copy number DNA template can render polymerase chain reaction error prone in a sequence-dependent manner. J Mol Diagn 2005;7:36-39. DOI: 10.1016/s1525-1578(10)60006-2

[17] Kapila SN, Boaz K, Natarajan S: The post-analytical phase of histopathology practice: Storage, retention and use of human tissue specimens. Int J Appl Basic Med Res 2016; 6:3-7. doi: 10.4103/2229-516X.173982

[18] García A, Cuello MT, dos Santos M, Elsner B, Avagnina A, Denninghoff V: Performance Assessment of Epidermal Growth Factor Receptor Gene Sequencing According to Sample Size in Daily Practice Conditions. Appl Immunohistochem Mol Morphol 2018;26:495-500. DOI: 10.1097/PAI.0000000000000455

[19] Dienstmann R, Elez E, Argiles G, Matos I, Sanz-Garcia E, Ortiz C, Macarulla T, Capdevila J, Alsina M, Sauri T, Verdaguer H, Vilaro M, Ruiz-Pace F, Viaplana C, Garcia A, Landolfi S, Palmer HG, Nuciforo P, Rodon J, Vivancos A, Tabernero J: Analysis of mutant allele fractions in driver genes in colorectal cancer – biological and clinical insights. Mol Oncol 2017; 11: 1263-1272. DOI: 10.1002/1878-0261.12099

[20] Do H, Dobrovic A: Limited copy number-high resolution melting (LCN-HRM) enables the detection and identification by sequencing of low level mutations in cancer biopsies. Mol Cancer 2009;8:82. DOI: 10.1186/1476-4598-8-82

[21] García-Foncillas J, Garrido P, Gómez J, Palacios J, Tarón M: Recomendaciones para la determinación de las mutaciones del gen EGFR en el carcinoma de pulmón no microcítico. Rev Esp Patol 2011;44:17-31. DOI: 10.1016/j.patol.2011.02.003

[22] Al-Soud WA, Radström P: Purification and characterization of PCR-inhibitory components in blood cells. J Clin Microbiol 2001;39:485-493. DOI: 10.1128/JCM.39.2.485-493.2001

[23] Kerr KM, Wistuba I, Yatabe Y. Sample Acquisition, Processing and General Diagnostic Procedures. In: Tsao MS, Hirsch FR, Yatabe Y, editors. IASLC Atlas of ALK Testing in Lung Cancer. International Association for the Study of Lung Cancer. IASLC Press: Colorado USA; 2013. p. 13-16.

[24] Jung CY: Biopsy and Mutation Detection Strategies in Non-Small Cell Lung Cancer. Tuberc Respir Dis 2013;75:181-187. DOI: 10.4046/trd.2013.75.5.181

[25] de Biase D, Visani M, Malapelle U, Simonato F, Cesari V, Bellevicine C, Pession A, Troncone G, Fassina A, Tallini G: Next-Generation Sequencing of Lung Cancer EGFR Exons 18-21 Allows Effective Molecular Diagnosis of Small Routine Samples (Cytology and Biopsy). Plos One 2013;8:e83607. DOI: 10.1371/journal.pone.0083607

[26] Kerr KM, Bubendorf L, Edelman MJ, Marchetti A, Mok T, Novello S, O'Byrne K, Stahel R, Peters S, Felip E, Panel Members: Second ESMO consensus conference on lung cancer: pathology and molecular biomarkers for non-small-cell lung cancer. Ann Oncol. 2014;25:1681-1690. DOI: 10.1093/annonc/mdu145

[27] Heydt C, Fassunke J, Künstlinger H, Ihle MA, König K, Heukamp LC, Schildhaus HU, Odenthal M, Büttner R, Merkelbach-Bruse S: Comparison of pre-analytical FFPE sample preparation methods and their impact on massively parallel sequencing in routine diagnostics. PLoS One 2014;9:e104566. DOI: 10.1371/journal.pone.0104566

[28] Rowlands V, Rutkowski AJ, Meuser E, Carr TH, Harrington EA, Barrett JC: Optimisation of robust singleplex and multiplex droplet digital PCR assays for high confidence mutation detection in circulating tumour DNA. Scientific Reports 2019;9:12620. DOI: 10.1038/s41598-019-49043-x

[29] Sanger F; Coulson AR (May 1975). A rapid method for determining sequences in DNA by primed synthesis with DNA polymerase. J Mol Biol 1975;94:441-448. DOI:10.1016/0022-2836(75)90213-2

[30] Sanger F; Nicklen S; Coulson AR: DNA sequencing with chain-terminating inhibitors. PNAS 1977;74:5463-5467. DOI:10.1073/pnas.74.12.5463

[31] Behjati S, Tarpey PS: What is next generation sequencing? Arch Dis Child Educ Pract Ed 2013;98:236-238. DOI: 10.1136/archdischild-2013-304340

[32] Hung SS, Maissner B, Chavez EA, Ben-Neriah S, Ennishi D, Jones MR, Shulha HP, Chun-Chan F, Boyle M, Kridel R, Gascoyne RD, Mungdall AL, Marra MA, Scott DW, Connors JM, Steidl C: Assessment of Capture and Amplicon-Based Approaches for the Development of a Targeted Next-Generation Sequencing Pipeline to Personalize Lymphoma Management. J Mol Diagn 2018;20:203-214. DOI: 10.1016/j.jmoldx.2017.11.010

[33] Sholl LM, Aisner DL, Varella-Garcia M, Berry LD, Dias-Santagata D, Wistuba II, Chen H, Fujimoto J, Kugler K, Franklin WA, Iafrate J, Ladanyi M, Kris MG, Johnson BE, Bunn PA, Minna JD, Kwiatkowski DJ, and on behalf of the LCMC Investigators. Multi-institutional Oncogenic Driver Mutation Analysis in Lung Adenocarcinoma: The Lung Cancer Mutation Consortium experience. J Thorac Oncol 2015;10:768-777. DOI: 10.1097/JTO.0000000000000516

[34] Kohno T, Nakaoku T, Tsuta K, Tsuchihara K, Matsumoto S, Yoh K, Goto K: Beyond ALK-RET, ROS1 and other oncogene fusions in lung cancer. Transl Lung Cancer Res 2015;4:156-164. DOI: 10.3978/j.issn.2218-6751.2014.11.11

[35] Devarakonda S, Morgensztern D, Govindan R. Genomic alterations in lung adenocarcinoma. Lancet Oncol 2015;16:e342-351. DOI: 10.1016/S1470-2045(15)00077-7

[36] The AACR Project GENIE Consortium: AACR Project GENIE:

powering precision medicine through an international consortium.Cancer Discov 2017;7:818-831. DOI: 10.1158/2159-8290. CD-17-0151

[37] Perazzo F, Piaggio F, Krupitzki H, García A, Avagnina A, Elsner B, Denninghoff V: Clinical-pathological features and gene profile in colorectal cancer Medicina (B Aires) 2013;73:417-422.

[38] Sherwood JL, Brown H, Rettino A, Schreieck A, Clark G, Claes B, Agrawal B, Chaston R, Kong BSG, Choppa P, Nygren AOH, Deras IL, Kohlmann A: Key differences between 13 KRAS mutation detection technologies and their relevance for clinical practice. ESMO Open 2017; 2:e000235. DOI: 10.1136/esmoopen-2017-000235

Section 3

Digital Pathology

Chapter 5

Fast Regions-of-Interest Detection in Whole Slide Histopathology Images

Junzhou Huang and Ruoyu Li

Abstract

Detecting and localizing pathological region of interest (ROI) over whole slide pathological image (WSI) is a challenging problem. To reduce computational complexity, we introduced a two-stage superpixel-based ROI detection approach. To efficiently construct superpixels with fine details preserved, we utilized a novel superpixel clustering algorithm which cluster blocks of pixel in a hierarchical fashion. The major reduction of complexity is attributed to the combination of boundary update and coarse-to-fine refinement in superpixel clustering. The former maintains the accuracy of segmentation, meanwhile, avoids most of unnecessary revisit to the 'non-boundary' pixels. The latter reduces the complexity by faster localizing those boundary blocks. Detector of RoI was trained using handcrafted features extracted from super-pixels of labeled WSIs. Extensive experiments indicates that the introduced superpixel clustering algorithm showed lifted accuracy on lung cancer WSI detection at much less cost, compared to other classic superpixel clustering approaches. Moreover, the clustered superpixels do not only facilitate a fast detection, also deliver a boundary-preserving segmentation of ROI in whole slide images.

Keywords: region of interest, whole slide histopathology images, superpixel, segmentation, detection, unsupervised learning

1. Introduction

At our age, many hazardous infectious diseases, e.g. bird flu, and many different kind of cancers, e.g. lung cancer, are still the top threats to our personal health and the public sanitation as well. Automatic searching and localizing Regions of Interest (ROIs) on histopathological images is a crucial intermediate step between large-scale images acquisition and the computer-aided automated diagnosis that we pursue. As the fast development of deep learning techniques and the introduction of neural network models, e.g. convolutional neural networks (CNNs), to medical image understanding area, we are finally able to extend the boundary of modern medical image saliency detection, classification and segmentation [1–3]. Whole Slide Images (WSIs) are the digitized histopathology images taken over an entire slide of tissue, which retrains as much intact pathological information as possible. Therefore, a typical WSI, that usually has resolution at scale of $10^6 \times 10^6$, is $1.5 \sim 2.0$ Gigabyte large on disk, which is thousands times larger than those images from deep learning benchmark datasets, like MNIST [4] and CIFAR [5].

Therefore, traditional fully convolutional networks, used to work perfectly for medical image segmentation [6], are no longer applicable, because of the parameter scale that may explode and the rising risk of under-fitting along with lack of labeled WSIs for training. We need a brand-new cost-efficient solution designed especially for WSIs to handle such magnificent scale of data without losing too much performance. As far as we know, there are no existing convolutional neural networks who claim themselves to directly work on raw images at WSI scale without any downsampling or patching. The most popular walk-around for extracting features from WSIs is to first sample a bag of patches over WSIs and then train and execute inference on patches respectively. Then, aggregating the prediction from patch level to WSI level is to give final model output. Patch-based network [2] successfully handled classification task on WSIs, [7] enabled survival time inference purely based on tumor tissue WSIs. Although, these models applied to WSIs successfully saved most of computational cost by patching, they also dumped lots of task-relevant information hidden in those patches not being sampled. Besides, losing topological spatial information of patches after being sampled from WSI makes predictor treat patches equally, which is obviously not the optimal strategy.

Considering the practical clinic scenarios for image detection and segmentation techniques applied to CT [6] and MRI [8] and the associated pathophysiological procedures, we summarized some challenging but necessary technical requirements for any ROI detection and segmentation solutions for WSIs:

1. High time and energy efficiency. To make it scalable, the ROI detection and localization is supposed to be accomplished within short period of time with high recall and acceptable precision.

2. High fidelity and high trustworthiness on generated ROIs of WSI. We need to quickly and correctly classify if a proposed ROI belongs to, at least partly, ground truth ROIs. Because the ROI prediction may largely affect downstream tasks, e.g. disease diagnosis decisions.

Regions of interest (ROI) could have different definition according to particular scenarios. In this article, we name ROIs as the local regions filled with tumor cell cluster or other cancer-related cells such as lymphocyte. In past related works, ROI detection and segmentation are usually treated separately as two different tasks. The former is to quickly search and localize any suspicious regions on image according to predefined patterns. The output of this task may not have to be fine-detailed at pixel level, due to computational efficiency concern, and sometimes a bounding box that surrounds, at least partly, the ground-truth ROI is enough satisfactory. While, the latter task is to give a pixel-accurate contour of each detected ROIs, which is significantly more expensive. In fact, detection and segmentation are not strictly isolated, and on the opposite, the two tasks could be combined as one under some circumstances. Many CNNs based image segmentation models are indeed end-to-end solutions directly extract and learn hierarchical feature pyramid from raw channels of images to execute pixel-clustering at different level of granularity. Semantic segmentation network [9] is to obtain object detection and segmentation in single forward-pass of network. The advantages of applying deep neural network is from treating the feature design work as an optimization problem, and therefore CNNs are able to discover hidden representations that better serve prediction tasks than handcrafted descriptors, who are either over-localized or not robust. The requirement on high recall rules out patch-based WSI solutions. And patch-based methods obviously cannot handle segmentation of entire WSIs. However, in order to directly work on WSI input, the networks either make the receptive field of convolutional operators large enough to cover any potential region of interest, or stack more layers with relatively small kernel to aggregate local features from entire ROI to form its high-level representations for classification. No matter what architecture is chosen, the total count of parameter in WSI segmentation network is going to be magnificent. Due to the expense of having quality annotation of all ROIs (i.e. tumor cells) on WSIs, the annotated ground-truths of segmentation for training models is quite constrained and very likely not enough to train a wide and deep network as described above that directly works on raw WSIs.

To work around this difficulty, in the method to be introduced, we first chose to still rely on handcrafted features as descriptors of patches to save massive feature aggregation calculations in CNNs, and in the meanwhile we also utilized the hierarchical pyramid structures appear between feature maps of consecutive convolutional layers of CNNs. While, different from what happened in CNNs, in the pyramid of introduced multi-level iterative method, feature vectors of descriptor are not changed along with level, because we did not have gradients back-propagated from loss to update feature formations, while the spatial segmentation did get updated at different granularity of patching. Without having ground-truth of segmentation of ROIs, we introduced superpixel clustering as an unsupervised way to learn spatial segmentation of image, since we do not have gradient to update the assignment of segmentations as well. At different level granularity, we divide the entire WSI into patches of different scale, then the introduced superpixel clustering method [10] is going to cluster patches based on several handcrafted local textual descriptors, preserving both topological consistency and appearance similarity. After superpixel constructed, we run a pre-trained classifier, e.g. SVM or CRF, to classify superpixels represented by the averaged descriptors of patches. Averaging of patch descriptors is to avoid additional difficulty of training a classifier for superpixels of different size and varying shape. This is also the biggest challenge for building an end-to-end fully convolutional network fed with clustered superpixels, since the shape of input tensor to any neural network cannot be undefined.

The main contributions of article is to decouple and reformulate ROI detection and semantic segmentation, that requires dense annotation, into an iterative execution of unsupervised superpixel clustering and classification at coarse-to-fine level of patching granularity. This semi-supervised approach largely replies on quality of superpixel clustering. To obtain better fine-detailed superpixels, we introduced a novel topology-preserved superpixel clustering algorithm to this problem. Besides, the approach introduced is also dependent on accurate classification of superpixels, especially at coarser levels, because any mistaken classification of coarse superpixel cannot be compensated in fine-grained superpixel refinement at next level of granularity. The recall of ROIs will benefit from the increased classification accuracy. Therefore, we trained compact but robust classifier, e.g. SVM, with minimal data requirement. On the other hand, without fine-tune, an improved segmentation of superpixels will automatically boost accuracy of a pre-trained classifier.

2. Related work

Superpixel is a common replacement of pixel with purposes more than saving computational cost. It clusters nearby pixels of similar attributes together as fundamental operational unit in downstream tasks, e.g. object detection, segmentation and even real-time tracking. In this session we introduced the state-of-the-art superpixel clustering algorithms and the combination of superpixel with deep neural networks (DNNs) in medical image understanding.

2.1 Superpixel clustering

One important feature of superpixel construction is that this is a pure unsupervised approach in which there are no annotated ground-truths in any format for guiding the label assignment on pixels. The pixels are clustered purely based on the attributes, such as appearance and physical location, etc. SLIC [11] is an iterative K-mean superpixel clustering that walk through all pixels. It is able to generate almost equally-sized superpixels with outstanding boundary adherence. And the time complexity could be further reduced by limiting search space to a small nearby area. While, iterating over entire pixels is still too expensive, stopping SLIC from being applied on large images like WSIs. If compromise part of accuracy, SEEDS [12], that started from randomly initialized superpixel partitions, focused on updating boundary pixel allocation only and proposed a fast energy function to evaluate each adaption of pixel label assignment by enforcing color homogeneity. Linear spectral clustering, a.k.a. LSC, combined normalized cut and K-mean clustering after discovering optimizing these two objective functions are in fact equivalent on the condition that defines similar function as inner product of feature vectors [13]. LSC also achieved satisfactory boundary adherence and color consistency within segmented superpixels with $\mathcal{O}(N)$ complexity, where N is the pixel number. Compared to SLIC, LSC saved computations from pre-allocation of pixel to large regions by eigenvector-based normalized cuts. And different from the two-stage Ncuts [14], LSC accomplished Ncuts and K-mean in one-stage. Similar to LSC, the computational complexity of SEEDS and SLIC is also approximated as $\mathcal{O}(N)$. Therefore, within visual comparison in **Figure 1**, we did not include expensive solutions such as ERS [15] with $\mathcal{O}(N^2 \log N)$ and EneOpt0 [16] with $\mathcal{O}(N^3)$ complexity. Because we only consider those approaches who are potentially feasible for segmenting whole slide images.

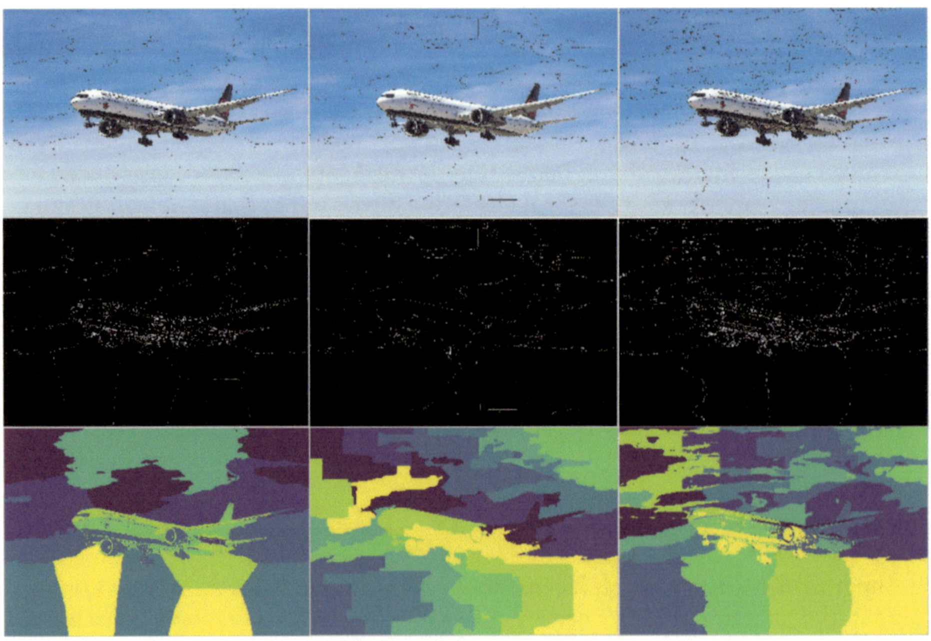

Figure 1.
Example of superpixel clustering on image with three classic solutions: LSC [13] (left), SEEDS [12] (middle) and SLIC [11] (right). The upper row is the edges of superpixels displayed on image. The middle row is the contours of superpixels. The bottom row is the segmentation mask filled with different color on different superpixel.

2.2 ROI and superpixel

Regions of interest (ROI) in histopathology whole slide images (WSIs) are usually those disease-related cells or the tissues of specific patterns, but they do not have descriptive definitions to form a category of objects. Due to the magnificent scale of WSI, the major challenge would be the scalability and the memory efficiency of algorithms. Bejnordi et al. [17] relied on cheap segmentation of superpixels on downsampled WSIs to filter out those regions irrelevant to ROIs. However, it did not correctly notice the inevitable influence of wrong classification of coarse superpixels, because the algorithm completely ruled out those regions from later more accurate segmentation and classification. Besides, the classifiers had to be trained multiple times with patches extracted from the superpixels of different magnification to work on different levels of granularity. Litjens et al. [18] reduced the workload of labeling and grading by two ways: by excluding the areas of definitely normal tissues within a single specimen or by excluding entire specimens which do not contain any tumor cells. Litjens et al. [18] presented a multi-resolution cancer detection algorithm to boost the latter. While it also suffered from the loss of recall as [17]. Another superpixel automated segmentation method is [19], which trained a classifier to predict where mitochondrial boundaries occurs using diverse cues from superpixel graph. While, because the selected superpixel clustering approach [11] did not offer satisfactory boundary adherence, the classifier encumber the overall detection performance. As summary, in order to accomplish a quick detection and segmentation of ROIs in WSI, a combination of superpixel clustering and pre-trained classifier seems a popular choice, while the performance bottleneck was the tradeoff between the efficiency and the quality of superpixel clustering, which directly determined classifier accuracy.

To reduce the intense computational cost in superpixel clustering, the algorithm to be introduced creatively combined the coarse-to-fine scheme [20] and the boundary-only update strategy proposed in SPSS [21]. In our method, clustering manipulated the rectangular blocks of pixel as basic unit and a coarse segmentation of superpixel would be constructed before a more fine-detailed refinement got executed. on each level of construction, only boundary blocks or their nearby neighbors got chance of label update. **Figure 2** illustrated the procedures of introduced superpixel clustering. Furthermore, the introduced boundary-only update strategy on next level would emphasize on differentiating foreground and background blocks, considering the boundaries between superpixels within ROIs are less important. The improvement brought by our algorithm on ROI detection accuracy has been proved and verified in [10, 22], where the method had quantitatively verify the improvement of the accuracy of ROI detection in histopathology images,

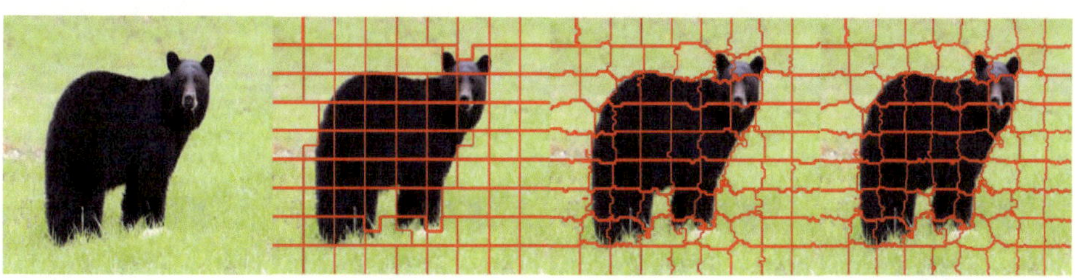

Figure 2.
An example of the coarse-to-fine/boundary-only update based superpixel segmentation algorithm first presented in [10]. The basic manipulation unit is the rectangular block instead of pixels during each stage. We start from a coarse segmentation and end with pixel-level refinement on superpixel boundary. The block size is respectively 10×10, 2×2, 1×1 *(single pixel) from left to right.*

e.g. lung cancer H&E-stained WSIs. **Figure 3** shows comparison of classic superpixel methods [11–13] on cancer patients WSI.

2.3 DNNs on superpixel

As success of deep neural networks in computer vision, many works have extended application of DNNs onto superpixel. Gadde et al. [23] introduced a bilateral inceptions module to accelerate convergence of CNNs with superpixel as network input for semantic segmentation. Kwak et al. [24] treated superpixels as "pooling" layer in neural network, but preserving low-level structures. Therefore, their framework trained semantic segmentation network without pixel-level ground-truth. To construct superpixels for small objects of complicated boundaries, [25] introduced a superpixel segmentation based on pixel features trained with affinity loss and segmentation error. In medical images domain, superpixels are also utilized as a topology-preserving simplification of data for deep network. The organ segmentation network in [26] worked on the descriptors extracted from superpixels clustered in CT images. And then CNN simply did a pixel-wise refinement based on the coarse segmentation given by superpixel. Different from previous works who simply utilized superpixels as reduction of image primitives, [27] proposed an end-to-end" Superpixel Sampling Network" (SSN) which contains differentiable superpixel construction together with learning a task-specific prediction.

The rest of article is organized as following: we first introduce the multi-resolution fast superpixel clustering with coarse-to-fine and boundary-only strategy to increase efficiency. Both mathematical explanation and illustrative examples will be given in Section 3. Then we elaborate the numerical results on classification accuracy and visual comparison of superpixels with classic methods on TCGA WSI dataset in Session 4. Lastly, conclusion and future work will be given in Session 5.

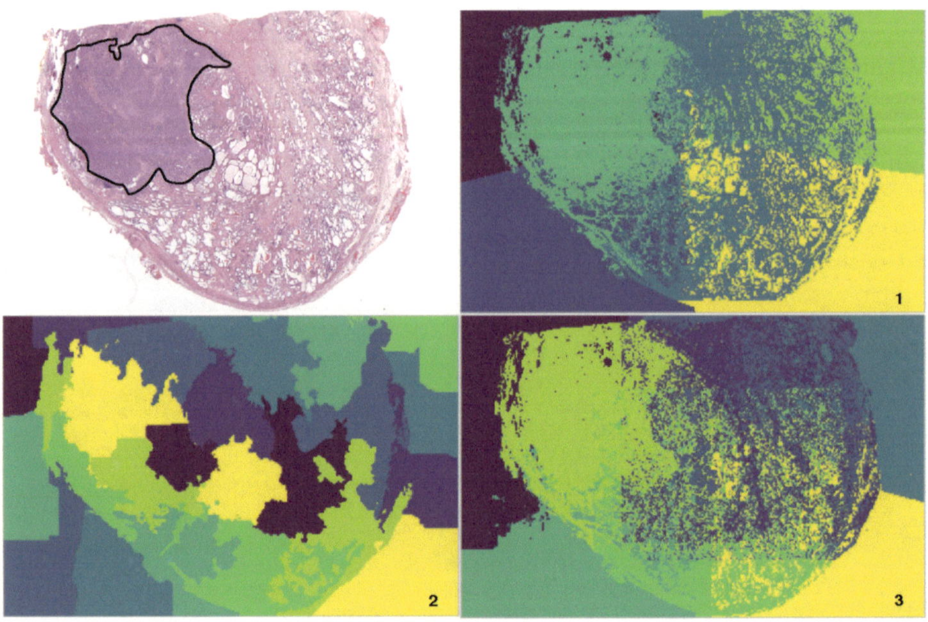

Figure 3.
Example of pathological whole slide image with ROI annotations and the superpixels generated by three classic solutions of linear complexity: (1) LSC [13], (2) SEEDS [12] and (3) SLIC [11].

3. Methodology

The detection framework introduced is not only going to propose bounding box to surround ROIs, but also is going to offer fine-detailed, boundary-adherent superpixel segmentation of them. On the other hand, an improved superpixel construction contributes the differentiation of ROI from background as well. Therefore, the proposed approach comprised two components: fine-detailed superpixel segmentation and superpixel classification. For reduction of computational expense, we chose not to accomplish superpixel segmentation at finest level in one shot. For instead, we first obtain a coarse superpixel segmentation from clustering big pixel blocks (e.g. 500×500). A pre-trained binary classifier then predicts label (ROI v.s. background) of superpixels. Afterwards, those superpixels labeled as ROI along with their neighbors will move to next round of segmentation at finer resolution. The process will be repeated until quality becomes satisfactory. Different from previous superpixel clustering methods [11, 21], the introduced algorithm gave topology-preserving superpixels. A better detection recall is expected as well, since our method did not completely rule out negatively labeled superpixel at coarse stage as [17, 18], and for instead we include negative neighbor superpixels to next level of segmentation.

3.1 Superpixel clustering and detection

3.1.1 Energy function

Think of superpixels of flexible number of blocks $\mathbf{S} = \{s_0, \cdots, s_{K-1}\}$, and the blocks belong to superpixel $\mathbf{S}_k$ as $\{b_0, \cdots, b_{M-1}\}$, we devised two representations of block: appearance and position. Appearance representation of block is the averaged RGB color over pixels in block as $\mathbf{C}$. Position representation of block is the relative position coordinates at center point of block as $\mathbf{P}$. At superpixel level, $\Theta = (\theta_0, \cdots, \theta_{K-1})$ and $\Xi = (\xi_0, \cdots, \xi_{K-1})$ are the center positions and the mean color vectors of superpixels. The objective function to be minimized consists of a series of energy functions and penalty terms. For appearance, total variance of three color channels are color energy function of superpixel $\mathbf{S}_k$ defined as:

$$E_{col}(\mathbf{S}_k) = \sum_{q=0}^{2} \frac{1}{\|s\|} \sum_{b \in \mathbf{S}_k} \left(c_b^q - \xi_k^q\right)^2, \tag{1}$$

also known as appearance coherence. For position, the averaged $l2$ distance from block position $\mathbf{P}_b$ to the center position of its superpixel is the position energy function, $E_{pos}(\mathbf{S}_k) = \frac{1}{\|S_k\|} \sum_{b \in \mathbf{S}_k} \|\mathbf{P}_b - \theta_k\|^2$. This is to ensure clustered blocks are geophysically close. Besides, to avoid seeing any superpixels with sophisticated boundary, we use the total boundary length as boundary penalty function. Furthermore, we constrain the minimal size of finalized superpixel to be at least 25% of initial size. If any update of block's belonging violates this constrain, we give infinity penalty to this update, therefore, the algorithm will reject such label assignment update.

$$P_{size}(\mathbf{S}_k) = \begin{cases} +inf, & size(\mathbf{S}_k) < 0.25 \times initialsize \\ 0, & otherwise. \end{cases} \tag{2}$$

Similar penalty would be applied, if the update causes any isolated blocks who are surrounded by blocks from other superpixels. This is to enforce all generated superpixels to be topologically connected.

3.1.2 Boundary-only update

To define boundary energy function, we need to define boundary block and length. If a block has any neighbor block from other superpixel, then it is a boundary block. The boundary length of block is the number of neighbor blocks that belong to other superpixel.

$$P_b(s) = \sum_{b \in \mathbf{S_k}} \sum_{b_n \in Neighbor(b)} S(\mathbf{S}_k, b_n), \quad (3)$$

where $S(\mathbf{S}_k, b_n)$ is the indicator function of superpixel belonging for block, which return 0 if $b_n \in S_k$, otherwise 1. In our algorithm, we first stack entire initial boundary blocks into a queue, then the iterative superpixel clustering algorithm will work on boundary blocks only for consideration of updating label (i.e. superpixel assignment) of block. This is so-called 'boundary-only update'. In other words, the non-boundary blocks will not be considered for label change until they become boundary blocks. When the algorithm decides to update the label of a block, its neighbor will be considered to become new boundary blocks. When using the boundary-only update, there are two things to notice: 1) when update the label of block, it definitely change the list of boundary blocks; 2) we need to append the new boundary block to the end of the list because and follow the FIFO principle when deciding the order of blocks for consideration of changing label, in order to avoid the risk of divergence given by correlated dimensions in coordinate descent optimization. The candidate superpixel labels for a boundary block to swap are limited to its neighbor superpixels, otherwise it will trigger the topology connectivity penalty by having an isolated block. Given a trial of label update, the algorithm compares the objective function values before and after the change to see whether and how much the change is able to drive energy down.

We elaborate objective function each step of updating block-wise superpixel label assignment as below:

$$E(\mathbf{S}) = \sum_s (E_{col}(s) + \lambda_{pos}E_{pos}(s) + \lambda_b P_b(s) + P_{topo}(s) + P_{size}(s)), \quad (4)$$

where λ_{pos}, λ_b are respectively the tradeoff coefficients for position energy function and boundary length penalty term. In practice, the regularization on superpixel size and topological connectivity will give infinite penalty on those superpixels of over-small size as $P_{size}(S_k) \approx inf$ and those of isolated blocks, i.e. $P_{topo}(S_k) \approx inf$. Therefore, the algorithm will always reject such label proposal that violates topology connectivity and size regularization. When superpixel assignment of a boundary block is updated, the algorithm will add its neighbor blocks to queue, because those non-boundary blocks are now next to other superpixels. The convergence will arrive when the queue is empty.

Algorithm 1 Multi-resolution ROI Detection (MROID).

---

superpixel number - K
for l = 1 to levelMax **do**
  if l = 1 **then**
    1. Initialize blocks **B** on level l size on entire image;
    2. Initialize K superpixels **S**; initialize Θ, Ξ
  else

---

1. Initialize blocks **B** on level l size within positive superpixels and their neighbor superpixels $\hat{\mathbf{S}}$. Initialize Θ, Ξ for $\hat{\mathbf{S}}$.
end if
Compute the mean color and position in each block;
Initialize L, the queue of boundary blocks on level l;
while length$(L) \neq 0$ **do**
Pop out block b_i^l from the queue;
$E_{before} = E(\mathbf{S})$;
for $b_n \in \text{Neighbor}(b_i^l)$ **do**
change label of b_i^l to neighbor b_n's label;
$E_{after}(b_n) = E(\mathbf{S})$;
end for
find the $\hat{b}_n = \arg\min_{b_n \in Neighbor(b_i^l)} E_{after}(b_n)$;
if $E_{after}(b_n) < E_{before}$ then update label of b_i^l to that of $\hat{b}_n$.
append $Neighbor\left(b_i^l\right)$ to L.
end while
run binary classifier on superpixels to predict ROI.
end for

3.1.3 Coarse-to-fine detection

Instead of processing WSI at different resolutions [17], we cluster superpixels at coarse-to-fine level of resolution. Yao et al. [10] adopted boundary-only update as well to save unnecessary revisit to non-boundary blocks, while the boundary blocks on WSI may still be too much for extensive iterations. To further reduce the amount of data brought to finer update with more intense computation, we utilized a pre-trained classifier, e.g. SVM, to predict whether the superpixel belongs part of ROI. For any superpixel moved to finer update, smaller blocks will be initialized within its region. For example, a 10×10 block will be divided into 25 block of size 2×2 arranged at 5×5 grid. Boundary block queue will be refilled with 2×2 blocks who sit on superpixel boundaries. The classifier was trained using features extracted from patches sampled from ROI and non-ROI regions over annotated WSIs. To deal with different cardinality of patch per superpixel, we use pooling patch features at inference time. Given that we did not downsample images, therefore, the classifier trained on raw WSIs is able to be reused with different level of superpixel. See **Figure 4** as illustration.

3.2 Complexity analysis

Pixel-wise superpixel constructions [11, 12] have $\mathcal{O}(N)$ complexity, where N is number of pixel, while it made them infeasible on WSIs of trillions of pixels. The introduced algorithm is able to reduce the complexity to scale of number of block i.e. $\mathcal{O}\left(\sum_{k=0}^{K-1} \|S_k\|\right) \ll \mathcal{O}(N)$. The boundary-only update, first presented in [10], further constrains involved blocks to those boundary blocks. Considering the purpose of clustered superpixel, our algorithm combined detection and superpixel clustering together, and it only executes finer segmentation within those coarse superpixels who were classified as ROI. It saved the calculations wasted on updating the superpixels that do not contribute to ROI detection. Due to the reduced dimensionality, the convergence comes faster than pixel-wise clustering methods.

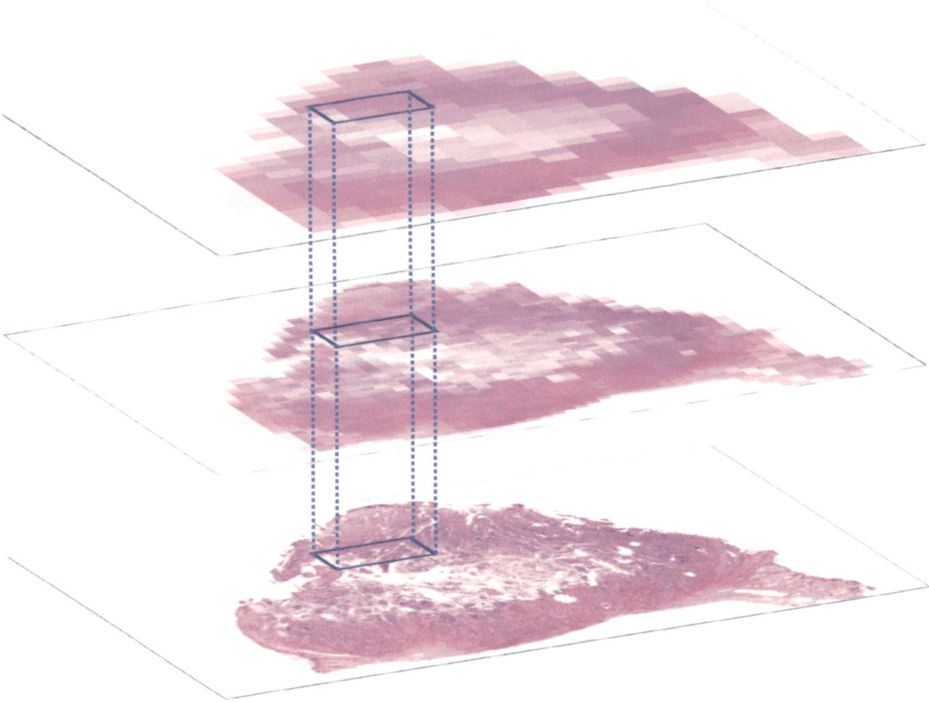

Figure 4.
An illustration of multi-resolution process of ROI detection on WSI. The example has 3 level of granularity in term of block size. Note that we did not downsample the WSI directly, which dump falsely many local details, and we still include neighbor superpixels close to positive ones at coarse classification to next level. If the bounding box is the ROI (a rough identifier), as resolution goes high, superpixels cover and surround the bounding box will get fine-detailed update.

4. Experiments

4.1 ROIs in lung cancer histopathology WSI

In histopathology images like lung cancer WSIs, the regions of interest are those areas consist of cancer cells or other tissues that may be related to tumor diagnosis. A fast detection approach of ROIs is to search and localize those regions on image at WSI scale, that usually have trillions of pixels. Traditional pixel-wise methods and neural network cannot directly work on WSI, due to the extraordinary data scale and image dimensionality. Downsampling of WSI reduces complexity but also loses local fine-detailed features. Superpixels first cluster those pixels of similar spacial, color and topological properties as whole, and then in downstream tasks e.g. detection and segmentation, the superpixels will act as minimal manipulatable unit, reducing image primitives and complexity. If superpixels were well constructed, the downstream will not be affected by the sparse representation of image. The tumor cells of lung cancer patients (not only for lung cancer, but also generally appear in other subtypes of cancer) infest as cell mass. If treat the regions where tumor cell mass appears as ROIs, we can easily see that the H&E stained histopathology images that those tumor cells are more deeply colored due to the massive reproduction of genetic materials inside tumor nuclei (See **Figure 5**).

4.2 Experimental setup

In the experimental stage, a random forest and a support-vector-machine (a.k.a. SVM) classifier were trained with local features extracted from regions defined by

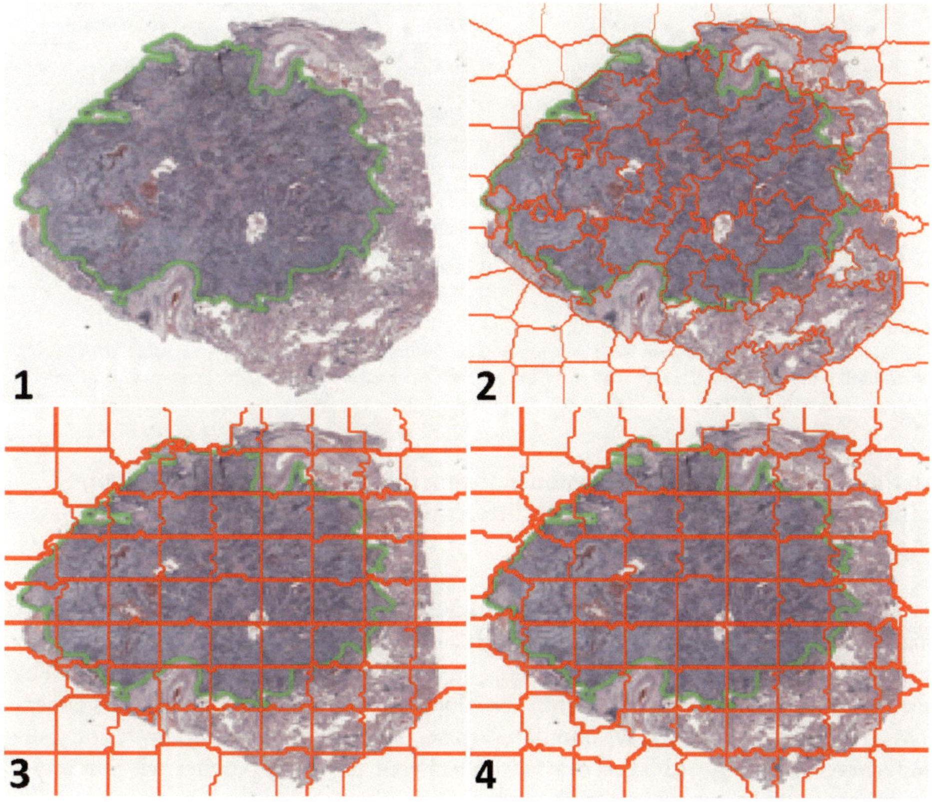

Figure 5.
The comparison of several superpixel clustering on lung cancer H&E stained WSI: 1) the origin (with ROI annotated), 2) SLIC [11], 3) SPSS [21], 4) our method. The ROI is contoured by green line.

the superpixels given by Algorithm 1. The total 384 dimensional features include local binary patterns and statistics derived from the histogram of the three-channel HSD color model as well as common texture features, e.g. color SIFT. The introduced method was compared against the superpixels generated by SLIC [11] and tetragonum (i.e. rectangular patches). The experiments used the adenocarcinoma and squamous cell carcinoma lung cancer WSIs from the NLST (National Lung Screening Trial) Data Portal1[1]. In superpixel classification, we executed feature extraction on the sampled patches (100×100) with 10% overlap with each other within each superpixel, we rule out patches sit across boundary avoiding noise. Lastly, we averaged the feature vectors of patches as representation of superpixel. When deciding ROI belonging for superpixel, if any part of ground-truth ROI fall into a superpixel, it will count as positive. The setup is rooted at the extremely high recall requirement for medical diagnosis. Given this setup, for better detection precision, superpixels should be better boundary adherent and clearly separated from background.

4.3 Experimental results

Due to the overwhelming fidelity of superpixels given by our algorithm, the classifier operated over the regions segmented by superpixels is able to deliver better classification results (See **Table 1**). Since the feature descriptors were built

---

[1] https://biometry. nci.nih.gov/cdas/studies/nlst/

Classifier	Metric	MROID	SLIC [11]	Tetragonum
Random Forest	Error rate	**0.1326**	0.1933	0.2047
	Precision	**0.7127**	0.6835	0.6740
	Recall	**0.7333**	0.6108	0.6450
SVM	Error rate	**0.3011**	0.3343	0.3061
	Precision	**0.6754**	0.6672	0.6723
	Recall	**0.7450**	0.6604	0.6972

Table 1.
The table presents the comparison results of the proposed solution, MROID (numbers in bold), SLIC and tetragonum (non-superpixel) in term of classification statistics including: the rate of error classification, precision and recall. Tetragonum: Sliding rectangular windows.

on the patches segmented by contours of superpixels, the better the superpixel adhere to the boundaries, the better differentiability the features have for superpixel classification.

Figure 6 demonstrated the introduced multi-resolution coarse-to-fine superpixel segmentation in a lung cancer histopathology images. The algorithm first manipulated large block (180× 180) to cluster superpixels, then move to finer segmentation with 10 × 10 blocks on the superpixels selected by the classifier. The recursive refinement continues until the block queue run out, which means energy loss converges. In **Table 1**, we compared the classification recall and precision using superpixels given by SLIC and our method as well as simply patches without any preprocessing like superpixel clustering. Our results showed that, compared to simple patching, utilizing superpixel may not always increase ROI recall but definitely lift precision. Compared to superpixel given by SLIC with sophisticated boundary, out method outperformed on both recall and precision. We also observed that, if superpixels do not adhere to boundary, a detection based on classification of superpixels of low segmentation accuracy leads to worse accuracy than a trivial patch based method. While, our method delivered best results at both recall and precision.

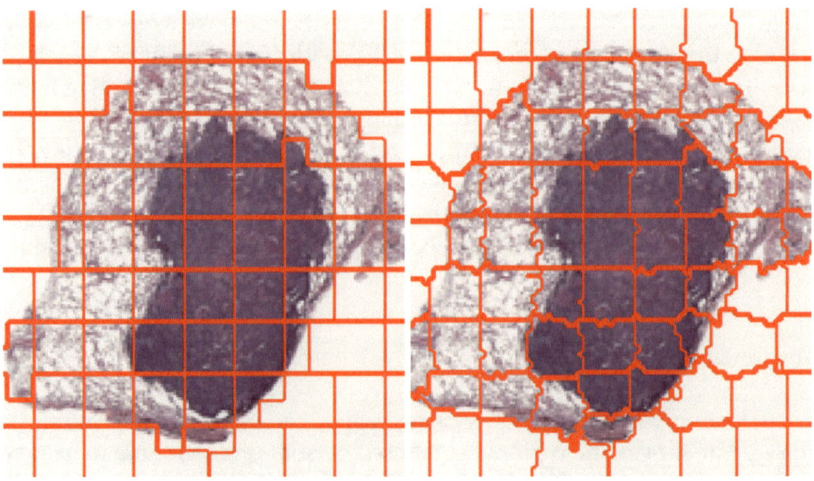

Figure 6.
A coarse-to-fine superpixel clustering on a lung cancer WSI from NLST. 1) coarse segmentation of superpixels using large blocks (180×180); 2) refined segmentation with small blocks within selected superpixels.

5. Conclusion

In the chapter, we presented a novel local feature based solution to fast search and detection of regions of interest (ROI) in whole slide lung cancer histopathology image. For superpixel clustering, we introduced coarse-to-fine multi-resolution segmentation of superpixel by manipulating blocks of different size. Besides, boundary-only update strategy also reduced the computational complexity to the scale of superpixel boundary length, irrelevant of image size.

We creatively embedded the ROI classification into superpixel clustering algorithm. Iteratively executing superpixel construction and ROI detection. A better superpixel will accelerate detection and lift accuracy, while on the other hand, a better classification of ROI on coarse superpixel guides superpixel segmentation at finer level. Our algorithm performed a faster and finer ROI detection and segmentation. The effectiveness and efficiency of our algorithm has been verified on large histopathology WSI database, e.g. NLST.

In future, as the development of neural network capable of flexible input size [28, 29], it is likely to merge superpixel construction and downstream tasks, e.g. semantic segmentation, classification together in neural network architecture, in which superpixels are clustered using hidden features, while superpixels boost feature learning as well.

Author details

Junzhou Huang* and Ruoyu Li
1 500 UTA Boulevard, The University of Texas at Arlington, Arlington, TX, United States

*Address all correspondence to: jzhuang@uta.edu

References

[1] Takács P, Manno-Kovacs A. MRI Brain Tumor Segmentation Combining Saliency and Convolutional Network Features. In2018 International Conference on Content-Based Multimedia Indexing (CBMI) 2018 Sep 4 (pp. 1–6). IEEE.

[2] Hou L, Samaras D, Kurc TM, Gao Y, Davis JE, Saltz JH. Patch-based convolutional neural network for whole slide tissue image classification. InProceedings of the ieee conference on computer vision and pattern recognition 2016 (pp. 2424–2433).

[3] Bándi P, van de Loo R, Intezar M, Geijs D, Ciompi F, van Ginneken B, van der Laak J, Litjens G. Comparison of different methods for tissue segmentation in histopathological whole-slide images. In2017 IEEE 14th International Symposium on Biomedical Imaging (ISBI 2017) 2017 Apr 18 (pp. 591–595). IEEE.

[4] LeCun Y, Cortes C, Burges CJ. MNIST handwritten digit database.

[5] Krizhevsky A, Hinton G. Convolutional deep belief networks on cifar-10. Unpublished manuscript. 2010 Aug;40(7):1–9.

[6] Zhou Z, Siddiquee MM, Tajbakhsh N, Liang J. Unet++: A nested u-net architecture for medical image segmentation. InDeep Learning in Medical Image Analysis and Multimodal Learning for Clinical Decision Support 2018 Sep 20 (pp. 3–11). Springer, Cham.

[7] Yao J, Zhu X, Jonnagaddala J, Hawkins N, Huang J. Whole slide images based cancer survival prediction using attention guided deep multiple instance learning networks. Medical Image Analysis. 2020 Jul 19:101789.

[8] Milletari F, Navab N, Ahmadi SA. V-net: Fully convolutional neural networks for volumetric medical image segmentation. In2016 fourth international conference on 3D vision (3DV) 2016 Oct 25 (pp. 565–571). IEEE.

[9] Chan L, Hosseini MS, Rowsell C, Plataniotis KN, Damaskinos S. Histosegnet: Semantic segmentation of histological tissue type in whole slide images. InProceedings of the IEEE International Conference on Computer Vision 2019 (pp. 10662–10671).

[10] Yao J, Boben M, Fidler S, Urtasun R. Real-time coarse-to-fine topologically preserving segmentation. InProceedings of the IEEE Conference on Computer Vision and Pattern Recognition 2015 (pp. 2947–2955).

[11] Achanta R, Shaji A, Smith K, Lucchi A, Fua P, Süsstrunk S. SLIC superpixels compared to state-of-the-art superpixel methods. IEEE transactions on pattern analysis and machine intelligence. 2012 May 29;34(11):2274–82.

[12] Van den Bergh M, Boix X, Roig G, de Capitani B, Van Gool L. Seeds: Superpixels extracted via energy-driven sampling. InEuropean conference on computer vision 2012 Oct 7 (pp. 13–26). Springer, Berlin, Heidelberg.

[13] Li Z, Chen J. Superpixel segmentation using linear spectral clustering. InProceedings of the IEEE Conference on Computer Vision and Pattern Recognition 2015 (pp. 1356–1363).

[14] Ren X, Malik J. Learning a classification model for segmentation. Innull 2003 Oct 13 (p. 10). IEEE.

[15] Liu MY, Tuzel O, Ramalingam S, Chellappa R. Entropy rate superpixel segmentation. InCVPR 2011 2011 Jun 20 (pp. 2097–2104). IEEE.

[16] Veksler O, Boykov Y, Mehrani P. Superpixels and supervoxels in an

energy optimization framework. InEuropean conference on Computer vision 2010 Sep 5 (pp. 211–224). Springer, Berlin, Heidelberg.

[17] Bejnordi BE, Litjens G, Hermsen M, Karssemeijer N, van der Laak JA. A multi-scale superpixel classification approach to the detection of regions of interest in whole slide histopathology images. InMedical Imaging 2015: Digital Pathology 2015 Mar 19 (Vol. 9420, p. 94200H). International Society for Optics and Photonics.

[18] Litjens G, Bejnordi BE, Timofeeva N, Swadi G, Kovacs I, Hulsbergen-van de Kaa C, van der Laak J. Automated detection of prostate cancer in digitized whole-slide images of H and E-stained biopsy specimens. InMedical Imaging 2015: Digital Pathology 2015 Mar 19 (Vol. 9420, p. 94200B). International Society for Optics and Photonics.

[19] Lucchi A, Smith K, Achanta R, Lepetit V, Fua P. A fully automated approach to segmentation of irregularly shaped cellular structures in EM images. InInternational Conference on Medical Image Computing and Computer-Assisted Intervention 2010 Sep 20 (pp. 463–471). Springer, Berlin, Heidelberg.

[20] Van den Bergh M, Roig G, Boix X, Manen S, Van Gool L. Online video seeds for temporal window objectness. InProceedings of the IEEE international conference on computer vision 2013 (pp. 377–384).

[21] Yamaguchi K, McAllester D, Urtasun R. Efficient joint segmentation, occlusion labeling, stereo and flow estimation. InEuropean Conference on Computer Vision 2014 Sep 6 (pp. 756–771). Springer, Cham.

[22] Li R, Huang J. Fast regions-of-interest detection in whole slide histopathology images. In: International Workshop on Patch-based Techniques in Medical Imaging 2015 Oct 9 (pp. 120-127). Springer, Cham.

[23] Gadde R, Jampani V, Kiefel M, Kappler D, Gehler PV. Superpixel convolutional networks using bilateral inceptions. InEuropean Conference on Computer Vision 2016 Oct 8 (pp. 597–613). Springer, Cham.

[24] Kwak S, Hong S, Han B. Weakly supervised semantic segmentation using superpixel pooling network. InAAAI 2017 Feb 4 (Vol. 1, p. 2).

[25] Tu WC, Liu MY, Jampani V, Sun D, Chien SY, Yang MH, Kautz J. Learning superpixels with segmentation-aware affinity loss. InProceedings of the IEEE Conference on Computer Vision and Pattern Recognition 2018 (pp. 568–576).

[26] Liu X, Guo S, Yang B, Ma S, Zhang H, Li J, Sun C, Jin L, Li X, Yang Q, Fu Y. Automatic organ segmentation for CT scans based on super-pixel and convolutional neural networks. Journal of digital imaging. 2018 Oct 1;31(5):748–60.

[27] Jampani V, Sun D, Liu MY, Yang MH, Kautz J. Superpixel sampling networks. InProceedings of the European Conference on Computer Vision (ECCV) 2018 (pp. 352–368).

[28] Li R, Wang S, Zhu F, Huang J. Adaptive graph convolutional neural networks. arXiv preprint arXiv: 1801.03226. 2018 Jan 10.

[29] Yang F, Sun Q, Jin H, Zhou Z. Superpixel Segmentation with Fully Convolutional Networks. InProceedings of the IEEE/CVF Conference on Computer Vision and Pattern Recognition 2020 (pp. 13964–13973).

Chapter 6

Approaches for Handling Immunopathological and Clinical Data Using Deep Learning Methodology: Multiplex IHC/IF Data as a Paradigm

Siting Goh, Yueda Chua, Justina Lee, Joe Yeong and Yiyu Cai

Abstract

Recent advancements in deep learning based artificial intelligence have enabled us to analyse complex data in order to provide patients with improved cancer prognosis, which is an important goal in precision health medicine. In this chapter, we would be discussing how deep learning could be applied to clinical data and immunopathological images to accurately determine survival rate prediction for patients. Multiplex immunohistochemistry/immunofluorescence (mIHC/IF) is a relatively new technology for simultaneous detection of multiple specific proteins from a single tissue section. To adopt deep learning, we collected and pre-processed the clinical and mIHC/IF data from a group of patients into three branches of data. These data were subsequently used to train and validate a neural network. The specific process and our recommendations will be further discussed in this chapter. We believe that our work will help the community to better handle their data for AI implementation while improving its performance and accuracy.

Keywords: immunopathology, deep learning, multiplex IHC/IF

1. Introduction

Improved cancer prognosis is a vital goal of precision health medicine. Advancements in Deep Learning (DL) based Artificial Intelligence (AI) technologies enable modelling of complex data providing deeper insights and patients with more reliable results. Machine Learning (ML) is the process of enabling machines to make predictions from data that is fed into it. This includes DL, a type of approach created from the development of artificial neural networks [1]. The DL network consists of multiple layers of artificial neural networks including an input, an output and multiple hidden layers [2, 3]. Predictions are made after datasets are generated from and trained against these hidden layers. Recent advancements in computational processing power has sparked interest in tapping into the vast research on DL and applying it to digital pathology. Digital pathology is the process of digitizing Whole-Slide Images (WSI) using advanced slide-scanning techniques and AI-based methods for detecting, segmenting, diagnosing and analysing digitized images [4].

DL is the engine of advancement in artificial learning in both computer and clinical sciences. It is a collection of computer learning algorithm layers that uses the raw data input to first generate generalise features that are subsequently used to progressively extract higher level features such as tumour stroma count, and assign them class labels. Eventually, the system will distinguish different interest categories via the identified ideal data features. The DL approaches are widely accepted due to the ability of discovering patterns and signals from data too large for human comprehension. Furthermore, the multiple layers allow modelling of highly complex non-linear problems. On top of having higher accuracy, the DL approaches are also easily applied.

1.1 The importance of deep learning in digital pathology and mIHC

In current clinical practice, pathologists base their medical diagnosis on the quantification and visual recognition of the analysed sample details, which could lead to diagnostic discrepancies and potential suboptimal patient care [5]. The increased adoption of non-invasive clinical procedures to acquire diagnostic samples has also severely reduced the quantity and quality of samples obtained, which compounds the workload of pathologists. In view of the inter-variabilities in analysing samples manually and the limitations of available samples, the use of DL analysis has thus been researched on and progressively applied in the clinical practice.

DL in digital pathology aims to improve the workload of pathologists by automating time-consuming tasks, hence allowing additional time to be spent on disease presentations with complex features. AI applications in digital pathology can also be applied to develop prognostic assays that evaluate the severity of diseases and make an accurate prognosis in response to therapy. This could be applied to various image processing and classification tasks, such as low-level jobs revolving around image recognition issues including detection and segmentation, as well as high-level tasks such as prognosis of response to therapy based on patterns of images [6, 7]. Such AI approaches are designed to extract relevant image renditions to train machines to be used as specific segmentation, diagnostic or prognostic tools.

One of the most extensively used DL models in pathology image analysis is the Convolutional Neural Networks (CNN). The CNN is a class of deep, feedforward networks, comprising several layers which extrapolate an output from an input and contains multiple convolutional sheets. These convolution sheets are the foundation of a CNN in which the network learns and extrapolates feature maps from images using filters between the input and output layers [4]. These layers in CNN are not connected as the neurons in one layer only interact with a specific region of the previous layer instead of all its neurons. The CNN also contains pooling layers which primarily function to scale down or reduce the dimensionalities of the features. CNN DL-based approaches are used for image-based detection and segmentation tasks to distinguish and quantify cells, histological features or highlight regions of interest [4]. CNN DL-based approaches have also been developed to automatically distinguish and segment blurry areas in digitised WSIs with high accuracy.

Another type of DL approach is the Fully Convolutional Network (FCN) which learns representations from every pixel and makes a potential feature detection that may occur sparsely in the entire pathology image [4]. FCNs uses co-registered Haemotoxylin and Eosin (H&E) images with multimodal microscopy techniques to classify WSIs into 4 classes: cancer, non-malignant epithelium, background and other tissues. When FCN was used to detect invasive breast cancer regions on WSIs, it had a diagnostic accuracy of 71% (Sørensen-Dice coefficient) when compared to an expert breast pathologist's assessment [8]. With better technologies and further research, FCNs can potentially automate these tasks with a higher accuracy, reducing the workload of pathologists.

AI-based approaches such as Generative Adversarial Network (GAN)-based approaches can be used for training to automatically score tumoral programmed cell death 1 ligand 1 (PD-L1) expression in biopsy sample images [4]. They reduce the number of inputs required from pathologists and make up for lack of tissue samples available in biopsy specimens. Novel GAN-based approaches propose converting H&E staining of WSIs to virtual immunohistochemistry staining, thus eliminating the need for destructive IHC tissue testing.

Many have also trialled DL in the field of immunohistochemistry (IHC). Traditional IHC is a common diagnostic tool used in pathology, but its application is significantly limited by its ability of only allowing single marker labelling per tissue section [9]. Alternatively, multiplex immunohistochemistry/immunofluorescence (mIHC/IF) technologies permit simultaneous detection of several markers on a single tissue section [9]. However, analysing large samples with multiple markers in conventional and manual ways by pathologists are highly time-consuming, laborious and susceptible to human error. By combining mIHC/IF with DL to analyse digitized WSIs, this will overcome the limitations.

In conclusion, the research and diagnostic fields have come a long way since the introduction of IHC. With the introduction of Al-based approaches in the application of IHC, higher accuracy and productivity could be achieved not just in the diagnostic level but also providing us with a platform to further venture into areas of medical knowledge yet to be fully understood.

1.2 mIHC/IF Technologies

To-date, our understanding of cancer immunotherapy has evolved and led to multiple studies investigating and refining strategies targeting negative regulators. Many have studied the use of checkpoint blockade immunotherapy such as programmed cell death receptor 1 (PD-1), PD-L1 and cytotoxic T-lymphocyte–associated protein 4 (CTLA-4) in a variety of cancers. The subsequent success of checkpoint blockade inhibition in clinical trials has led to the Food and Drug Administration's approval of various drugs such as Ipillimumab and Prembrolizumab for melanoma treatment of non-small cell lung cancer (NSCLC) respectively [10]. Furthermore, trial of combination immunotherapy has shown clinical efficacy in various cancers [11, 12]. However, other studies have also suggested that efficacy of these immunotherapy in various cancers may depend on the expression of biomarkers. For example, PD-L1 is suggested as a useful predictive marker in patients with NSCLC receiving Prembrolizumab [13]. However, this is not the case in patients with stage III melanoma [14]. To further discover potential biomarkers that could determine the efficacy of immunotherapy in various cancers, IHC has been introduced as a platform for these clinical studies.

Since its introduction in the 1940s [15], conventional IHC has been widely used in field of pathology and research. It involves the process of staining tissues samples using antibodies specific to antigens present within the samples. This specificity allows microscopic visualisation for diagnosis of neoplasm and obtaining valuable prognostic information. Despite this, it does have several limitations. The inability of labelling more than one marker per tissue sample has resulted in loss of potential information for analysis. For instance, the prediction of prognosis to an immunotherapy such as PD-L1/PD-1 checkpoint blockade may depend on the expression of an individual biomarker or in combination with other biomarkers [16–18]. Furthermore, the immune system can potentially be better understood, if the analysis of various biomarkers' expression patterns are done simultaneously, or cellular interactions within the tumour microenvironment can be visualised [19].

Moreover, IHC involves many critical steps which have high inter-user variability. For instance, antigens such as Ki-67 are more vulnerable to ischemia. As such, over fixation could result in irreversible damage to these antigens [20]. The concern of IHC's reproducibility such as for Ki-67 and its implications was also mentioned in the 2017 St. Gallen International Expert Consensus Conference [21]. However, multiple studies have since demonstrated that analytical variability can be negated with the use of digital analysis to calculate biomarkers index [22, 23].

Although conventional IHC is a cost-effective diagnostic and prognostic tool, it has been replaced with the introduction of mIHC. mIHC has been used to overcome the shortcoming of single biomarker labelling in conventional IHC. The use of mIHC has proven to provide an even more accurate analysis as seen in the study by Yeong *et al.,* where the simultaneous quantification of three different PD-L1 antibodies (22C3, SP142 and SP263) by mIHC scoring had moderate-to-strong correlation (with 67%–100% individual concordance rates and Spearman's rank correlation coefficient values up to 0.88 [24]) when compared with manual scoring from four different pathologists.. This demonstrated the use of mIHC as a promising tool for an even more accurate analysis.

The use of mIHC has played a significant role in both research and clinical studies of cancer immunotherapy. mIHC is a relatively new tool to study the spatial tumour microenvironment especially those of limited tissue specimens. It has great potential in clinical and translational application. This was demonstrated by Halse *et al.*, who used mIHC to reveal a close relationship between the presence of $CD8^+$ T cells within the tumour and the expression of PD-L1 in melanoma [25]. A systemic review and meta-analysis of studies also reported that mIHC improved results in predicting responses to PD-1/PD-L1 checkpoint blockade immunotherapy in various solid tumour types when compared to using conventional IHC analysis [26]. Several studies have also used various types of mIHC to obtain data for analysis. For instance, TSA-based mIHC was used to profile PD-1 to PD-L1 proximity in 166 metastatic melanoma samples and 42 Merkel cell carcinoma samples in two respective studies [27, 28]. As aforementioned, understanding the tumour microenvironment could potentially provide a foundation upon which interpretation of immunotherapy response could be made.

1.3 Use of mIHC in combination with digital pathology

mIHC can be powered by digital pathology analysis software, such as inForm (Akoya Biosciences, California, USA) [29–31] and HALO TM (Indica Labs) [28, 32].

	Digital pathology software		
	InForm	**HALO**	**Oncotopix**
Developer	**Akoya Biosciences**	**Indica Labs**	**Visiopharm**
Compatibility with multiplex IHC platforms	Yes	Yes	Yes
Co-localisation of markers	Yes	Yes	Yes
Tissue segmentation	Yes	Yes	Yes
Spatial analysis	No	Yes	Yes
Ready solution for interrogation of breast cancer markers	No	No	Yes (Ki-67, HER2, ER, PR)
Use in breast cancer research	Yes	Yes	Yes

Table 1.
Digital pathology softwares, InForm, HALO, and Oncotopix and their software features for multiplex IHC/IF.

These software resolve the restrictions of labeling a single marker per tissue section by precisely evaluating the unique localization of multiple simultaneously detected biomarkers and their co-expressions or interactions between cells [33].

For example, although Ki-67/PD-L1 labeling is useful by itself, a multiplex approach enables several markers to be interrogated simultaneously [34–36]. However, only analytical digital pathology solutions for Ki67 and PD-L1 scoring are currently commercially available as listed in **Table 1** [33, 37]. The involvement of digital pathology has also decreased intra- and inter-observer variability seen in manual scoring as previously highlighted. Consequently, using mIHC in conjunction with digital analysis software will resolve the restrictions of conventional IHC, thus providing us with an accurate and powerful tool in the interpretation of immune response in various fields.

2. Proposed deep learning framework for analysing immunopathological and clinical data

This section presents a holistic guiding framework to select and develop a DL architecture for multi-dimensional analysis. The entire pipeline can be broken down into 3 parts: [1] data pre-processing, [2] feature engineering and [3] model selection, validation, and evaluation (**Figure 1**). This includes treating the data input, selecting the appropriate model for the type of data and using the preferable method to validate the selected model.

To demonstrate the clinical application of the framework, a total of 107 clinical as well as mIHC/IF data from patients with breast cancer (BC) previously published [37]. The clinical data consists of parameters such as age and tumour grade as stated in **Table 2** Row 1, while the mIHC data comprised of antibody-based spectral unmixing result obtained from stained mIHC image of tumour section labeling markers such as cytokeratin, CD68, CD8, CD20, FOXP3, PD-L1, and CK/EpCAM (**Figure 2**).

2.1 Data pre-processing

The first step in data pre-processing involves analysis of the dataset. This process consists of four main components: [1] one-hot encoding, [2] data normalization, [3] data enhancement and [4] data shape conformity.

2.1.1 One-hot encoding

One-hot encoding is the process of converting any non-numerical data existing in the clinical dataset to a categorical numerical representation that is readable by

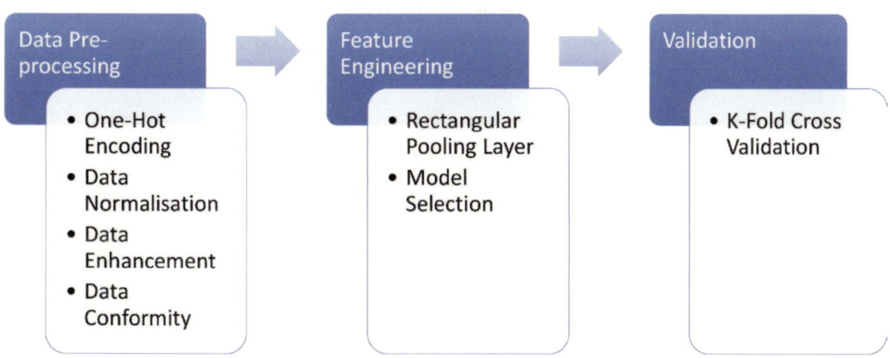

Figure 1.
General overview of the DL framework.

Age at Diagnosis	Tumour Grade	Tumour Size	Lymphovascular Invasion	Lymph Node Positive	Lymph Node Stage	Disease Free (month)	Overall Survival (month)
Integer	Ordinal Integer	Integer	Categorical (positive/possible/negative)	Integer	Ordinal Integer	Integer	Integer

Table 2.
Data of Clinical Dataset.

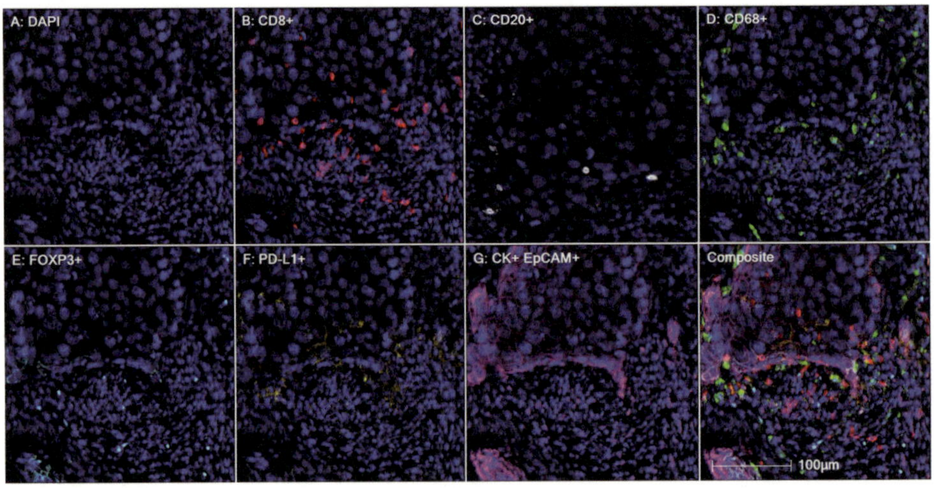

Figure 2.
Representative images of breast tissue stained using multiplex immunohistochemistry/immunofluorescence (mIHC/IF) [DAPI (blue), CD8 (red), CD20 (white), CD68 (green), FOXP3 (cyan), PD-L1 (yellow), CK/EpCAM (magenta)]. (Magnification, 200X).

the computer. Any non-numerical data within each category is split into the number of categories it has and encoded with a binary 0/1. For example, in the case of our clinical data, the columns, "Lymphovascular Invasion" contains 3 possible values: positive, possible, negative (**Table 3**). This represents 3 categories and is the prime candidate to be one-hot encoded. The input column is subsequently expended to 3 columns, one for each category in this input as shown in **Tables 3** and **4**.

2.1.2 Data normalisation

Most CNN research and models are developed with the intention for application in Computer Vision, where an entire input image data points are all pixels with ranges from zero to 255. Non-imaging datasets are more complicated as each input parameters have different units of measurements that might range from ones

Lymphovascular Invasion
Absent
Present
Absent
Absent
Possible

Table 3.
Lymphovascular invasion data before One-hot encoding.

Lymphovascular Invasion Absent	Lymphovascular Invasion Possible	Lymphovascular Invasion Present
1	0	0
0	0	**1**
1	0	0
1	0	0
0	**1**	0

Table 4.
Lymphovascular invasion data after One-hot encoding.

to hundreds of thousands. Using such models with disparate values meant that a model with a large input parameter could easily outweigh another with a smaller value range. Therefore, data normalisation is needed to ensure that the dataset has comparable values across the data inputs while still maintaining their distribution within each data input. Data normalisation was done by scaling each input column to carry a mean of 0 and a standard deviation, by applying the following formula:

$$X_{New} = \frac{X - \mu}{\sigma}$$

An example of a segment of clinical dataset following one-hot encoding is as shown in **Table 5**. A notable feature of the clinical dataset is the disparate values across the columns which arose due to the different units of measurements used across the columns, such as categorical numbers, months, and millimetres. As such, these numbers could not be directly compared. To obtain a more comparable data, normalisation of these values was done, while maintaining the distribution within each column (**Table 6**).

2.1.3 Data enhancements

When working with a medical dataset, it will be advantageous to have medical insights augment the data, as it can improve the result. The use of medical insights is however dependent on the context of the problem and is subjective to the augmentation or removal of features and/or any dataset. In this study, clinically relevant data was augmented to the cell dataset to count the number of stroma and cancer cells of each patient. Subsequently this was evaluated with a simple 12-layer dense neural network and the obtained results were compared with and without data enhancements on 10000 epochs. It was discovered that there was a marked improvement in the reduction of mean absolute error by 14.8% when the clinical dataset was enhanced with more relevant information. However, the reduction in mean absolute error was highly dependent on clinical dataset used and thus varies with its application.

2.1.4 Ensuring data conformity

The CNN requires the dataset to be homogeneous in its shape, which is achievable in the classical Computer Vision problems where images could be resized to a uniform rectangular shape. However, in the case of medical dataset, the dimensions are mostly dependent on the source of the data, which is usually 3-dimensional or more. There are two ways to homogenise medical dataset, either by appending non-meaningful data to the clinical dataset, or selectively removed data until the shape is uniform. This process requires a higher dimensional visualisation which is best explained using a tangible example as follows:

Age at Diagnosis	Tumour Grade	Tumour Size (mm)	Lympho-vascular Invasion (Present)	Lymph Node Positive	Lymph Node Stage	tumour count	stroma count	Disease Free Survival (month)	Overall Survival (month)
54	3	25	0	0	0	1550	667	39.90322581	48.5483871
43	3	30	1	0	0	4236	1144	27.5483871	32.12903226
47	3	30	0	1	1	3132	1715	140.8666667	140.8666667
36	3	50	0	0	0	6264	777	139.3225806	139.3225806
49	3	24	1	0	0	3404	1504	139.1	139.1
65	2	32	0	0	0	3338	5237	50.6	139.2666667

Table 5.
Original Sample Cell Data Before Normalisation.

Age at Diagnosis	Tumour Grade	Tumour Size (mm)	Lymphovascular Invasion (Present)	Lymph Node Positive	Lymph Node Stage	tumour count	stroma count	Disease Free Survival (month)	Overall Survival (month)
0.01679224	0.35540932	0.32887951	0.69721667	0.09712858	0.37974281	0.65319726	0.83253395	0.85909418	0.75847927
0.91517705	0.35540932	0.15397838	1.4342743	0.09712858	0.37974281	0.65319726	0.93975876	0.37551795	1.00897651
0.58849167	0.35540932	0.15397838	0.69721667	0.09712858	0.21114331	0.43886691	0.21131083	0.20335423	1.28857808
1.48687648	0.35540932	0.54562614	0.69721667	0.09712858	0.37974281	0.65319726	2.27788594	0.74757765	1.25727138
0.42514897	0.35540932	0.36385973	1.4342743	0.09712858	0.37974281	0.65319726	0.39078351	0.01055475	1.25275851
0.88159257	2.81365708	0.08401793	0.69721667	0.09712858	0.37974281	0.65319726	0.34723499	3.77391084	0.54159967

Table 6.
Sample Cell Data After Normalisation.

In this study, the cell dataset has the attributes of a 3D feature shape, where each patient has a list of cell inputs. This gives it a general 3D shape consisting of (Patients x No of Cells x Cell Parameters x 1). However, as each patient has a different number of cells, this results in a non-uniform dataset shape of (104 patients x χ cells x 144 Cell Parameters x 1), whereχ denotes the patient dependent number of cells in the dataset which ranges from 991 cell inputs to 10720 cell inputs.

Two strategies were evaluated to assess for the best approach of ensuring data conformity. The first method involves keeping the model and parameters constant. A dataset (Complete Cell Data) of "ghost cells" with value 0 were appended to the data to ensure regular shape of (107 x 10720 x 144). Alternatively, a dataset (Random Sampled Cell Data) with cells that were sampled randomly are pegged to the patient with the least number of markers to create a shape of (107 x 991 x 10720) (**Table 7**). Random sampled cell data are also employed for the training and evaluation of the DL model in this study. Following evaluation, no difference in the accuracy between both sets of data were observed. However, it was found that the smaller dataset required a smaller DL network that requires less computational power.

2.2 Feature engineering

In retrospect, there is no definitive answer when selecting a DL model. However, there is a wide array of models including the basic dense layers or CNN that could be applied. In view of multi-dimensional datasets, CNN is the most versatile in its ability to accommodate multi-dimensionality and has a strong community of research & development from Academics to Corporations. Despite so, CNN may be unsuitable for a non-imaging problem, as most CNN research is based on imaging problems where many of its tools such as max pooling may only work for spatial data. However, if harnessed correctly, CNN offers a highly flexible and advanced architecture that works for many types of data.

To understand the limitations of CNN on non-imaging dataset, it is essential to understand the fundamental difference between a spatial and non-spatial data. In spatial data like an image, a data point in one position is highly related to its surrounding pixels. Whereas for purely numerical data, one data point may not be related to its surrounding data points. It could instead be related to another data that is located at a different position, or more succinctly, is position independent.

2.2.1 Model selection and parameters

Most CNN tools assume that data points are position dependent. In this study, we looked at the dataset at hand to select a suitable CNN model and to adapt a powerful CNN tool called *Pooling Layer* to the non-spatial data. To select a suitable model that best fits the dataset and problem at hand, one should consider the general dimensions of the dataset which dictates the type of CNN to be used as listed in **Table 8**. For models that involve interaction with the environment, agent-based

Name	Size [patients*cell entries*markers]	Description
Base Dataset	107 x **12347** x 144	Full patient cell data, where patients with lacking cell entries are appended with "ghost cells" to form a regular shaped dataset
Random Row	107 x **991** x 144	Patients cell entries randomly selected via algorithm based on the patient with the least cell entries

Table 7.
Overview of Cell Data Size of Both Approaches.

Dimension	Probable Features (In imaging terms)	Best CNN Type
1D - Vector	(sample x features)	—
2D – Time Series/ sequence	(samples x timestamp x feature)	1D CNN
3D – Image Data	(samples x height x width x channels)	2D CNN
4D – Video Data	(samples x frames x channels x height x width)	3D CNN

Table 8.
Overview of Different Data Dimension and Suitable CNN Type.

Problem Type	Output Node Configuration	Objective Function	Equation
Scalar Regression	1 Node - Sigmoid Function	Mean Squared Error/ Mean Absolute Error	$MAE = \frac{1}{n}\sum \left\| y - \hat{y} \right\|$
Binary Classification	1 Node - Sigmoid Function	Cross Entropy	$BCE = \frac{1}{N}\sum_{i=1}^{N} y_i * \log(p(y_i)) + (1 - y_i) * \log(1 - y_i)$
Multi-Class Classification	1 Node for each class - SoftMax	Cross Entropy	$CE = -\sum_{i=N}^{N} y_i \log(f(s_i))$

Table 9.
Overview of Objective Function of Different Problems.

models may be used. Furthermore, one should consider if the problem is a prediction or classification problem and if additional correlational features are necessary. As for a complex problem, the use of a deeper model may be more appropriate. Nevertheless, using a deeper model could lead to additional problems that require new architecture to overcome. Lastly, the objective of the problem and if it is a scalar prediction or classification problem must also be deduced (**Table 9**).

In this study, 2D CNN is used as the dataset is 3D and image-like. The problem type is a prediction model thus a plain 2D CNN with no agent-based is used. Given that the problem is complex, a Wide Residual Neural Network (WRN) identity mapping may help with modelling its complexity. Lastly, as this is a scalar prediction problem, the model should end with 1 sigmoid function and mean absolute error (MAE) objective function (**Table 9**).

The model selection process must be carefully chosen as it dictates the basis of the model and its result. To illustrate, an early stage proof-of-concept of application of DL on this dataset, a categorical approach was taken, where the patients were split into categories based on their survival rate in years. In designing it this way, the aim was to apply categorisation as the objective function [38]. However, this approach introduced an unintended consequence, a fixed error of the range of each category that could not be rid of regardless of how accurate the model is. This was because of framing a scalar problem as a categorical problem. Even though the resulting model achieved an accuracy of 90% [38], it did not show the in-built error of the prediction that was hidden by the range of each category.

Pooling layers progressively achieve spatial invariance by reducing the resolution of the feature maps, which reduces the number of parameters and computation in the network. This presents one with the ability to create a much deeper network with limited computational cost and overfitting. In a pooling layer, a simple function could be applied. The two conventional functions available are [1] maximization function, which find the maximum value of the region as a representation, and [2] average pooling function that aims to find an average representation of the region, where p is the resultant value of the pooling operation (**Figure 3**).

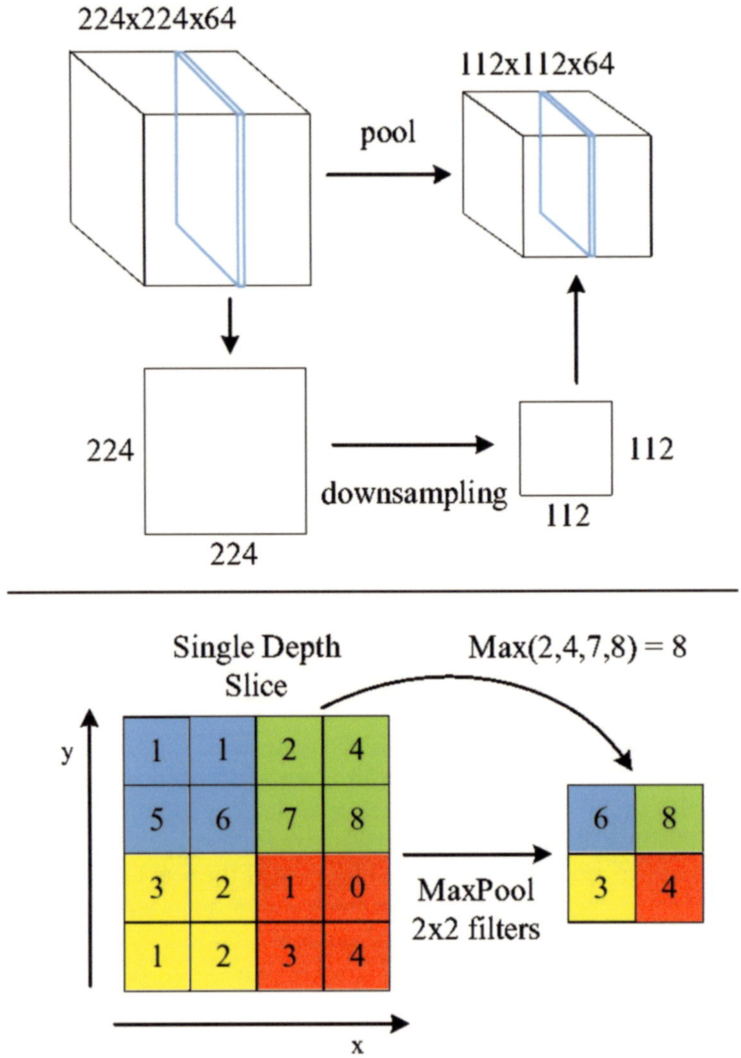

Figure 3.
Pooling Layer Computation & Representation- Pooling provides a form of abstraction of our data by down-sampling an input representation. There are two common rules for downsampling. Max-Pooling- which picks the input with the largest value. Average-Pooling – which averages out the input in the region. This prevents over-fitting by reducing noise in the data, also to reduce computational cost by reducing the number of parameters to learn. In the figure, a 4 x 4 matrix with 16 parameters is down-sampled to a 2 x 2 matrix of 4 parameters.

However, conventional form of a rectangular pooling layer is not applicable in datasets with only vertical relations. Pooling is mainly done in the context where all data in a 2D array are spatial, where any integers within the array size are related spatially. Such techniques help to compact representations, which could greatly influence the model's performance. With regards to this study, a 2D non-spatial cell dataset, each row has a different unit such as size (mm) or standard deviations. Pooling together variables of different types would result in an invalid representation. Thus, a different form of a pooling layer for non-spatial data could be created instead. Such rectangular pooling seeks to pool between data of the same type to create a representative value of the region, while reducing data noise, and the parameter size of the network.

Furthermore, the operation of the study aims to take a sample of group of nine cell markers of the BC dataset and to obtain the maximum value of each set. A graphical representation of the operation of max rectangular pooling layer (RPL) is shown in **Figure 4**.

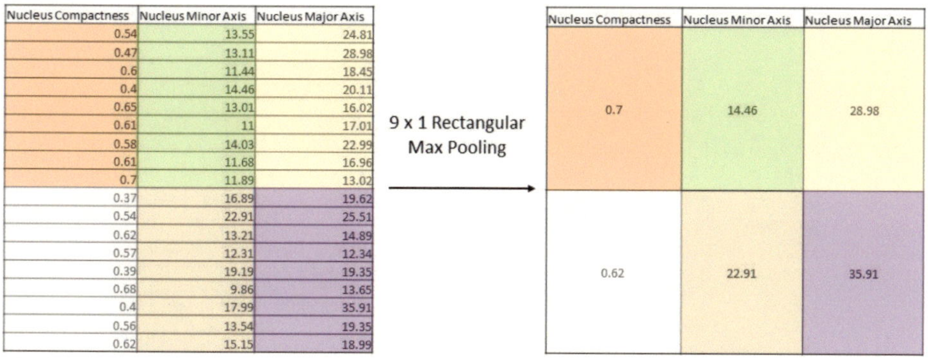

Figure 4.
Max Rectangular Pooling Layer Operation Representation – This shows a sample of how Rectangular Pooling Layer affects our input dataset. With a rectangular pool matrix, we ensure that non-related columns are not pooled together, unlike in a conventional square pooling layer. The transformation is a smaller dataset, with no loss in representation. This reduction in data size, results in faster learning generalisation and computation of the model.

In another experiment comparing a plain vanilla 2D CNN with RPL of 9 x 1 dimension and a conventional square pooling layer (SPL) of 3 x 3 dimension, it showed both having the same max function (**Table 10**). Comparing the training record of both pooling shapes, the RPL generalised at a much faster rate, of about 500 epochs ahead of SPL to achieve the same MAE. The former also achieved a lower MAE at the end of the training. In the context of a large dataset and DL network, using RPL in a non-spatial 2D dataset could achieve significant reduction in computational time.

2.2.2 Validation and evaluation

2.2.2.1 Validation

In the context of medical dataset, one common hampering factor is having a small dataset. This results in a validation process that is not robust enough as there may be an uneven distribution of data across the dataset. Traditional holdout validation is not rigorous enough to negate this effect and may result in an unfair representation of the efficacy of the model. This could be overcome with the use of K-Fold cross validation (K-cv), which is done by splitting the dataset by *k* iteratively holding out the sections of the data and evaluating the model with an average prediction error of all *k* evaluations (**Figure 5**).

Epochs	Rectangular Max Pooling MAE (months)	Square Max Pooling MAE (months)	Difference between Square Max Pooling and Rectangular Max Pooling (% Base using Rectangular Max Pooling)
500	81.341	81.869	0.65
1000	73.678	76.340	3.61
1500	67.018	71.577	6.80
2000	60.403	65.921	9.14
2500	53.717	58.351	8.63
3000	48.375	52.431	8.38
3500	45.761	49.085	7.26

Table 10.
Result of Rectangular Pooling Layer (RPL) vs. Square Pooling Layer (SQL).

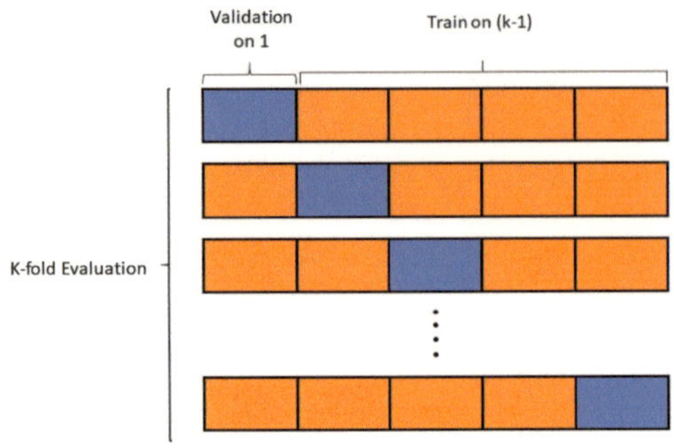

Figure 5.
K - Fold Cross Validation – By splitting our dataset into k folds, we can evaluate our model across the entire dataset independently. This is especially critical for small datasets (as is the case in medical context).

K-cv provides a more robust way of validating a model by validating a model with the entire data set. A study by Rodriguez et al. confirmed that K-cv reduces variance in prediction error and recommends implementing a K-cv whenever computationally possible [39]. In this study, the BC dataset was split into four groups of 23 patients and the standard deviation σ of each group is evaluated. It was discovered that the σ across all four groups was 8.43 months, which is a substantial amount in its ability to misrepresent the efficacy of the dataset.

2.2.2.2 Evaluation

The evaluation step acts as a feedback loop to the development of the CNN model. An iterative approach must be taken to analyse these results from a DL and a medical point of view to understand how further improvements could be made to the CNN model. Firstly, a model was built to evaluate clinical dataset followed by another model to evaluate the cell dataset. In an experiment with 107 patients, an adaptation of Dense ResNet [40] to the clinical data was used. A 2D CNN Wide Residual Network (WRN) [41] was also adapted for the cell data (**Figure 6**). A benchmark was developed on the dataset as a starting point for comparison, as this was a greenfield application. A simple vanilla dense network was used as a starting point to benchmark the results for the clinical dataset containing patients' information such as age, ethnicity, and tumour size. For the immunopathological dataset, we use a benchmark CNN model from the imaging domain as our starting point. MobileNet50 V2 [42] was chosen for the starting benchmark for

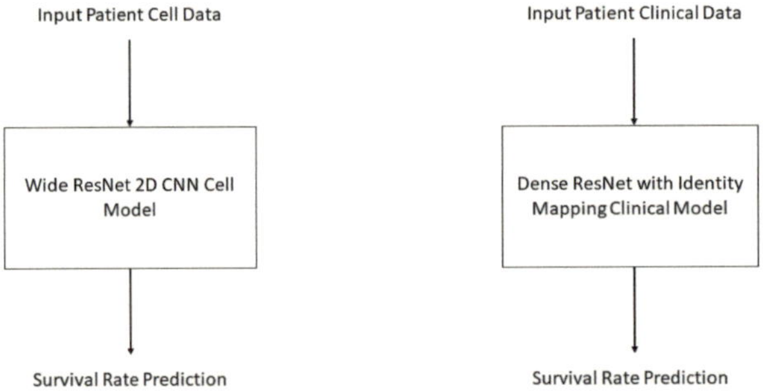

Figure 6.
Proposed Network Layout – Two independent model first learn representation from their respective dataset, which will have their weights combined together to create a unified model to create a single prediction from both datasets.

immunopathological dataset due to its accuracy, and training speed secondary to its small size (**Table 11**).

A sample k-fold training record as shown in **Figure 7**, shows the overfitting tendencies as the training error is minimised, but the validation error is not minimised. This could be attributed to the unsuitability of the models in the imaging domain without adaptation, which emphasises the importance of using the framework to adapt available CNN models to specific needs. In this study, a more suitable model was developed to clean up, augment, and enhance our dataset following the steps of the framework.

As shown in **Table 12**, the clinical dataset results were augmented from ±15.69 to ±8.24 by the immunopathological data from mIHC/IF with two additional information: number of stromal immune cells and cancer cells of each patients quantitated from the cell dataset. The results were subsequently normalised and iteratively developed to form a new Dense Neural Network based on the ResNet architecture that was better suited to the dataset. With regards to the cell dataset, the results

Clinical Vanilla MAE (months)	Cell MobileNet50 V2 MAE (months)	Unified Model MAE (months)
± 15.69	± 81.66	± 97.34

Table 11.
Benchmark Results for Both Dataset.

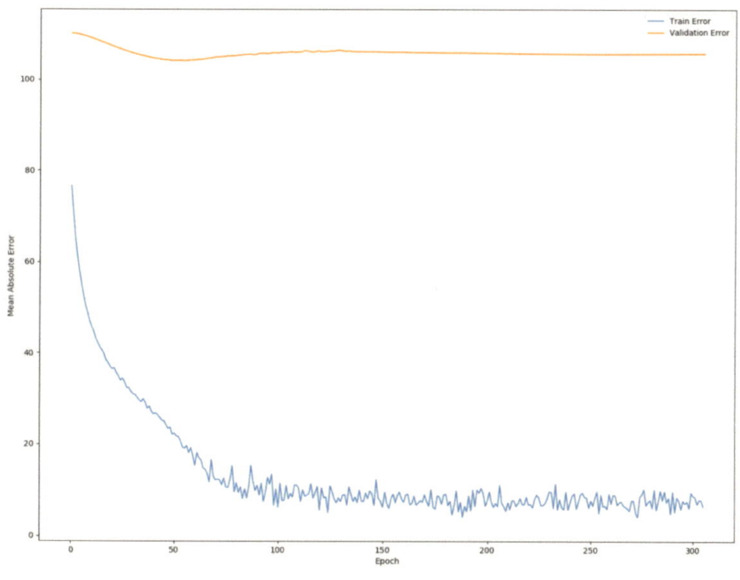

Figure 7.
Training History of MobileNet V2 – Benchmarking using a conventional general CNN model. Without adapting the model from imaging domain to our specific use case, we see a tendency to overfit by the divergence decreasing training error (Blue line) and the constant validation error (red line). This shows that there is no generalisation in the model, which serves as a good starting point, and a reminder of the need to adapt CNN to our specific use case.

Clinical ResNet MAE (months)	Cell WRN MAE (months)	Unified Model MAE (months)
± 8.24	± 40.23	± 55.23

Table 12.
Result for Both Dataset and Unified Model Using Adapted Models which factored in immunopathological data from mIHC/IF.

Survival Rate Cut-Off (Months)	No. of Patients	Combined MAE (Months)	Clinical + immunopathological data
Full Dataset (Benchmark)	107	± 55.23	± 8.24
≥12	96	± 52.17	± 8.78
≥16	92	± 35.11	± 10.67
≥20	88	± 25.86	± 11.42

Table 13.
MAE of dataset of Cut-Off Survival Rate.

were normalised to develop a more suitable CNN using WRN with RPL. Significant improvements in both the cell and clinical dataset were seen, which is appended with immunopathological data. The results were further improved by including a threshold based on the patients' survival rate.

A filter of patients with lower survival rate was experimented where the dataset was split with an arbitrary cut-off of ≥12 months, ≥16 months, and ≥ 20 months. Evaluating using the same unified model, **Table 13** showed the following MAE on 5-fold K-cv for each cut-off, where comparison of the combined clinical dataset and cell dataset were made after applying cut-off filter. The clinical dataset augmented with the stroma and tumour count from the cell dataset is also reflected in **Table 13** for reference. The increased in cut-off threshold meant that the model had a smaller dataset. Therefore, an increased in MAE of the model was expected, which was in line with the results shown in **Table 13**.

3. Limitations

Some limitations of this study should be noted. Firstly, this study uses a small dataset, which meant that the results could be less robust and of a lower confidence level. Although, this was minimised with the use of k-fold cross validation, more advanced techniques such as semi-supervised learning could be explored to augment the dataset. Secondly, there is currently no medical evidence to support using a cut-off to segregate patients as a valid approach. The approach used in this study is solely from a DL standpoint and therefore requires more medical based research to prove its validity. Moreover, given the novelty of the proposed framework, there is currently limited literature to support its application in other medical domains.

4. Conclusions

The adaptation of DL technology with the use of mIHC in the analysis of complex data is in the upcoming alternative approach of analysis in the field of immunopatholgy. However, given its novelty, further studies are needed to optimised the framework to enable application in varies medical field. Nevertheless, the framework proposed in this chapter serves to provide a starting foundation for application in clinical studies.

Author contributions

Conceptualization and design, Y. Chua and J. Yeong; literature review, S. Goh and Y. Chua; writing-original draft, S. Goh and Y. Chua; intellectual input and critical review, J. Lee, J. Yeong and Y. Cai.; writing-review and final editing, S. Goh and J. Lee. All authors have read and agreed to the published version of the manuscript.

Author details

Siting Goh[1], Yueda Chua[4], Justina Lee[3], Joe Yeong[1,2,3]* and Yiyu Cai[4]

1 Division of Pathology, Singapore General Hospital, Singapore

2 Duke-NUS Medical School, Singapore

3 Institute of Molecular Cell Biology (IMCB), Agency of Science, Technology and Research (A*STAR), Singapore

4 Nanyang Technological University (NTU), Singapore

*Address all correspondence to: yeongps@imcb.a-star.edu.sg

References

[1] Xin Yao, "Evolving artificial neural networks," in *Proceedings of the IEEE*, vol. 87, no. 9, pp. 1423-1447, Sept. 1999, doi: 10.1109/5.784219.

[2] Deng, L., & Yu, D. (2014). Deep learning: methods and applications. Foundations and trends in signal processing, *7*(3-4), 197-387.

[3] LeCun, Y., Bengio, Y., & Hinton, G. (2015). Deep learning. *nature*, *521*(7553), 436-444.

[4] Bera, K., Schalper, K. A., Rimm, D. L., Velcheti, V., & Madabhushi, A. (2019). Artificial intelligence in digital pathology—new tools for diagnosis and precision oncology. Nature reviews Clinical oncology, *16*(11), 703-715.

[5] Elmore, J. G., Longton, G. M., Carney, P. A., Geller, B. M., Onega, T., Tosteson, A. N., ... & O'Malley, F. P. (2015). Diagnostic concordance among pathologists interpreting breast biopsy specimens. Jama, *313*(11), 1122-1132.

[6] Bejnordi, B. E., Veta, M., Van Diest, P. J., Van Ginneken, B., Karssemeijer, N., Litjens, G., ... & Geessink, O. (2017). Diagnostic assessment of deep learning algorithms for detection of lymph node metastases in women with breast cancer. Jama, *318*(22), 2199-2210.

[7] Chen, J., & Srinivas, C. (2016). Automatic lymphocyte detection in H&E images with deep neural networks. *arXiv preprint arXiv:1612.03217*.

[8] Cruz-Roa, A., Gilmore, H., Basavanhally, A., Feldman, M., Ganesan, S., Shih, N., Tomaszewski, J., Madabhushi, A., & González, F. (2018). High-throughput adaptive sampling for whole-slide histopathology image analysis (HASHI) via convolutional neural networks: Application to invasive breast cancer detection. PloS one, *13*(5), e0196828. https://doi.org/10.1371/journal.pone.0196828

[9] Tan, W., Nerurkar, S. N., Cai, H. Y., Ng, H., Wu, D., Wee, Y., Lim, J., Yeong, J., & Lim, T. (2020). Overview of multiplex immunohistochemistry/immunofluorescence techniques in the era of cancer immunotherapy. Cancer communications (London, England), *40*(4), 135-153. https://doi.org/10.1002/cac2.12023

[10] Gong J, Chehrazi-Raffle A, Reddi S, Salgia R. Development of PD-1 and PD-L1 inhibitors as a form of cancer immunotherapy: a comprehensive review of registration trials and future considerations. J Immunother Cancer. 2018 Jan 23;6(1):8.

[11] Hellmann MD, Ciuleanu T-E, Pluzanski A, Lee JS, Otterson GA, Audigier-Valette C, et al. Nivolumab plus Ipilimumab in Lung Cancer with a High Tumor Mutational Burden. New England Journal of Medicine. 2018;378(22):2093-2104.

[12] Yau T, Zagonel V, Santoro A, Acosta-Rivera M, Choo SP, Matilla A, et al. Nivolumab (NIVO) + ipilimumab (IPI) + cabozantinib (CABO) combination therapy in patients (pts) with advanced hepatocellular carcinoma (aHCC): Results from CheckMate 040. Journal of Clinical Oncology. 2020;38(4_suppl):478-478.

[13] Garon EB, Rizvi NA, Hui R, Leighl N, Balmanoukian AS, Eder JP, et al. Pembrolizumab for the Treatment of Non–Small-Cell Lung Cancer. New England Journal of Medicine. 2015;372(21):2018-2028.

[14] Eggermont AMM, Blank CU, Mandala M, Long GV, Atkinson V, Dalle S, et al. Adjuvant Pembrolizumab versus Placebo in Resected Stage III Melanoma. N Engl J Med. 2018 May 10;378(19):1789-1801.

[15] Coons AH, Creech HJ, Jones RN. Immunological Properties

of an Antibody Containing a Fluorescent Group. Proceedings of the Society for Experimental Biology and Medicine. 1941 1941/06/01 [cited 2020/07/13];47(2):200-202.

[16] Ahmadzadeh M, Johnson LA, Heemskerk B, Wunderlich JR, Dudley ME, White DE, et al. Tumor antigen-specific CD8 T cells infiltrating the tumor express high levels of PD-1 and are functionally impaired. Blood. 2009 Aug 20;114(8):1537-1544.

[17] Muenst S, Hoeller S, Willi N, Dirnhofera S, Tzankov A. Diagnostic and prognostic utility of PD-1 in B cell lymphomas. Dis Markers. 2010;29(1): 47-53.

[18] Yeong J, Lim JCT, Lee B, Li H, Chia N, Ong CCH, et al. High Densities of Tumor-Associated Plasma Cells Predict Improved Prognosis in Triple Negative Breast Cancer. Front Immunol. 2018;9:1209.

[19] Hainaut P, Plymoth A. Targeting the hallmarks of cancer: towards a rational approach to next-generation cancer therapy. Curr Opin Oncol. 2013 Jan;25(1):50-51.

[20] Kim S-W, Roh J, Park C-S. Immunohistochemistry for Pathologists: Protocols, Pitfalls, and Tips. Journal of Pathology and Translational Medicine. 2016 10/13 04/18/received 08/05/rev-recd 08/08/accepted;50(6):411-418. Available from: ScienceCentral

[21] Curigliano G, Burstein HJ, Winer EP, Gnant M, Dubsky P, Loibl S, et al. De-escalating and escalating treatments for early-stage breast cancer: the St. Gallen International Expert Consensus Conference on the Primary Therapy of Early Breast Cancer 2017. Ann Oncol. 2017 Aug 1;28(8):1700-1712.

[22] Tay TKY, Thike AA, Pathmanathan N, Jara-Lazaro AR, Iqbal J, Sng ASH, et al. Using computer assisted image analysis to determine the optimal Ki67 threshold for predicting outcome of invasive breast cancer. Oncotarget. 2018;9(14):11619-11630. Available from: PubMed

[23] Koopman T, Buikema HJ, Hollema H, de Bock GH, van der Vegt B. Digital image analysis of Ki67 proliferation index in breast cancer using virtual dual staining on whole tissue sections: clinical validation and inter-platform agreement. Breast Cancer Res Treat. 2018 May;169(1):33-42.

[24] Yeong J, Tan T, Chow ZL, Cheng Q, Lee B, Seet A, et al. Multiplex immunohistochemistry/immuno-fluorescence (mIHC/IF) for PD-L1 testing in triple-negative breast cancer: a translational assay compared with conventional IHC. J Clin Pathol. 2020 Jan 22.

[25] Halse H, Colebatch AJ, Petrone P, Henderson MA, Mills JK, Snow H, et al. Multiplex immunohistochemistry accurately defines the immune context of metastatic melanoma. Scientific Reports. 2018 2018/07/24;8(1):11158.

[26] Lu S, Stein JE, Rimm DL, Wang DW, Bell JM, Johnson DB, et al. Comparison of Biomarker Modalities for Predicting Response to PD-1/PD-L1 Checkpoint Blockade: A Systematic Review and Meta-analysis. JAMA Oncol. 2019 Jul 18;5(8):1195-1204.

[27] Johnson DB, Bordeaux J, Kim JY, Vaupel C, Rimm DL, Ho TH, et al. Quantitative Spatial Profiling of PD-1/PD-L1 Interaction and HLA-DR/IDO-1 Predicts Improved Outcomes of Anti-PD-1 Therapies in Metastatic Melanoma. Clin Cancer Res. 2018 Nov 1;24(21):5250-5260.

[28] Giraldo NA, Nguyen P, Engle EL, Kaunitz GJ, Cottrell TR, Berry S, et al. Multidimensional, quantitative assessment of PD-1/PD-L1 expression in patients with Merkel cell carcinoma

and association with response to pembrolizumab. J Immunother Cancer. 2018 Oct 1;6(1):99.

[29] Fiore C, Bailey D, Conlon N, Wu X, Martin N, Fiorentino M, et al. Utility of multispectral imaging in automated quantitative scoring of immunohistochemistry. Journal of Clinical Pathology. 2012;65(6):496-502.

[30] Abel EJ, Bauman TM, Weiker M, Shi F, Downs TM, Jarrard DF, et al. Analysis and validation of tissue biomarkers for renal cell carcinoma using automated high-throughput evaluation of protein expression. Hum Pathol. 2014;45(5):1092-1099.

[31] Feng Z, Bethmann D, Kappler M, Ballesteros-Merino C, Eckert A, Bell RB, et al. Multiparametric immune profiling in HPV– oral squamous cell cancer. JCI Insight. 2017 07/20/;2(14).

[32] Mascaux C, Angelova M, Vasaturo A, Beane J, Hijazi K, Anthoine G, et al. Immune evasion before tumour invasion in early lung squamous carcinogenesis. Nature. 2019 Jun 26.

[33] Parra ER, Francisco-Cruz A, Wistuba, II. State-of-the-Art of Profiling Immune Contexture in the Era of Multiplexed Staining and Digital Analysis to Study Paraffin Tumor Tissues. Cancers (Basel). 2019 Feb 20;11(2).

[34] Tan AS, Yeong JPS, Lai CPT, Ong CHC, Lee B, Lim JCT, et al. The role of Ki-67 in Asian triple negative breast cancers: a novel combinatory panel approach. Virchows Arch. 2019 Dec;475(6):709-725.

[35] Yeong J, Lim JCT, Lee B, Li H, Ong CCH, Thike AA, et al. Prognostic value of CD8 + PD-1+ immune infiltrates and PDCD1 gene expression in triple negative breast cancer. Journal for ImmunoTherapy of Cancer. 2019 2019/02/06;7(1):34.

[36] Tan WCC, Nerurkar SN, Cai HY, Ng HHM, Wu D, Wee YTF, et al. Overview of multiplex immuno-histochemistry/immunofluorescence techniques in the era of cancer immunotherapy. Cancer Commun (Lond). 2020 Apr;40(4):135-153.

[37] Yeong J, Thike AA, Lim JC, Lee B, Li H, Wong SC, Hue SS, Tan PH, Iqbal J. Higher densities of Foxp3+ regulatory T cells are associated with better prognosis in triple-negative breast cancer. Breast Cancer Res Treat. 2017 May;163(1):21-35.

[38] Z. Jin Yan, "INVESTIGATION OF ARTIFICIAL INTELLIGENCE FOR MEDICAL IMAGE BASED DIAGNOSIS USING DEEP LEARNING," B.Eng Aerospace Engineering Final Year Project, Mechanical and Aerospace Engineering, Nanyang Technological University, Singapore 2018.

[39] J. D. Rodriguez, A. Perez, and J. A. Lozano, "Sensitivity analysis of k-fold cross validation in prediction error estimation," IEEE transactions on pattern analysis and machine intelligence, vol. 32, no. 3, pp. 569-575, 2009.

[40] K. He, X. Zhang, S. Ren, and J. Sun, "Deep residual learning for image recognition," in *Proceedings of the IEEE conference on computer vision and pattern recognition*, 2016, pp. 770-778.

[41] S. Zagoruyko and N. Komodakis, "Wide residual networks," *arXiv preprint arXiv:1605.07146,* 2016.

[42] M. Sandler, A. Howard, M. Zhu, A. Zhmoginov, and L.-C. Chen, "Mobilenetv2: Inverted residuals and linear bottlenecks," in *Proceedings of the IEEE conference on computer vision and pattern recognition*, 2018, pp. 4510-4520.

Section 4

Liquid Biopsy

Chapter 7

Liquid Biopsy: A New Diagnostic Strategy and Not Only for Lung Cancer?

Stefania Scarpino and Umberto Malapelle

Abstract

Targeted molecular therapies have significantly improved the therapeutic management of advanced lung cancer. The possibility of detecting lung cancer at an early stage is surely an important event in order to improve patient survival. Liquid biopsy has recently demonstrated its clinical utility in advanced non-small cell lung cancer (NSCLC) as a possible alternative to tissue biopsy for non-invasive evaluation of specific genomic alterations, thus providing prognostic and predictive information when the tissue is difficult to find or the material is not sufficient for the numerous investigations to be carried out. Several biosources from liquid biopsy, including free circulating tumor DNA (ctDNA) and RNA (ctRNA), circulating tumor cells (CTCs), exosomes and tumor-educated platelets (TEPs), have been extensively studied for their potential role in the diagnosis of lung cancer. This chapter proposes an overview of the circulating biomarkers assessed for the detention and monitoring of disease evolution with a particular focus on cell-free DNA, on the techniques developed to perform the evaluation and on the results of the most recent studies. The text will analyze in greater depth the liquid biopsy applied to the clinical practice of the management of NSCLC.

Keywords: liquid biopsy, NSCLC, cfDNA, ctDNA, biomarkers

1. Introduction

In the era of precision medicine, the management of cancer patients has dramatically changed. An increasing number of prognostic and predictive biomarkers are being implemented in order to ensure the best treatment option for advanced stage cancer patients and pathologists have learned to refine their reports [1]. To date, the analysis epidermal growth factor receptor (EGFR) gene mutations, anaplastic lymphoma kinase (ALK), and ROS 1 proto-oncogene (ROS1) rearrangements and schedules the state of death-ligand 1 (PD-L1) is capital for clinical decision making [2, 3]. In addition to these biomarkers, other activating mutations harbored by other clinically relevant genes are under investigation in clinical trials. However, despite the rapid development of this field in terms of discovered predictive biomarkers and platforms, tissue still remains an issue. To date, tissue samples represent the "gold standard" starting material to obtain nucleic acids (DNA and RNA) for molecular purposes and the only matherial available for morphological diagnosis and molecular analisys is often represented by paucicellular samples (cytological speciments or small tissue histological biopsies) [4]. However, a not negligible percentage, about 30%, of advanced stage NSCLC patients, cannot be tested because tissue sample is not adequate both for anatomo pathological revision and for molecular analysis [5]. In addition, even in high expertise centers, the percentage of inadequate molecular results, in particular when small tissue samples are adopted, may be significant [6]. In this setting, and in order to avoid to leave patients behind, liquid biopsy represents a valid option as a rapid, noninvasive and accurate clinical option. Several biosources from liquid biopsy, including free circulating DNA (cfDNA) and RNA (cfRNA), circulating tumor cells (CTCs), exosomes and tumor-educated platelets (TEPs), can be isolated. While each of these modalities has the potential to provide new diagnostic information and their exploration is highly encouraged, ctDNA certainly represents the most mature example of the survey on liquid biopsy in clinical practice for lung cancer patients. Therefore, this chapter will mainly focus on the clinical value of the free circulating tumor DNA (ctDNA), a small fraction of cfDNA extracted from plasma samples and we will review the available data that suggest the role of liquid biopsy in the management of NSCLC.

To date, Food and Drug Administration (FDA) has approved the analysis of ctDNA in two different NSCLC patients settings: naïve advanced stage NSCLC (basal setting), when tissue is not available or inadequate for molecular analysis of the Epidermal Growth Factor Receptor (EGFR) in order to select patients for first or second generation EGFR tyrosine kinase inhibitor (TKI) administration; acquisition of somatic resistance mechanism after first or second EGFR TKI administration (resistance setting), in order to detect the EGFR exon 20 p.T790M resistance point mutation and select patients for third generation EGFR TKIs [7].

Here we will report the potential of liquid biopsy to help manage NSCLC throughout all stages: cancer screening, minimal residual disease detection to guide adjuvant treatment, early detection of relapse, systemic treatment initiation and monitoring of response (targeted or immune therapy), and resistance genotyping. Moreover, we will also carefully analyze each step of the pre-analytical management of liquid biopsy specimen, (sample collection, ctDNA extraction, and molecular analysis) and the advantages and disadvantages found in the use of liquid biopsy respect the adoption of gold standard tissue sample in the context of clinical practice.

2. Liquid biopsy: definition

The term liquid biopsy refers to the use of biological fluids as a surrogate for neoplastic tissue to obtain information useful for diagnostic, prognostic purposes or to predict the response to therapy with specific anticancer drugs. In the biological fluids (blood, urine, saliva, cerebrospinal fluid, pleural effusions, ascites or cytology specimen-derived supernatant [8–10] of tumor patients are contained cell-free DNA (cfDNA), circulating tumor DNA (ctDNA)circulating tumor cells, circulating RNA, microRNAs (miRNA), platelets and exosomes, which can be a valuable source of information about molecular assessment of cancer. Analysis of ctDNA contained in the free circulating DNA (cfDNA) that can be isolated from peripheral blood, represents to date the main liquid biopsy approach employed in clinical practice. In healthy patients, cfDNA is released in low quantity from normal cells during cellular turnover and is represented by small DNA fragments (150–200 base pairs). On the otherwise cancer patients show an increased levels of cfDNA [11, 12] with a consistent release of ctDNA generally represented, by more small fragment, with sizes ranging from 90 to 150 base pairs [13]. The amount of ctDNA is variable in cancer patients, ranging from less than 0.1% to more than 90% [11, 12]. The cf./ctDNA ratio can depends on the time of sample collection and clinical condition of the patient and is influenced by total tumor burden, location and extent of metastases, proliferation rate, apoptotic potential and genome instability [14]. ctDNA can enter the bloodstream through two different mechanisms: by a passive mechanism derived from apoptosis and necrosis or by an active mechanism derived from a spontaneous release of DNA fragment from primary tumor tissues or from circulating tumor cells or tumor-associated macrophages [15, 16].

2.1 Liquid biopsy versus traditional biopsy

The new College of American Pathologists (CAP), International Association for the Study of Lung Cancer (IASLC)/Association for Molecular Pathology (AMP) guideline for molecular testing of patients with NSCLC, although did not recommend the performance of molecular analysis when tissue is available, they strongly suggest liquid biopsy in those cases where tissue sample is not adequate to perform molecular analysis [17] In fact, a significant subgroup of patients cannot undergo a biopsy or rebiopsy for several reasons such as unsuitable clinical conditions or an unfavorable tumor site such as bone or central nervous system or multiple small pulmonary nodules that are not safely amenable to biopsy [18].

Let us see what are the advantages and disadvantages of using liquid biopsy.

Liquid biopsy shows several advantages over that traditional biopsy:

- the procedure is not invasive, as it is a simple blood sampling and than may spare the patient an invasive procedure with the incumbent risks of major complications. Often occurs that patient need a rebiopsy due to the scant tumor tissue to obtain new tissue for further tests and to performing all the required analyses;

- the ability to represent more comprehensively than tissue biopsy the molecular heterogeneity of the disease. Several studies have compared mutational profiles of different sites of metastatic disease from the same patient and have established the intratumoral heterogeneity and spatial and temporal tumor heterogeneity of solid tumors [19, 20]. While tissue only offers a snapshot of the tumor at a given time and location, may not represent the complex genetic profile of a patient's tumor and can introduce the hypothesis of false-negative results, ctDNA that is shed into the periphery from multiple sites of disease has the potential to overcome both spatial and temporal tumor heterogeneity. Circulating markers are more effective in depicting the emergent biology in actively growing metastatic lesions which may be missed [21, 22].

- can follow subclonal evolution through iterative noninvasively blood draws taking into account different clones present within all metastatic sites as a surrogate for more invasive tissue biopsies. It can be usefull to monitor molecular evolution of the disease, although there is no evidence to date that addresses a modify the therapeutic choice, in the absence of clinical progression of disease;

- as a cost-effective alternative for patients considering that performing a tissue biopsy is considerably more expensive than a blood draw;

- turnaround time may be shorter considering the scheduling time involved [23].

- However, ctDNA suffers of several limitations that may impact on the adoption in routine predictive laboratory practice:

- the amount of ctDNA in the context of cfDNA is often extremely limited, (<0.5% of the total circulating cell free DNA) [24] depending on both the volume and the localization of the disease and this can lead to misinterpret molecular results (false negatives);

- ctDNA has a very low half-life (about 15 minutes) and this is a crucial limitation [24]. This aspect lead to reduce of 50% cfDNA molecules each 15 minutes from the withdrawn.

The International Association for the Study of Lung Cancer (IASLC) established in a statement paper the guideline when considering to adopt liquid biopsy samples for molecular analysis [7].

3. What are the methods for ctDNA analysis? Pre-analytical consideration: from blood collection to ctDNA

CtDNA can be extracted from various biological fluids. However, the procedures more standardized in clinical practice concern isolation of ctDNA from peripheral blood. ctDNA can be isolated from serum or plasma. Several studies compare cfDNA levels in plasma and serum samples and have shown significantly higher cfDNA concentrations in serum [25, 26] but shown that the use of plasma is preferable to serum. In the latter, in fact, the coagulation process causes the release of genomic DNA deriving from leukocytes and leads to a contamination of germline DNA that causes a ctDNA dilution.

Isolation and enrichment of ctDNA is a great challenge given the high degree of cfDNA fragmentation and its low concentration in the bloodstream to the extent of a few ng/ml, of which the ctDNA is alone a fraction [15]. Several factors affect the quality and quantity of ctDNA including: the burden of disease, the rate of release of the ctDNA in the bloodstream and the levels of DNA released by non- transformed cells. Therefore, for these reasons the pre-analytical phase must be carefully checked. to achieve superior quality results.

3.1 Sample collection

A first problem that can affect the quality of the sample is constituted from hemolysis that can occur during phlebotomy. It is necessary, therefore, that blood sampling is carried out by highly qualified personnel.

The sample can be collected in standard EDTA tubes or using tubes containing special fixatives, capable of stabilizing the blood and the cfDNA for several days. If the sampling is carried out using standard tubes, one important factor must be taken into account. cfDNA has a short half-life, estimated at around 2.5 hours therefore tubes can be stored before plasma isolation for a maximum of 3 hours at room temperature (**Figure 1**). Several studies have shown that after three hours of sampling, the wild-type cfDNA concentration could increase due to lysis of hematological cells thus reduce the relative percentage of tumor-specific ctDNA [27]. The storage of blood at a temperature of 4°C it does not prevent leukocyte lysis. Operators dealing with blood collection, handling, and eventual shipping should be cognizant of these time constraints. Blood should never be frozen before plasma extraction.

3.2 Extraction, quantification and storage of cfDNA

There are many methods for extracting cfDNA, which include both the use of commercial kits and protocols developed by laboratories.

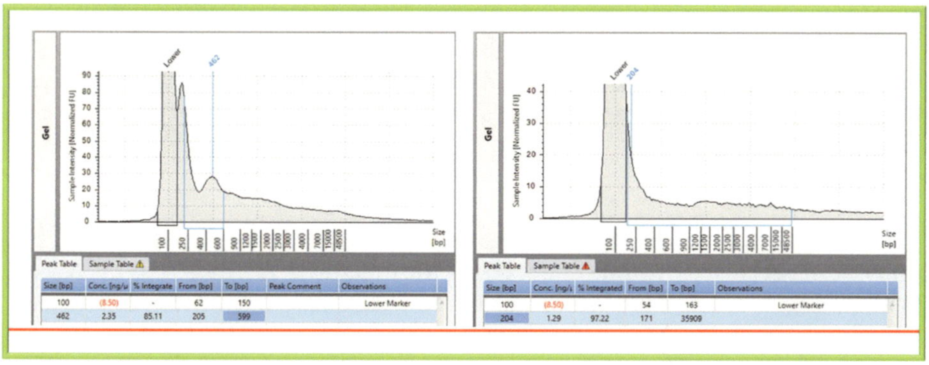

Figure 1.
Incidence of time withdrawn in the managment of liquid biopsy specimen. The figure shows the comparison between electhropherograms performed by nanofluidic platform Tapestation 4200, (Agilent, Santa Clara, California, USA) on a sample immediately and after 1 h processed to isolate cfDNA respect time of withdrawn. In the left profile, ctDNA peak of 180–200 bp is inspected; on the right profile the peak is not detected.

The extraction method must be very reliable and must generate as much possible DNA of the sample under examination. For the extraction and purification of cfDNA from plasma they are now available various commercial kits dedicated to this specific use. These kits are generally based on the use of columns equipped with silica membranes in association with a vacuum pump, or on the use of magnetic balls for the capture of nucleic acids.

Once extracted, the cfDNA must undergo quantification in order to optimize the amplification process and to know if the subsequent molecular analyzes may be possible starting from the cfDNA extract [28].

Optimal storage of cfDNA is very important as it allows its use also a time to carry out further molecular investigations, The process takes adequate equipment, including –20° C/ -80° C freezers, devices graphic temperature control, acoustic alarm systems, quality controls of the biological material stored [28].

4. Analytical methods for detecting ctDNA

Until recently, the available technology was not sensitive enough to detect ctDNA and use it in a meaningful way but in recent years highly sensitive blood-based assays have been developed to test cfDNA at very low concentrations for most genomic abnormalities and advances in pre-analytical processes and purification methods have enabled the capture, amplification and sequencing of ctDNA to be successful. A good molecular ctDNA test should retain an acceptable concordance to molecular testing in the tumor tissue. However, even with the increased sensitivity, a negative result from ctDNA analisys is not sufficient to exclude the potential existence of a driver alteration; therefore, in these circumstances tissue analysis should be performed.

The methods currently used to detect or measure ctDNA are numerous and can be divided into two categories: polymerase chain reaction (PCR)-based techniques and next-generation sequencing (NGS) technologies.

4.1 Polymerase chain reaction (PCR)-based techniques

Within the PCR-based techniques are included real time PCR, digital PCR (dPCR), droplet digital PCR (ddPCR), peptide nucleid acid (PNA) clamp-based PCR assay (Taqman assay), beads, emulsions, amplification and magnetics

(BEAMing). PCR-based approaches, can detect mutations in cfDNA at allele frequencies of 0.01% or lower. Although there are numerous platforms currently for ctDNA evaluation, the gold standards in pcr-based technologies are basically quantitative PCR (qPCR) and digital PCR.

4.1.1 PCR real time

PCR-based tests generally have faster response times and are less expensive, but can typically evaluate only one or a few specific mutations at a time. The analysis of point mutations or small insertions/deletions on ctDNA it can be often conducted through the use of Real Time technologies PCR, often modified to increase the sensitivity of the test. There are commercially available ctDNA kits based on different amplification technology (e.g. Refractory Mutation System ARMS/SCORPION) which detect mutations against EGFR exons 19, 20 and 21. These kits allow the co-amplification of one or more mutated alleles and of an endogenous control gene. The analysis with these kits allows to detect low percentages of mutated allele in the presence of high amounts of wild-type genomic DNA and can reach an even lower limit of detection (LOD) 0.5%. The main limitation related to the adoption of this approach is related to the annealing step where probes may not able to target corresponding genomic region (**Figure 2**).

4.1.2 Digital PCR (dPCR)

Digital PCR (dPCR) is a next-generation evolution of PCR of which there are two technological platforms: "digital droplet PCR - ddPCR" and "BEAMing dPCR" (Beam, Emulsion, Amplification, Magnetics).

Both methods, utilize emulsion technology to quantify the amount of mutant cfDNA in patient plasma and are based on the limiting dilution of DNA with a distribution of the sample in thousands of homogeneous "droplets" in an oil–water

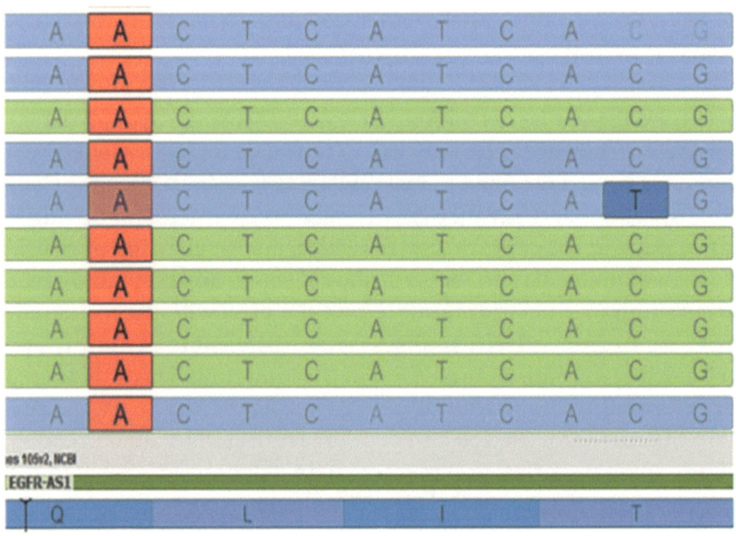

Figure 2.
Visual inspection of p.T790M EGFR acquired resistance mutations by using NGS system. The figure shows the manual count of aligned reads generated by Golden helix genome browse 1.1.2 (Golden helix genome browse Inc). In the red box is reported a polymorphism in the genomic region near p.T790M base change (blue box). Although the presence of this polymorphic alteration, NGS platform is able to p.T790M resistance mutation while RT-qPCR based approaches report a false negative result.

emulsion. These characteristics are of great importance in the context of the analysis of ctDNA, where it is necessary to search for and amplify rare molecules of tumor DNA in the presence of a large excess of wildtype germline DNA.

In fact, the breakdown of the sample into droplets has the function of reduce competition between mutated tumor DNA and wild-type DNA increasing the specificity and sensitivity of the analysis.

Both of these experimental approach is very useful for the identification of rare variants since only a small concentration of template is required for the analysis.

The sensibility and the specificity of the tests with ddPCR and BEAMing dPCR are, respectively 0.1% and 0.01%.

Several studies have compared multiple platforms for detecting EGFR mutations in plasma ctDNA. In one study, two non-digital platforms (cobas®EGFR mutation test and therascreen EGFR amplification refractory mutation system test) and two digital platforms (Droplet Digital PCR and BEAMing digital PCR) were compared in their ability to identify sensitizing mutations and the results support the potential use of both platforms in a clinical development program [29].

The limit of these technologies is that of their limited ability to detect complex genomic alterations and perform multiplex testing.

4.2 NGS in liquid biopsy

In contrast to PCR-based methods, NGS is a fascinating technology able to analyze different biomarkers for different patients, simultaneously [30] and detect rare and previously uncharacterized alterations. NGS are capable of detection of mutations, indels, copy number variations and genomic rearrangements such as oncogenic fusions. Another advantage of an NGS approach is the possibility to quantify the amount of DNA that brings a particular alteration.

This technology, based on massive and parallel sequencing, ensures a high sequencing throughput, by generating from hundreds of thousands to millions of sequences (reads) [30]. To overcome the limitations of ctDNA, next generation sequencing (NGS) may be a viable option. The use of NGS for liquid biopsy requires changes to the protocols normally used for blood and tissue analysis. Operational protocols dedicated to liquid biopsy.

Different NGS platforms are commercially available and validated on liquid biopsy samples [31]. Among these, Illumina (San Diego, California) platform adopts a sequencing-by-synthesis chemistry able to identify DNA bases, while introducing them into a nucleic acid strand, by adopting a system of fluorescently labeled nucleotides; Ion Torrent (ThermoFisher Scientifics, Waltham, Massachusetts) platform adopts a sequencing-by-synthesis chemistry able to identify DNA bases, while introducing them into a nucleic acid strand, by adopting a semiconductor system useful to measure a change in pH due to the release of an H+ ion [32]. Important differences exist between these various platforms with respect to the number of genomic alterations included in a single panel, the ability to multiplex these assays, the turnaround time of the test, and its ability to detect complex genomic alterations.

Different NGS gene panels have been adopted for ctDNA analysis and numerous studies have been carried out in recent years to validate concordance to molecular testing in the tumor tissue. A higher sensitivity and specificity was obtained by Reckampet al by using a short footprint mutation enrichment NGS assay to analyze ctDNA samples extracted from plasma of NSCLC patients [8]. On the overall, taking into account the results obtained on matched tissue samples, a sensitivity of 93, 100, and 87% for EGFR exon 20 p.T790M, EGFR exon 21 p.L858R, and EGFR exon 19 deletions, was reached. The specificity, for the same mutations was 94, 100, and 96% [8]. In the experience of Paweletz et al. a high sensitivity (86% and 79%) and specificity (100% and 100%) was obtained by using a targeted NGS approach on NSCLC patients for EGFR and KRAS mutations [33]. Another valid approach is represented by the use of narrow gene panels. In the experience of the Predictive Molecular Pathology Laboratory at the University of Naples Federico II a custom, narrow NGS gene panel (named SiRe®), that cover 568 clinical relevant mutations in six genes (EGFR, KRAS, BRAF, NRAS, KIT and PDGFRA), was routinely employed for both tissue and liquid biopsy testing [34, 35]. In the validation study on different tumor types, a sensitivity of 90.5% and a specificity of 100% was reached by comparing results obtained on ctDNA extracted from serum and plasma with those obtained on matched tissue samples. In addition, this panel may be useful to detect EGFR and KRAS actionable mutations in basal setting NSCLC patients [35].

Ultra-sensitive NGS techniques dedicated to analysis have been developed of the ctDNA. The characterizing element of Cancer custom profiling deep sequencing (Capp-Seq), its is a selector that identifies different classes of somatic mutations with sensitivity and specificity greater than 90%. Similar results in terms of sensitivity and specificity were achieved with Tagged-amplicon deep sequencing (Tam-Seq) and Safe-Sequencing techniques System (Safe-SeqS).

What was once a limitation of ngs technology, the turnaround time is now acceptable for clinical management — approximately 13 days — and costs have been significantly reduced [36]. Also the difficulty of analyzing the numerous information deriving from the multigene panels has also been overcome since a variety of publically available and proprietary bioinformatics tools have been developed to assist in these calculations.

4.3 New emerging technologies to the study of liquid biopsy

Several studies today aim to overcome the current limits of sensitivity for liquid biopsy, to support extensive research and clinics applications. Although for the evaluation of the ctDNA the gold standards are basically quantitative PCR (qPCR), digital PCR and NGS to these have been added many technologies such as whole genome sequencing (WGS) [37], Rare Ep iAlleles by Melt qPCR (DREAMing) [38] and bidirectional pyrophosphorolysis activated polymerization (bi-PAP).

Moreover, of great interest in biomedicine applied to the study of liquid biopsy are the PCR-free methods [39]. Several articles have been published dealing with PCR-free methods for the detection of point mutations [40]. These methods applied alternative isothermal-amplification methods whitch do not require thermal cycling to avoid heating and cooling steps. About the smetods include those based on nucleic acid sequences polymerization (NASBA), loop-mediated amplification (LAMP, helicase-dependent amplification (HAD), rolling - circle amplification (RCA), recombinase-polymerase amplification (RPA) and multi-displacement amplification (MDA), isothermal displacement of the circular filament polymerization (ICSPD).

Among these methods of sure interest is surface plasmon resonance imaging (SPR-I). This tecnology are able to detected Attomolar concentrations of target genomic DNA, demonstrating the ultra-sensitivity of the new method [39].

Thanks to these new ultra-sensitive technologies, several authors are pushing towards new horizons. In some studies differences in fragment lengths of circulating DNA could be exploited to enhance sensitivity for detecting the presence of ctDNA and for noninvasive genomic analysis of cancer. Mouliere et al. [13] argue that cfDNA fragment size analysis improved the discrimination between samples from patients with cancer and those from healthy individuals.

All these technologies are now supported by different platforms and have already been approved for clinical use [41]. However, the lack of standardization limit the clinical implementation for most of these methodologies.

5. Liquid biopsy in clinical practice

There are two main scenarios in which the liquid biopsy might confer an advantage to NSCLC advanced patients:at initial molecular profiling and at progression during targeted therapy. To date, Food and Drug Administration (FDA) has approved the analysis of ctDNA extracted from plasma samples in two different patient settings: in treatment naïve advanced stage NSCLC (basal setting), when tissue is not available or inadequate for molecular purposes, for the Epidermal Growth Factor Receptor (EGFR) gene assessment in order to select patients for first or second generation EGFR tyrosine kinase inhibitor (TKI) treatments and in advanced stage NSCLC resistant to a first or second EGFR TKI (resistance setting), in order to detect the EGFR exon 20 p.T790M resistance point mutation and select patients for third generation EGFR TKIs [7].

5.1 Tumor molecular profiling of naïve patients (basal setting)

Liquid biopsy should be taken into consideration at the time of initial diagnosis in all patients who need tumor molecular profiling, but:

- tumor tissue is insufficient or unavailable;
- in patients for whom invasive procedures may be risky or contraindicated;
- in those cases where the biopsy scheduling time exceeds two weeks causing a serious delay in diagnosis;
- in the case of bone biopsies where the decalcification processes of the sample irreversibly damage the nucleic acids and therefore invalidate any molecular investigation;
- moreover, indications for choosing treatment-naive patients for ctDNA molecular testing are all patients with advanced/metastatic nonsquamous NSCLC and patients with squamous NSCLC if never smoker and/or younger age.

In clinical practice, liquid biopsy is currently mainly used for analysis of mutational status of the epidermal growth factor receptor (EGFR) in advanced NSCLC patients. Several studies and meta-analyzes [42, 43] have evaluated the diagnostic accuracy of ctDNA analysis for the identification of the most frequent activating mutations of the EGFR gene (deletions of exon 19, L858R of exon 21) in patients naïve with advanced NSCLC proving a good specificity greater than 90%. Sensitivity results instead be lower, with fluctuations between 50% and 80% depending on the technology used. On the basis of these evidences the evaluation of the mutational status of the EGFR gene on liquid biopsy is currently recommended as a possible alternative to analysis on tumor tissue.

A positive finding of an actionable mutation in ctDNA, if using a validated assay, is sufficient to initiate targeted treatment. However, a negative result it cannot be trusted and it should be followed up with a secondary test or conventional tumor testing. A negative result can be negative for several factors. The amounts of DNA into peripheral circulation of patients with indolent slow-growing tumors is often insufficient for detection and these patient may be at more risk of a false negative compared to patients with a more disseminated cancer. Therefore, it is imperative that operators are aware of the possibility of a false negative result from the liquid biopsy.

For this reason the liquid biopsy at diagnosis is far from being able to replace the traditional analysis of the tissue which therefore remains the standard goal in patient's diagnosis.

5.1.1 Other oncogenic drivers in NSCLC have been detected in ctDNA isolated from plasma

In addition to EGFR mutations a wide range of potentially actionable alterations are of particular interest clinically and are detectable in patients with NSCLC, including ROS1, fibroblast growth factor receptor 3 (FGFR3), and neurotrophic receptor tyrosine kinase (NTRK) rearrangements and ALK, MEK, AKT, BRAF, HER2, MEK1/2, NRAS, KRAS mutations and MET receptor tyrosine kinase mutations and amplification. All of these abnormalities have been detected in ctDNA isolated from plasma and could therefore be used for screening naive patients.

As regards the study of rearrangements, which is carried out at the ctRNA level, some technical difficulties may arise due to the low stability of the circulating plasma RNA which easily undergoes degradation. The most commonly used techniques to identified ALK at the time of diagnosis, are qPCR and digital PCR or next-generation sequencing (NGS) approaches [44, 45].

The sensitivity of the techniques for studying this alteration is less high than those that can normally be used on the tissue (e.g., immunohistochemistry or Fluorescent in situ Hybridization (FISH).

5.1.2 The liquid biopsy in other fluids

Although plasma is the most widely used fluid sample for liquid biopsy, other samples are available such as urine, sputum, cerebrospinal fluid or pleural effusion as a source of ctDNA.

Sputum is an important source of nucleic acids and different studies investigated EGFR status in NSCLC patients. Wu et al. [46] identified a high concordance between sputum and tissue samples (74%). In a recent study it has been identified the potential role as a diagnostic biomarker for NSCLC of P16INK4 gene promoter methylation in both bronchoalveolar lavage (BAL) and sputum [47]. A recent study showed that sensitivity of EGFR mutation detection in the urine is comparable to that found in the plasma of the same patient [48] and concordance of mutations in the driver gene may increase when compared to plasma alone to combination of plasma, urine and sputum [49].

The ability to use ctDNA obtained from cerebrospinal fluid (CSF) to study genetic alterations and monitor response to treatment is very important as brain metastases are difficult to reach.

5.2 Monitoring therapeutic resistance

Resistance inevitably arises in almost all patients undergoing treatment for metastatic disease [50]. The ability to detect the presence of multiple resistance mechanisms is critical. Acquired resistance to therapy is often driven by presence of one or more tumor subclones that harbor resistance alterations [51]. These subclones drive disease progression and may reside in the same tumor lesion or in different metastatic lesions [52]. Therefore, a standard tumor biopsy of a single lesion at the time of disease progression may fail to capture resistance mechanisms present in tumor cells outside of the biopsied region [53]. This is where the liquid biopsy comes into play overcomes the limit of tumor heterogeneity.

p.T790M gatekeeper resistance identification in liquid biopsy is currently employed as a first diagnostic approach in all patients with EGFR-positive advanced NSCLC in progression after EGFR-TKI treatment. However, due to the risk of "false negatives" associated with such method, all patients in whom the mutational analysis on ctDNA results "negative" and even the initial sensitizing mutation is not detected must be subjected to test tumor tissue taken by re-biopsy, in order to define the best therapeutic strategy. However before proceeding with the tissue biopsy, it would be advisable to repeat liquid biopsy. In the absence of such a mutation, the test should be considered non-informative as the sample contains no sufficient ctDNA. In this regard, multiple studies, and a recent meta-analysis, have clearly highlighted as the site of metastases cancer significantly affects the diagnostic accuracy of the mutation analysis of the EGFR gene performed on ctDNA. The sensitivity of that method in determining both activating and p.T790M mutation can in fact vary from 80% in presence of extra-thoracic metastases at 50% in the presence of exclusively intra-thoracic localizations [28]. In order to increase the chances of success of the liquid biopsy, the test should be performed at the time of obvious progression of disease, when the probability that the tumor DNA is released into the circulation is higher.

Liquid biopsy is also utilized to detected additional coexisting resistance alterations, such as MET amplification that predicts decreased benefit from subsequent therapy with third-generation EGFR inhibitors and EGFR p.C797S mutation following therapy with the third-generation EGFR inhibitor osimertinib [52].

6. How should the results of liquid biopsy be reported? The reporting

European Society of Pathology Task Force on Quality Assurance in Molecular Pathology and the Royal College of Pathologists published standards of molecular diagnostics reporting [54].

Reporting is an integral part of the diagnostic procedure and should contain the following information: patient identifiers, specimen type, assay methodology and the platform used including sensitivity and limit of detection, date of collection of the material used for the analysis and date of arrival of the sample in the laboratory that performs the analysis, methods of conservation of the sample investigated mutations, results of the test, data interpretation and an overall evaluation of the analysis specifying whether a detected alteration is clinically relevant.

The report must be completed on a predetermined form, dated and signed by the service manager.

7. Emerging application and future direction of liquid biopsy

Liquid biopsy is a rapidly growing field in oncology and ctDNA analysis is considered to be very promising as a biomarker for early stage detection, identification and monitoring of minimal residual disease (MRD), immuno-oncology, assessment of treatment response, and monitoring tumor evolution. Currently, several trials are ongoing in this field.

7.1 Potential applications in early stage NSCLC: screening

Detection of lung cancer at an earlier stage of disease, potentially susceptible of curative resection, can be critical to improve patients survival. Current screening and diagnostic tests, such as computed tomography (CT) scans and cytological/histological analyzes could be supplemented by the specificity of cfDNA [55]. The evaluation of genomic anomalies, including specific mutations, in cfDNA could offer a promising, non-invasive approach for the early diagnosis of lung cancer, considering the high specificity of these related tumors alterations. A limitation is due to the low frequency of some mutations and the fact that the mutant cfDNA can be obscured by an excess of background wild-type DNA. However, highly sensitive approaches have been developed to analyze low-level mutants cfDNA, including NGS-based options.

Many studies have focused on assessing the quantities of cfDNA. In a study carried out on smoking patients it was shown that the concentration in cfDNA, of the human telomerase reverse transcription (hTERT) gene was eight times higher in lung cancer patients than in controls and correlate with a strong risk factor for the development of lung cancer [56]. In other studies it has been shown that a greater amount of cfDNA during surgery correlates with a worse prognosis at 5 years survival, selecting a more aggressive disease [57]. Using a very sensitive quantitative test [57] it was demonstrated the possibility of discriminate between healthy subjects and NSCLC patients by measuring the quantities of cfDNA [58, 59]. cfDNA were significantly higher in NSCLC patients compared to healthy controls.

Methylation is an early and frequent epigenetic alteration that can be detected in cfDNA, including in plasma [60, 61]. Epigenetic modifications, regulate the expression of a large number of genes involved in malignant transformation and carcinogenesis. DNA alterations in methylation occur early in carcinogenesis and are remarkably more stable than other potentials diagnostic biomarkers.

Several studies have evaluated the methylation levels of single or panels of tumor suppressor genes in plasma or serum from lung cancer patients. Several genes have been found to be differentially methylated in cfDNA between patients with lung cancer and controls including MGMT, p16, RASSF1A, DAPK, RAR-β, DCLK1, SHOX2 and septin9 [62, 63]. In a recent study, a methylation panel of six genes showed a sensitivity of 72% for the detection of stage Ia NSCLC [64].

However though, methylation changes can also occur in the DNA of peritumor normal tissue which can therefore interfere with the analysis of tumor DNA generating a false positive result [65]. Considering together the fact that ctDNA is absent or very low in the early stages, the possibility to detect mutations in cfDNA derived from non tumor cells and the lack of standardized methods and large validation studies the analysis of ctDNA has not been introduced in the clinic screening yet.

7.2 Identification and monitoring residual disease

Measurement of residual disease after primary tumor treatment is an area of active investigation.

Efficient methods of identifying MRD in patients treated with surgery or adjuvant chemotherapy are currently lacking. Mutation monitoring can be a significant predictor of early relapses and MRD. Several studies have focused on detecting these mutations in ctDNA as an early indicator of relapse and a potential marker of residual disease.

Monitoring of ctDNA for residual disease has been used in several studies in lung cancer. Presence of ctDNA after local treatment was highly predictive of disease recurrence in a small cohort of lung cancer patients with stage I-III lung undergoing local treatment with radiation, surgery, or both [66].

DOI: http://dx.doi.org/10.5772/intechopen.94838

A prospective trial is ongoing to investigate the ability of ctDNA mutations and methylation monitoring to detect MRD after surgery for stage Ia–III NSCLC [67].

The limit of the use of ctDNA in detect MRD in clinical practice beyond is the lack of circulating tumor specific alterations.

7.3 Monitoring treatment response and cancer progression

CtDNA analysis could be a way to monitor cancer status in real time. Methods for monitoring treatment response and changes in tumor burden with cfDNA involve the identification of genomic alterations specific to an individual patient's tumor and the relationship between changes in ctDNA levels, that can be monitored in real time during therapy (**Figure 3**).

In one study, long-term monitoring of a patient with NSCLC for analysis of EGFR mutations (p.L858R and p.T790M) using ctDNA isolated from serum and plasma a close correlation with the onset of metastasis was identified. In another study carried out with NGS technology on plasma-derived ctDNA from 168 patients with different types of cancer, the molecular alterations identified correlated to which of tissue [68].

ctDNA levels drop dramatically after one to two weeks in patients responding to treatment [69, 70]. Some authors suggested that a rise in ctDNA levels may precede radiographic progression.

Data obtained by several studies, conducted on different tumor type [71] using very sensitive new technologies involving multiplexed mutation-specific PCR and NGS suggest that the additionof ctDNA monitoring into clinical care could be a valuable tool to more accurately predict patient response and detect progression.

7.4 Liquid biopsy and immuno-oncology

Cancer immunotherapy is certainly the most profound innovation recorded in recent years in the fight against cancer. The recent use of anti-programmed death

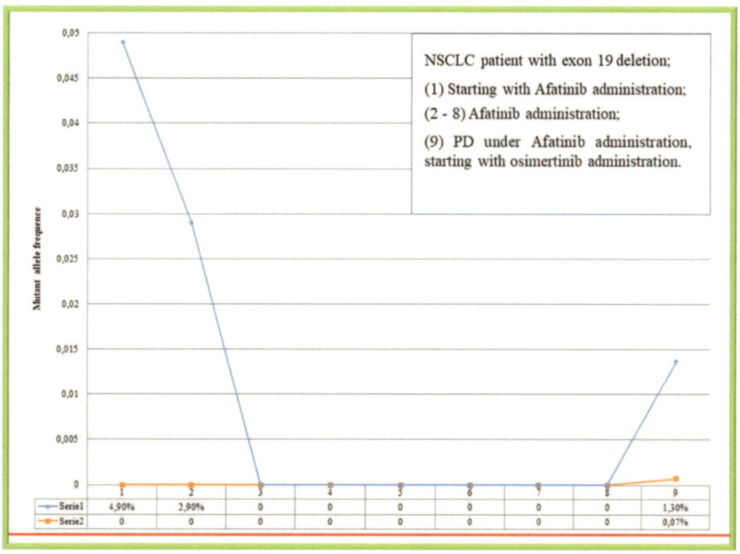

Figure 3.
Molecular follow up of a NSCLC patient. The figure shows the behavior of inspected molecular alterations [exon 19 deletion (blue line) and p.T790M point mutation (red line)] analyzed by serial liquid biopsy specimens in relation to the clinical outcome of a NSCLC patient.

receptor-1 (PD-1) /PD-1 ligand 1 immune checkpoint inhibitors (IC) in clinical trials indicates their efficacy in immune therapy against cancer.

These immune checkpoint inhibitors have been shown to have an effective therapeutic response, particularly in tumors with high tumor mutation burden (TMB) [72]. If the ctDNA can be used to guide and monitor immune therapy is just beginning to be evaluated [73].

In several studies, tumor mutation burden (TMB) can be estimated from ctDNA with good concordance with tissue results [74, 75]. Moreover, the identification of a high TMB in the ctDNA correlates closely with the two inhibitors of programmed cell death (PD)1 and its ligand (PD-L1) [74].

In a recent study it was shown that ctDNA TMB it has a closer correlation with metastatic tissue than primary tumor. Furthermore, this concordance is greater in cases with high ctDNA concentrations [76].

Another possible application of ctDNA in immunotherapy is in response monitoring. Has been proven a good correlation between ctDNA modification and clinical response. Some studies show indeed that the amount of cfDNA correlate with the response to immunotherapy and a decrease of cfDNA was an indicator of good response. Moreover, also chromosomal instability, predictive for immunotherapy response canbe evaluated by NGS in cf-DNA [77, 78].

A new interesting area is represented by the evaluation of tumor microenviroment adopting liquid biopsy specimen in the clinical administration of lung cancer patients. Cai et al. compared IC positive outcome and inflammation markers (INFγ, lymphocites ratio CD4/CD8) in relation to the conventional target biomarkers (PD-L1, CTLA4) for the selection of lung cancer patients to IC administration. They showed that a wide range of inflammatory biomarkers may integrate clinical outcome in NSCLC patients clinical administration [79].

Other applications of cfDNA are likely to emerge in the near future, in the field of immuno oncology such as the detection of minimal residual disease for adjuvant immunotherapy, and the identification of resistance mechanisms linked to the onset of new mutations such as the acquired JAK1/2 or B2M mutations [73].

However, in this context it is not yet possible to think of a complete replacement of the liquid tissue biopsy. The tumor biopsy will have more and more value, both in the evaluation of PD-L1 expression on tumor cells and in the analysis of the tumor microenvironment.

And while it is possible to identify resistance mechanisms as acquired mutations in the blood, however, acquired resistance could be linked to dynamic changes in the microenvironment, which cannot be detected by a simple blood draw.

7.5 Liquid biopsy in the management of other tumors

Several pre clinical studies were performed in order to evaluate the role of cfDNA in the management of other tumor patients.

Wang et al. [80] demonstrated that ctDNA may be considered a diagnostic biomarker in head and neck squamous cell carcinoma (HNSCC) patients. 93 saliva and matching blood specimens were collected from HNSCC patients to identify somatic mutations in genes (TP53, PIK3CA, CDKN2A, HRAS, NRAS) that could play a potential clinical role in the management of this patient cohort. Results showed that ctDNA was successfully isolated from 76% and 87% of saliva and plasma samples, respectively. The authors, highlighting a percent detection rate for hot spot mutations of 100% and 76% for saliva and blood specimens respectively, defined how cfDNA extracted from saliva samples may be considered a reliable tool to identify HNSCC malignant lesions in early stage setting. Similarly, Salvi et al. [81] discussed how cfDNA may be adopted in early stage section for prostate cancer patients by elucidating an accuracy of 80% to discriminate cancer patients from benign lesions. In addition, Christensen et al. [82] showed how a digital droplet PCR approach is suitable to identify somatic alterations in urine cell free DNA (Ucf-DNA) by demonstrating how a correlation between Ucf-DNA alteration and tumor stage, size and grade, were statistically significant. In relation to this section, stool DNA also represents a promising diagnostic tool to early detect colorectal carcinoma patients in the early stage. According to this point, Imperiale et al. [83] showed that the sensitivity of novel technical approach DNA-based were characterized by higher analytical performance in the analysis of both CRC (92.3%) and advanced precancerous lesions (42.4%) respect the conventional screening test commercially available.

8. Conclusion

Is tissue still the issue?

One of the key questions facing oncologists today is whether ctDNA can replace biopsy or ribiopsy in clinical practice.

Liquid biopsy resulted improvements in the management of patients with NSCLC, offering an alternative to standard procedures in cases where tissue biopsy samples are insufficient or not feasible and providing a quick and dynamic assessment of emerging resistance mechanisms that can be used for guide treatment decisions so has been suggested to be included in clincal practice. However the fields of investigation using liquid biopsy are still restricted in routine practice. To date, FDA has approved the analysis EGFR gene assessment that is currently based on standardized and international practices recommendations and authorizes the administration of TKI. Recently, a document of the IASLC, stated that an EGFR, ALK, ROS1 or BRAF positive result of an NGS liquid biopsy analisys should be considered adequate for initiating first-line therapy in advanced NSCLC.

Although we can firmly state that liquid biopsy is a great help in NSCLC patient managing, however, in our opinion, for now it cannot replace tissue biopsy, which will remain the gold standard. Especially in the context of diagnosis where the definition of the tumor subtype can only be clarified through a cytomorphological analysis and immunohistochemical criteria. Furthermore, even the exact stage of cancer can only be obtained with tissue sampling. Moreover, in the setting of detect EGFR-sensitizing alterations in peripheral blood a negative plasma test it should be considered non-informative and will always need tissue confirmation.

Moreover, results of clinical studies have highlighted the existence of significant critical issues in the execution of a mutational test on liquid biopsy, either in the pre-analytical phase both in the analytical phase. Standardization of the various stages of the process is fundamental. It is certainly important that the analysis be performed in laboratories highly specialized, who already have experience in using highly sensitive molecular techniques in order to avoid false positives or false negatives results.

As indicated, there are numerous methods of studying circulating nucleic acids. In view of the large number of actionable targets in NSCLC, guidelines support the position that broad-based testing by NGS. The NGS technique requires workflow complex and use of multigene panels also requires the use of sophisticated software and, sometimes, the help of bioinformatics.

So it is therefore evident that the choice between the different technologies must hold account of their sustainability and the clinical use required in the context in which you operate.

In conclusion we think that ctDNA can play complementary roles in the management of patient NSCLC and act as a prognostic or predictive biomarker as a part of a thorough clinical evaluations to assess the disease, that include comparative sequence analyses of plasma DNA, and biopsies in combination with imaging studies and detailed functional studies.

Conflict of interest

The authors declare no conflict of interest.

Author details

Stefania Scarpino[1*†] and Umberto Malapelle[2†]

1 Pathology Unit, Department of Clinical and Molecular Medicine, Sapienza University, Sant'Andrea Hospital, Rome, Italy

2 Department of Public Health, University Federico II of Naples, Italy

*Address all correspondence to: stefania.scarpino@uniroma1.it

† Both authors contributed equally to this manuscript.

References

[1] Goossens N, Nakagawa S, Sun X, Hoshida Y. Cancer biomarker discovery and validation. Transl Cancer Res. 2015;4(3):256-269. doi: 10.3978/j.issn.2218-676X.2015.06.04.

[2] Gerber DE, Gandhi L, Costa DB. Management and future directions in non-small cell lung cancer with known activating mutations. Am SocClinOncolEduc Book. 2014;353-365. doi: 10.14694/EdBook_AM.

[3] Saito S, Espinoza-Mercado F, Liu H, Sata N, Cui H, Soukiasian HJ. Current status of research and treatment for non-small cell lung cancer in never-smoking females. Cancer BiolTher. 2017;18(6):359-68. doi: 10.1080/15384047.2017.1323580.

[4] Bellevicine C, Malapelle U, Vigliar E, Pisapia P, Vita G, Troncone G. How to prepare cytological samples for molecular testing. J ClinPathol. 2017;70:819-826. doi: 10.1136/jclinpath-2017-204561.

[5] Malapelle U, Bellevicine C, De Luca C, Salatiello M, De Stefano A, Rocco D et al EGFR mutations detected on cytology samples by a centralized laboratory reliably predict response to gefitinib in non-small cell lung carcinoma patients. CancerCytopathol. 2013;121:552-60. doi: 10.1002/cncy.21322.

[6] Ofiara LM, Navasakulpong A, Ezer N, Gonzalez AV. The importance of a satisfactory biopsy for the diagnosis of lung cancer in the era of personalized treatment. CurrOncol. 2012 Jun;19(Suppl 1):S16-23. doi: 10.3747/co.19.1062.

[7] Rolfo C, Mack PC, Scagliotti GV, Baas P, Barlesi F, Bivona TG et al Liquid Biopsy for Advanced Non-Small Cell Lung Cancer (NSCLC): A Statement Paper from the IASLC. J ThoracOncol. 2018;13:1248-1268. doi: 10.1016/j.jtho.2018.05.030.

[8] Reckamp KL, Melnikova VO, Karlovich C, Sequist LV, Camidge DR , Wakelee H et al. A highly sensitive and quantitative test platform for detection ofNSCLC EGFR mutations in urine and plasma. J ThoracOncol. 2016; 11: 1690-1700. doi: 10.1016/j.jtho.2016.05.035.

[9] Kimura H, Fujiwara Y, Sone T, Kunitoh H, Tamura T, Kasahara K et al. EGFR mutation status in tumour-derived DNA from pleural effusion fluidis a practical basis for predicting the response to gefitinib. Br J Cancer 2006; 95: 1390-1395.

[10] Siravegna G, Marsoni S, Siena S, Bardelli A. Integrating liquid biopsies into the management of cancer. Nat Rev ClinOncol. 2017;14:531-548. doi: 10.1038/nrclinonc.2017.14.

[11] C. Bettegowda M, Sausen RJ, Leary I, Kinde Y, Wang N, Agrawal B et al. Detection of Circulating Tumor DNA in Early- and Late-Stage Human Malignancies SciTransl Med 2014; 6 (224): 224ra24. doi: 10.1126 / scitranslmed.3007094.

[12] Diehl F, Schmidt K, Choti MA, Romans K, Goodman S, Li M et al. 2008. Circulating mutant DNA to assess tumor dynamics. Nat.Med. 14:985-90doi: 10.1038 / nm.1789

[13] Mouliere F, Chandrananda D, Piskorz AM, Moore EK, Morris, Ahlborn LB et al. Enhanced detection of circulating tumor DNA by fragment size analysis. SciTransl Med 2018;10 (466): eaat4921. doi: 10.1126/scitranslmed.aat4921.

[14] Abbosh C, Birkbak NJ, Wilson GA, Hanjani MJ, Constantin T, Salari R et al. Phylogenetic ctDNA analysis

depicts early-stage lung cancer evolution Nature. 2017; 545 (7655): 446-451. doi: 10.1038/nature22364.

[15] Crowley E, Di Nicolantonio F, Loupakis F, Bardelli Liquid biopsy: monitoring cancer-genetics in the blood. Nat Rev ClinOncol. 2013; 10 (8): 472-84. doi: 10.1038/nrclinonc.2013.110.

[16] Jahr S, Hentze H, Englisch S, Hardt S, Fackelmayer FO, Hesch RD, R Knippers DNA fragments in the blood plasma of cancer patients: quantitations and evidence for their origin from apoptotic and necrotic cells. Cancer Res 2001; 61: 1659-1665

[17] Zill OA, Greene C, Sebisanovic D, Siew LM, Leng J, Leng J et al. Cell-free DNA next- generation sequencing in pancreatobiliary carcinomas. Cancer Discov. 2015; 5:1040-48 DOI: 10.1158/2159-8290.CD-15-0274

[18] Chouaid C, Dujon C, Do P, Monnet I, Madroszyk A, Caer HL et al. Feasibility and clinical impact of re-biopsy in advanced non small-cell lung cancer: a prospective multicenter study in a real-world setting (GFPC study 12-01). Lung Cancer (Amsterdam,Netherlands). 2014;86(2):170-3.doi: 10.1016/j.lungcan.2014.08.016.

[19] Valdes, M, Nicholas, G, Goss, G, Wheatley-Price P Chemotherapy in recurrent advanced non-small-cell lung cancer after adjuvant chemotherapy. CurrOncol. 2016;23(6):386-90.doi.org/10.3747/co.23.3191

[20] Sirohi, Matakidou A, Ashley S, Popat S, Saka W, Priestet K et al. Early response to platinum-based first-line chemotherapy in non-small cell lung cancer may predict survival. J Thoracic Oncol. 2007;2(8):735-40. doi.org/10.1097/JTO.0b013e31811f3a7d

[21] Cai W, Lin D, Wu C, Li X, Zhao C, Zheng L et al. Intratumoral heterogeneity of ALK-rearranged and ALK/EGFR coaltered lung adenocarcinoma.J ClinOncol. 2015;33(32):3701-9. doi:10.1200/JCO.2014.58.8293.

[22] Jamal-Hanjani M, Wilson GA, McGranahan N, Birkbak NJ, Watkins TBK, MCIT et al. Tracking the evolution of non-small-cell lung cancer. Cancer. 2017;376: 2109-2121 DOI: 10.1056/NEJ Moa1616288

[23] Sacher AG, Paweletz C, Dahlberg SE, Alden RS, O'Connell A, Feeney N et al. Prospective validation of rapid plasma genotyping for the detectionof EGFR and KRAS mutations in advanced lung cancer. JAMA Oncol. 2016;2 (8): 1014-22. doi: 10.1001 / jamaoncol.2016.0173

[24] Malapelle U, Pisapia P, Rocco D, Smeraglio R, di Spirito M, Bellevicine C et al. Next generation sequencing techniques in liquid biopsy: focus on non-small cell lung cancer patients. Transl Lung Cancer Res. 2016;5:505-510. doi: 10.21037/tlcr.2016.10.08.

[25] Lee TH, Montalvo L, Chrebtow V, Busch MP. Quantitation of genomic DNA in plasma and serum samples: higher concentrations of genomic DNA found in serum than in plasma. *Transfusion*. 2001;41(2):276-82. doi: 10.1046 / j.1537-2995.2001.41020276.x.

[26] Jung M, Klotzek S, Lewandowski M, Fleischhacker M, Jung K. Changes in concentration of DNA in serum and plasma during storage of blood samples. *Clin Chem*. 2003;49(6 Pt 1)1028-9. doi: 10.1373/49.6.1028.

[27] Norton SE, Lechner JM, Williams T, Fernando MR. A stabilizing reagent prevents cell-free DNA contamination by cellular DNA in plasma during blood sample storage and shipping as determined by digital PCR. ClinBiochem. 2013;46:1561-1565.

[28] Beretta G, Capoluongo E, Danesi R, Del Re M, Fassan M, Giuffrè G et al. Raccomandazioni 2020 per l'esecuzione di Test Molecolari su Biopsia Liquida in OncologiaAIOM - SIF - SIAPEC-IAP - SIBioC2020

[29] Thressa KS, Brantb R, Carrc TH, Deardend S, Jenkinse S , Brownd H, et al EGFR mutation detection in ctDNA from NSCLC patient plasma: Across-platform comparison of leading technologies to support the clinical development of AZD9291Lung Cancer 90 (3): 509-15. doi: 10.1016 / j.lungcan.2015.10.004.

[30] Rothberg JM, Hinz W, Rearick TM, Schultz J, Mileski W et al. An integrated semiconductor device enabling non-optical genome sequencing. Nature. 2011;475:348-52. doi: 10.1038/ nature10242

[31] Vendrell JA, Mau-Them FT, Béganton B, Godreuil S, Coopman P, Solassol J. Circulating Cell Free Tumor DNA Detection as a Routine Tool forLung Cancer Patient Management. Int J Mol Sci. 2017;18:264. doi: 10.3390/ ijms18020264.

[32] Roy S, LaFramboise WA, Nikiforov YE, Nikiforova MN, Routbort MJ, Pfeifer J et al. Next-Generation Sequencing Informatics: Challenges and Strategies for Implementation in a Clinical Environment. Arch Pathol Lab Med. 2016;140:958-75. doi: 10.5858/ arpa.2015-0507-RA.

[33] Paweletz CP, Sacher AG, Raymond CK, Alden RS, O'Connell A, Mach SL et al. Bias-Corrected Targeted Next-Generation Sequencing for Rapid, Multiplexed Detection of Actionable Alterations in Cell-Free DNA from Advanced Lung Cancer Patients. Clin Cancer Res. 2016;22:915-22. doi: 10.1158/1078-0432.CCR-15-1627-T.

[34] Pisapia P, Pepe F, Smeraglio R, Russo M, Rocco D, Sgariglia R et al. Cell free DNA analysis by SiRe® next generation sequencing panel in non small cell lung cancer patients: focus on basal setting. J Thorac Dis. 2017;9(Suppl 13):S1383-S1390. doi: 10.21037/ jtd.2017.06.97.

[35] Nacchio M, Sgariglia R, Gristina V, Pisapia P, Pepe F, De Luca C et al. KRAS mutations testing in non-small cell lung cancer: the role of Liquid biopsy in the basal setting. J Thorac Dis. 2020;12:3836-3843. doi: 10.21037/ jtd.2020.01.19.

[36] Pereira AAL, Morelli MP, Overman M, Kee B, Fogelman D, Vilar E et al. Clinical utility of circulating cell-free DNA in advanced colorectalcancer. PloSONE. 2017;12. doi.org/10.1371/ journal.pone.0183949

[37] Mohan S, Heitzer E, Ulz P, Lafer I, Lax S, Auer M et al. Changes in colorectal carcinoma genomes under anti-EGFR therapy identified by whole-genome plasma DNA sequencing. PLoS Genet 2014;10:doi: 10.1371 / journal. pgen.1004271.

[38] Pisanic TR, Athamanolap P, Poh W, Chen C, Hulbert A, Brock MV et al. THDREAMing: A simpleand ultrasensitive method for assessing intratumor epigenetic heterogeneity directly from liquid biopsies. NucleicAcids Res43: e154, 2015.e154. doi: 10.1093/nar/gkv795.

[39] D'Agata R, Breveglieri G, Zanoli LM, Borgatti M, Spoto G, Gambari R. Direct detection of point mutations in non amplified human genomic DNA. Anal Chem2011;83: 8711-8717, doi: 10.1021 / ac2021932

[40] Guo Q, Yang X, Wang K, Tan W, Li W, Tang H et al. Sensitive fluorescence detection of nucleic acids based on isothermal circular strand-displacement polymerization reaction. Nucleic Acids Res 2009:37: e20, doi:10.1093/nar/gkn1024

[41] Kloten V, Rüchel N, Brüchle NO, Gasthaus J, Freudenmacher N, Steib F *et al*: Liquid biopsy in colon cancer: Comparison of different circulating DNA extraction systems following absolute quantification of KRAS mutations using Intplex allele-specific PCR.Oncotarget 2017.8: 86253-86263, doi:10.18632/oncotarget.21134.

[42] Qiu M, Wang J, Xu Y, Ding X, Li M, Fet J al. Circulating tumor DNA is effective for the detection of EGFR mutation in non-small cell lung cancer: a meta-analysis. Cancer Epidemiol Biomarkers Prev. 2015;24(1):206-212. doi: 10.1158/1055-9965.EPI-14-0895.

[43] Rosell R, Moran T, Queralt C, Porta R, Cardenal F, Camps Cet al. Screening for epidermal growth factor receptor mutations in lung cancer. N Engl J Med 2009; 361: 958-967. doi: 10.1056 / NEJMoa0904554

[44] Hofman, P. ALK status assessment with liquid biopsies of lung cancer patients. Cancers (Basel) 2017; 9 (8): 106. doi: 10.3390/cancers9080106.

[45] Vendrell, J., Taviaux, S, Béganton B, Godreuil S, Audran, P, Det G et al. Detection of known and novel ALK fusion transcripts in lung cancer patients using next-generation sequencing approaches. Sci. Rep. 2017, 7, 12510. doi: 10.1038 / s41598-017-12679-8.

[46] Wu Z, Yang Z, Li CS, Zhao W, Liang ZX, Dai Y et al. Differences in the genomic profiles of cell-free DNA between plasma, sputum, urine, and tumor tissue in advanced NSCLC. Cancer Med. 2019;8(3):910-9. doi: 10.1002 / cam4.1935

[47] Tuo L, Sha S, Huayu Z, Du K*P16INK4a* gene promoter methylation as a biomarker for the diagnosis of non-small cell lung cancer: an updated meta-analysis. Thorac Cancer. 2018;9(8):1032-40. doi.org/10.1111/1759-7714.12783

[48] Huang Z, Huang D, Ni S, Peng Z, Sheng W, Du X: Plasma microRNAs are promising novel biomarkers for early detection of colorectal cancer. Int J Cancer 2010:127: 118-126. doi:org/10.1002/ijc.25007

[49] Lin CC, Huang WL, Wei F, Su WC, Wong DT: Emerging platforms using liquid biopsy to detect EGFR mutations in lung cancer. Expert Rev MolDiagn 2015:15:1427-1440, doi:10.1586/14737159.2015.1094379.

[50] Garraway LA, Janne PA. Circumventing cancer drug resistance in the era of personalized medicine 2012; 2 (3): 214-26. doi: 10.1158 / 2159-8290. CD-12-0012.

[51] Turke AB, Zejnullahu K, Wu YL, Song Y, Dias-Santagata D, Lifshits E et al. Preexistence and clonal selection of MET amplification in EGFR mutant NSCLC. Cancer Cell 2010; 17 (1): 77-88. doi: 10.1016/j.ccr.2009.11.022.

[52] Goyal L, Saha SK, Liu LY, Siravegna G, Leshchiner I, Get AG et al. Polyclonal secondary FGFR2 mutations drive acquired resistance to FGFR inhibition in patients with FGFR2 fusion-positive cholangiocarcinoma. Cancer Discov. 7:252-63Journal of Thoracic Oncology 2017; 7 (3): 252-263. doi: 10.1158/2159-8290.CD-16-1000.

[53] Russo M, Siravegna G, Blaszkowsky LS, Corti G, Crisafulli G, Ahronian LG et al. Tumor heterogeneity and lesion specific response to targeted therapy in colorectal cancer. Cancer Discov. 2016;6:147-53. doi: 10.1158/2159-8290.CD-15-1283

[54] Van Dessel LF, Beije N, Helmijr JC, Vitale SR, Kraan J, Look MP et al. Application of circulating tumor DNA in prospective clinical oncology

trials— standardization of preanalytical conditions. MolOncol. 2017;11:295-304. doi: 10.1002/1878-0261.12037

[55] National Lung Screening Trial Research Team, Aberle DR, Adams AM, et al. Reduced lung-cancer mortality with low-dose computed tomographic screening. N Engl J Med 2011; 365:395-409. doi: 10.1056/NEJMoa1102873

[56] Sozzi G, Conte D, Leon M, Ciricione, R., Roz, L., Ratcliffe et al. Quantification of free circulating DNA as a diagnostic marker in lung cancer. J Clin Oncol 2003;21:3902-8. doi.org/10.1200/JCO.2003.02.006

[57] Sozzi G, Roz L, Conte D, Mariani L, Andriani F, Lo Vullo S et al. Plasma DNA quantification in lung cancer computed tomography screening: five-year results of a prospective study. Am J RespirCrit Care Med 2009;179:69-74. doi: 10.1164/rccm.200807-1068OC.

[58] Paci M, Maramotti S, Bellesia E, Formisano D, Albertazzi L, Ricchetti T et al. Circulating plasma DNA as diagnostic biomarker in non-small cell lung cancer. Lung Cancer 2009;64:92-7. doi: 10.1016/j.lungcan.2008.07.012.

[59] Catarino R, Coelho A, Araújo A, Gomes M, Nogueira A, Lopes C et al. Circulating DNA: diagnostic tool and predictive marker for overall survival of NSCLC patients. PLoS One 2012;7:e38559. doi: 10.1371/journal.pone.0038559

[60] Esteller M, Herman J.G. Cancer as an epigenetic disease: DNA methylation and chromatin alterations in human tumours. J Pathol 2002;196:1-7. doi: 10.1002/path.1024.

[61] Shivapurkar N, Gazdar AF. DNA methylation based biomarkers in non-invasive cancer screening. CurrMol Med 2010;10:123-32. doi:10.2174/156652410790963303

[62] Konecny M, Markus J, Waczulikova I, Dolesova L, Kozlova R, Repiska V et al. The value of SHOX2 methylation test in peripheral blood samples used for the differential diagnosis of lung cancer and other lung disorders. Neoplasma 2016;63:246-53. doi: 10.4149/210_150419N208

[63] Powrózek T, Krawczyk P, Kucharczyk T, Milanowsk J Septin 9 promoter region methylation in free circulating DNA-potential role in noninvasive diagnosis of lung cancer: preliminary report. Med Oncol 2014;31:917. doi:10.1007/s12032-014-0917-4

[64] Ooki A, Maleki Z, Tsay J-CJ, Goparaju C, Brait M, Turaga N et al. A panel of novel detection and prognostic methylated DNA markers in primary non-small cell lung cancer and serum DNA. Clin Cancer Res 2017; 23: 7141-7152. doi: 10.1158/1078-0432.CCR-17-1222.

[65] Santarpia M, Karachaliou N, González-Cao M, Altavilla G, Giovannetti E, Rosell R Feasibility of cell-free circulating tumor DNA testing for lung cancer. Biomark Med 2016;10:417-30. doi: 10.2217/bmm.16.6.

[66] Chaudhuri AA, Chabon JJ, Lovejoy AF, Newman AM, Stehr H, Azad TD et al. Early detection of molecular residual disease in localized lung cancer by circulating tumor DNA profiling. Cancer Disc. 2017;7:1394-1403. doi: 10.1158/2159-8290.CD-17-0716

[67] Kang G, Chen K, Yang F, Chuai S, Zhao H, Zhang K et al. Monitoring of circulating tumor DNA and its aberrant methylation in the surveillance of surgical lung cancer patients: protocol for a prospective observational study. BMC Cancer 2019; 19: 579. doi: 10.1186/s12885-019-5751-9.

[68] Schwaederle M, Husain H, Fanta PT, Piccioni DE, Kesari S, Schwab RB et al. Use of liquid biopsies in clinical oncology: pilot experience in 168 patients. *ClinCancer Res*. 2016;22(22):5497-5505. doi: 10.1158/1078-0432.CCR-16-0318.

[69] Husain H, Melnikova VO, KoscoK, Woodward B, More S, et al. Monitoring daily dynamics of early tumor response to targeted therapy by detecting circulating tumorDNA in urine. *Clin. Cancer Res. 2017*. 23:4716-23. doi: 10.1158/1078-0432.CCR-17-0454

[70] Corcoran RB, Andre T, Atreya CE, Schellens JHM, Yoshino T, Bendell JC et al. Combined BRAF, EGFR, and MEK inhibition in patients with *BRAF*V600E-mutant colorectal cancer. *Cancer Discov*. 2018;8:428-43. doi: 10.1158/2159-8290.CD-17-1226.

[71] Dawson SJ, Tsui DW, Murtaza M, Biggs H, Rueda OM, Chin SF et al. 2013. Analysis of circulating tumor DNA to monitor metastatic breast cancer.*N. Engl. J. Med*. 368:1199-209. doi: 10.1056/NEJMoa1213261.

[72] Chalmers ZR, Connelly CF, Fabrizio D, Gay L, Ali SM, Ennis R et al. Analysis of 100,000 human cancer genomes reveals the landscape of tumor mutational burden. Genome Med. 2017, 9, 34. doi: 10.1186/s13073-017-0424-2.

[73] Cabel L, Proudhon C, Romano E, Girard N, Lantz O, Stern MH et al. Clinical potential of circulating tumour DNA in patients receiving an ticancer immunotherapy. Nat Rev ClinOncol 2018; 15: 639-650. doi: 10.1038/s41571-018-0074-3.

[74] Fabrizio D, Lieber D, Malboeuf C, Silterra J Abstract 5706: a blood-based next-generation sequencing assay to determine tumor mutational burden (bTMB) is associated with benefit to an anti-PD-L1 inhibitor, atezolizumab. Cancer Res 2018; 78: 13 Suppl., 5706-5717. doi: 10.1158/1538-7445.AM2018-5706

[75] Koeppel F, Blanchard S, Jovelet C Whole exome sequencing for determination of tumor mutation load in liquid biopsy from advanced cancer patients. PLoS One 2017; 12: doi:10.1371/journal.pone.0188174

[76] Yang N, Li Y, Liu Z, Qin H, Du D, Caoet X et al. The characteristics of ctDNA reveal the high complexity in matching the corresponding tumor tissues. BMC Cancer 2018; 18: 319.doi: 10.1186/s12885-018-4199-7

[77] Guibert N, Jones G, Beeler JF, Plagnol V, Delaunay M, Casanova A et al. Early prediction of outcomes to PD1 inhibitors in non-small cell lung cancer (NSCLC) using next generation sequencing (NGS) of plasma circulating tumor DNA (ctDNA). J ClinOncol 2018;36:Suppl.15,9078.doi: 10.1200/JCO.2018.36.15

[78] Cabel L, Riva F, Servois V, Livartowski A, Daniel C, Rampanou A et al. Circulating tumor DNA changes for early monitoring of anti-PD1 immunotherapy: a proof-of-concept study. AnnOncol2017; 28: 1996-2001. doi: 10.1093/annonc/mdx212.

[79] Cai LL, Wang J. Liquid biopsy for lung cancer immunotherapy. Oncol Lett. 2019 Jun;17(6):4751-4760. doi: 10.3892/ol.2019.10166.

[80] Wang Y, Springer S, Mulvey CL, Silliman N, Schaefer J, Sausen M et al. Detection of somatic mutations and HPV in the saliva and plasma of patients with head and neck squamous cell carcinomas. Sci Transl Med. 2015 Jun 24; 7(293): 293ra104. doi: 10.1126/scitranslmed.aaa8507

[81] Salvi S, Gurioli G, Martignano F, Foca F, Gunelli R, Cicchetti, G et al. Urine cell-free DNA integrity analysis for early detection of

prostate cancer patients. Dis. Markers 2015, |Article ID 574120 doi.org/10.1155/2015/574120574120.

[82] Christensen E, Nordentoft I, Vang S, Birkenkamp-Demtröder K, Jensen JB, Agerbæk M et al. Optimized targeted sequencing of cell-free plasma DNA from bladder Cancer patients. 2018 Sci Rep. Jan 30;8(1):1917. doi: 10.1038/s41598-018-20282-8.

[83] Imperiale TF, Ransohoff DF, Itzkowitz SH, Turnbull BA, Ross ME, Colorectal Cancer Study Group. Fecal DNA versus fecal occult blood for colorectal-cancer screening in an average-risk population. N. Engl. J. Med. 2004;351(26):2704-2714 DOI: 10.1056/NEJMoa033403

Chapter 8

Diagnosis of Non-Small Cell Lung Cancer via Liquid Biopsy Highlighting a *Fluorescence-in-situ-Hybridization* Circulating Tumor Cell Approach

Xin Ye, Xiao Zheng Yang, Roberta Carbone, Iris Barshack and Ruth L. Katz

Abstract

Lung cancer (LC), is the most common and lethal cancer worldwide. It affects both sexes and in its early stages is clinically silent, until it reaches a more advanced stage, when it becomes highly incurable. In order to improve the high mortality associated with LC there has been an urgent need for screening high risk patients by low dose CT scan (LDCT) for the early detection of small resectable malignant tumors. However, while highly sensitive to detect small lung nodules, LDCT is non-specific, resulting in a compelling need for a complementary diagnostic tool. For example, a non-invasive blood test or liquid biopsy, (LB), could prove quite useful to confirm a diagnosis of malignancy prior to definitive therapy. With the advent of LB becoming increasingly clinically accepted in the diagnosis and management of LC, there has been an explosion of publications highlighting new technologies for the isolation of and detection of circulating tumor cells (CTCs) and cell free tumor DNA (cfDNA). The enormous potential for LB to play an important role in the diagnosis and management of LC to obtain valuable diagnostic information via an approach that may yield equivalent information to a surgical biopsy, regarding the presence of cancer and its molecular landscape is described.

Keywords: Circulating Tumor Cells (CTCs), Cell Free Tumor DNA (ctDNA), *Fluorescence in situ hybridization (FISH)*, Multiplex FISH, Cytogenetically Abnormal Cells (CACs), Liquid biopsy (LB), Lung Cancer (LC), Low Dose CT Scan (LDCT), Artificial intelligence (AI), PD-L1, *ALK*

1. Introduction

Until recently, the clinical application of CTCs had been largely confined to an FDA approved test, CellSearch®, for testing patients with advanced breast, colorectal and prostate cancer, which relies on immuno-magnetic capture of circulating cells expressing EpCAM. However, this test has not been proved to be optimal for sensitive recovery of CTCs in early stage LC. Currently, in order to make real-time decisions on how to manage LC, there are several new and emerging label-free technologies for detecting CTCs which are more sensitive than the FDA approved test. While each platform differs in the methods that are employed for CTC enrichment and capture, all aim to accurately detect and enumerate CTCs [1]. In this chapter we present an overview of the current applications of LB, including both CTCs and cell free DNA (cfDNA) or circulating tumor DNA (ctDNA) for the detection, diagnosis and treatment of LC from early to advanced stages. We highlight the use of *fluorescence in situ hybridization* (FISH) to detect CTCs, in order to use these as adjunctive biomarkers, in conjunction with indeterminate nodules detected by LDCT scan, as a confirmatory test for early LC.

2. Incidence of lung cancer

Lung cancer (LC) is the leading cause of cancer incidence and mortality globally, with an estimation of 2.09 million new cases and 1.76 million deaths in 2018 [2]. GLOBOCAN Data shows that in industrialized nations, there is no substantial difference in LC deaths in males due to high cigarette consumption rates, but that there is a higher mortality rate in females. In developing countries, LC remains the second highest cancer-related mortality for women, behind breast cancer [3]. The LC incidence rate of women ranks from the highest in Northern America (30.7 per 100,000) and Western Europe (25.7 per 100,000) to the lowest in Western Africa (1.1 per 100,000). Even though women in China have a low prevalence of tobacco use, because of indoor pollution and occupational exposure [2, 4, 5], the incidence of LC in Chinese women also remains high (22.8 per 100,000) [2].

Because early-stage LC cases are asymptomatic, the majority of the patients are diagnosed with advanced disease [6]. The survival rate of stage I LC at 10 years is 92% [7], but the five-year survival rate of advanced LC with distant metastases is only 5% [8]; thus, early detection is critical in reducing lung cancer mortality rate.

3. Screening by LDCT

Lung cancer screening had become a controversial topic since the late 1990s, due to the fact that the risks, effectiveness, and procedures of screening, including the Early Lung Cancer Action Program and screening programs in Japan [9–11], were not verified. In 2002, a randomized trial, the National Lung Cancer Screening Trial (NLST) was initiated in the United States. The primary study goal was to compare the lung-cancer mortality rate between a large cohort of subjects screened for LC by conventional chest radiography versus low-dose computed tomography (LDCT). Follow up data until 2010 indicated that screening with LDCT can significantly reduce the death rate from LC, compared with the radiography group, and that, for the high-risk population [12] the lung cancer mortality rate was reduced by 20% in the LDCT group. The 10-year follow-up result of the Dutch Belgian Randomized Lung Cancer Screening trial (NELSON) that started in 2003 also successfully demonstrated a 26% mortality reduction of the high-risk population in the LDCT screening group, compared with the usual care group without screening [13]. These two studies have become the pivotal studies in LC screening history that have linked the utility of LDCT to reduced LC mortality amongst high-risk populations [14]. A growing list of organizations has established guidelines for LC screening with LDCT based on the evidence showed by the NLST and NELSON [15–17].

However, the benefits of LC screening with LDCT have been diminished by the high false-positive rate, as only 3.6% of the participants with positive LDCT screening results were diagnosed with lung cancer in NLST [12]. The substantial application of LDCT to lung cancer has resulted in a dramatic increase in pulmonary nodule detection in adults at high risk, without a corresponding rise in lung cancer incidence [18]. About 80% of the patients with positive LDCT results are classified as intermediate risk of LC, thus requiring follow-up to rule out malignancy [19]. For patients in this category, most will be required to undergo invasive biopsy to further evaluate the risk of malignancy. Also, more than one-third of these patients will not be diagnosed with LC, subjecting them to potential biopsy-related complications such as pneumothorax and hemorrhage [20]. For patients who are at low-risk, repeated LDCT scans are required, which may be potentially harmful due to frequent radiation exposure [21]. In the case of ground glass nodules [GGNs], which may have an unpredictable clinical course, current diagnostic methods including biopsy and positron emission tomography (PET) are insufficient to differentiate malignant from benign nodules [22, 23]. Consequently, there is an urgent need for a non-invasive diagnostic tool such as a blood test or liquid biopsy (LB) that can evaluate the malignancy of pulmonary nodules in individuals with positive LDCT screening results (**Figure 1a** and **b**) by demonstrating the presence of circulating tumor cells (CTCs) in the blood.

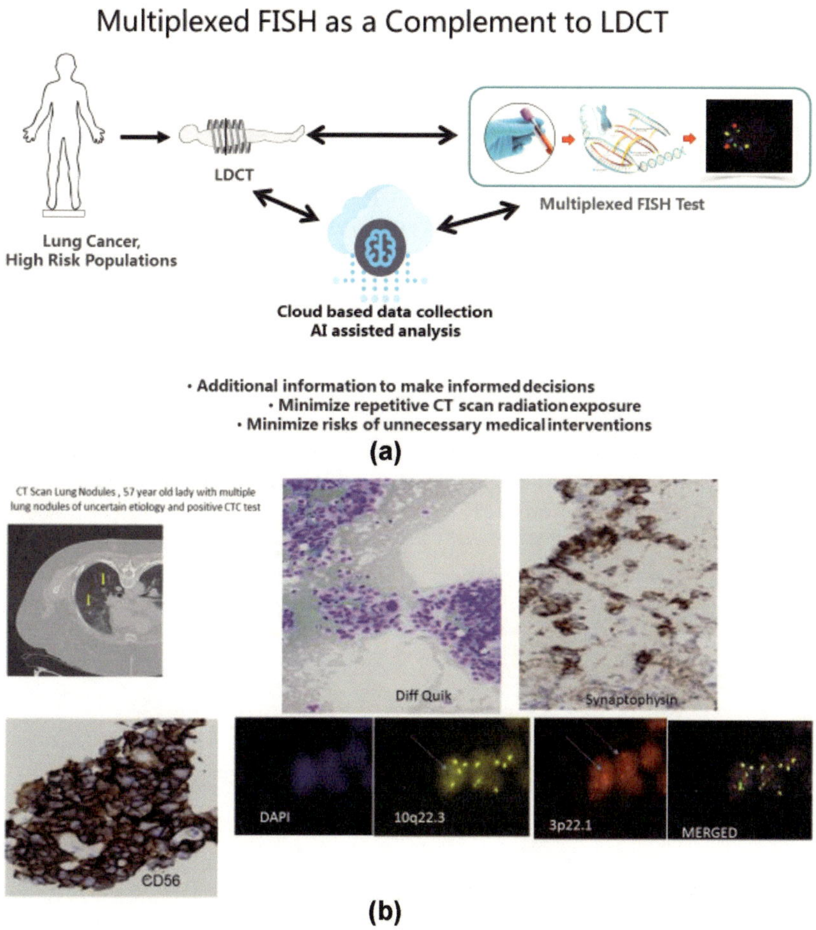

Figure 1.
(a) Schematic diagram demonstrating a hypothetical risk/benefit for lung cancer individual, undergoing LDCT scan with discovery of indeterminate lung nodule and complementary multiplexed FISH test performed on peripheral blood mononuclear cell fraction, to confirm presence of CTCs. (b) Real life example of a 55 year old lady with multiple nodules of uncertain etiology, and a fungal infection such as histoplasmosis was suspected. Multiplex 4 color FISH CTC assay performed on peripheral blood liquid biopsy showed more than 8 CTCs. Figure demonstrates CTCs stained with DAPI, and polysomy for 3p22.1 (three red signals) and polysomy 10q22.3 (3 gold signals) in same cells (merged images). Subsequent fine needle aspiration and cell block showed a well differentiated neuroendocrine tumor (diff Quik), which was positive with synaptophysin and CD56. [24].

4. Components of liquid biopsy

Liquid biopsies (LB) comprise circulating tumor cells (CTCs) from the cellular fraction of blood, and circulating tumor DNA (ctDNA), derived from the plasma fraction of blood (**Figure 2**). ctDNA originates directly from the tumor or CTCs, that are thought to release ctDNA via apoptosis and necrosis from dying cells, or active release from viable tumor cells. Both fractions have been shown to have potential for detecting, monitoring, and treating a variety of different cancers across all stages of disease. The term LB is not just confined to the use of tumor derived material from the blood stream and may also be applied to other biofluids such as urine, saliva, cerebro-spinal fluid, pleural fluid or bile from cancer patients, however for the purpose of this review, LB refers to the blood stream. Use of LB obviates the need for invasive tissue biopsies, which are frequently from inaccessible organ sites, and usually require the use of anesthesia. Complications are not unusual, and may include hemorrhage and infection, while for lung biopsies, pneumothorax is not uncommon. LB is an easy to use approach, as a simple blood draw, requiring only 10 ml of blood, may reveal circulating tumor cells (CTCs), or cancer specific mutations or aberrant methylation patterns [26] in the ctDNA portion of the plasma, that are consistent with malignancy [27, 28].

LB may be used in order to diagnose early LC and can be easily repeated over time to detect relapse of cancer or minimal residual disease (MRD) following surgery, or to monitor a patient's response to various chemo- biological or immune checkpoint therapies. The constant replenishment of CTCs and cell free ctDNA from the primary tumor and/or metastatic sites, enables LB to detect and monitor the development of new clones of CTCs that express different mutations, as compared to an original tissue biopsy or a preceding LB, which may have arisen as a response to a targeted therapy. The rate -limiting factor for the widespread use of LB especially in early-stage LC, has been the scarcity of recovery of CTCs and ctDNA. In addition, due to the wide range of different methodologies for detecting and capturing CTCs, as well as the lack of standardization and clinical validation of different platforms, it is difficult to know which is the optimal platform to choose [1].

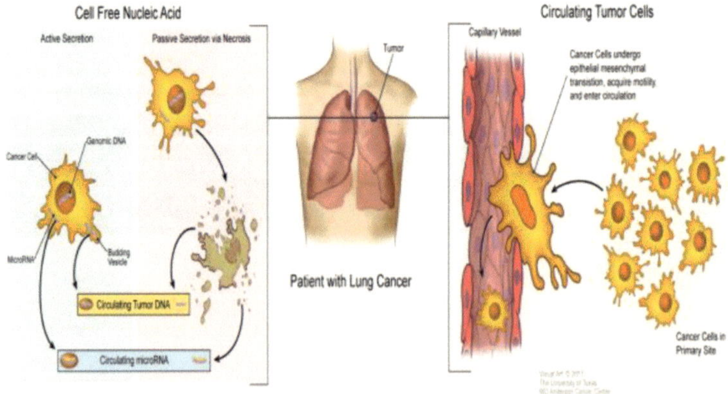

Figure 2.
Mechanism of extravasation of CTCs and circulating tumor DNA from primary lung carcinoma into the blood stream. The left-hand panel shows the source of circulating tumor DNA derived from necrosis and apoptosis of CTCs. The right-hand panel shows the mechanism of extravasation into the blood stream via EMT [25].

5. Scenarios in which LB may be indicated preferentially over tissue biopsy

First, as a complementary test in the face of abnormal images acquired by LDCT screening for lung cancer, where in order to determine the etiology of an indeterminate pulmonary nodule, a simple blood draw demonstrating the unequivocal presence of circulating tumor cells (CTCs) may be useful as a decision-making tool for the further clinical management of the patient. In this situation, tissue biopsy such as fine needle aspiration (FNA), needle biopsy or endoscopic ultra-sound guided biopsy, may be performed, however, occasionally may be both difficult and dangerous to the patient due to the small size and location of the mass and may be non-diagnostic because of the inability to procure representative tissue for pathological assessment. A positive CTC test (**Figure 1**) will lead to the procurement of an excisional surgical biopsy for standard pathological examination with curative intent or in other cases, patients may be candidates for stereotaxic radiation therapy. A negative CTC test will require follow up by LDCT, until the clinicians have determined that the nodule is stable and benign. However, in this scenario the patient will have been spared an invasive procedure for a non-malignant lesion.

Until now, current methods for detection and quantitation of CTCs have been time consuming and complex and require expensive instrumentation as well as a great deal of expertise available only at limited sites. As a result, large scale clinical trials involving thousands of patients at high risk for LC, evaluating the accuracy of screening for CTCs have not been possible. As an example, a large prospective multi-institutional study was performed using filtration of blood samples (ISET) to detect CTCs in COPD patients at high risk to develop lung cancer [29, 30]. Unfortunately, this study failed to confirm the initial promise of accurate early LC detection, due to difficulties in scaling up such technologies at multiple different sites [30]. Therefore, there is an urgent need for the establishment of platforms that can isolate CTCs from patients with early LC that are capable of producing reliable and reproducible results that are comparable amongst different populations.

Second, LB may be used as a minimally invasive, fairly rapid way, to obtain information on actionable mutations in order to deliver targeted therapies, especially in the case of advanced malignancy, where obtaining a tissue biopsy would be difficult. For advanced stage NSCLC, international guidelines have been developed by different pathology, molecular and oncology organizations, including amongst others the International Association for the Study of Lung Cancer (IASLC) and the Association for Molecular Pathology (AMP), the National Comprehensive Cancer Network (NCCN) and ASCO regarding a minimum panel of genes that should be tested to inform treatment decisions [27].

The recent introduction of comprehensive genomic profiling by NGS using ctDNA from LB in patients with advanced stage cancers, including NSCLC, has revolutionized the ability of oncologists to treat actionable mutations in this population in real time and sequentially, without resorting to invasive tissue biopsies, which frequently could not be performed due to lack of tissue or the poor state of health of the patient. Thus, in many cases, the convenience and quick turn-around time of LB may have significantly prolonged the overall survival of patients in this category, who were discovered to have developed actionable mutations following first and second -line therapies with conventional chemotherapy regimens or biological agents [27, 31].

Third, the ultimate aim or “the holy grail” of LB, is to prescreen at risk populations for the development of potentially lethal malignancies such as LC, in order to monitor these patients and institute rapid treatment if necessary.

6. Pathogenesis of CTCs

Cancers develop in epithelial cells as a result of chronic exposure to inflammation or carcinogens, such as tobacco smoke or air pollution. In the lungs, exposed tissues, such as vulnerable epithelial cells in the upper and lower bronchial tracts, may manifest both dysplastic epithelial changes as well as concomitant molecular abnormalities, resulting in a "field -cancerization" effect (**Figure 3**). In these areas, certain cells may undergo unregulated proliferation due to the acquisition of tumor-suppressor genes and oncogenes as well as methylation of tumor suppressor genes. Other factors, including increased glucose uptake, angiogenesis, an altered tumor microenvironment (TME) and a cell's ability to avoid immune surveillance via masking of checkpoint inhibitors such as PD-L1, may allow invasion of these genetically and phenotypically abnormal cells into the blood stream where they present as circulating tumor or CTCs. One of the hallmarks of CTCs is genetic heterogeneity and genomic or chromosomal instability (CIN) [33]. CIN includes microsatellite instability (MSI), chromosome structural variations such as deletions, duplications and translocations, as well as chromosome number. Aneuploidy, due to errors in chromosomal segregation, is a consequence of CIN and is implicated in tumorigenesis as evidenced by the increased rate of malignancies found in patients with global or mosaic aneuploidies. The knowledge that aneuploidy is a *sine qua non* or essential element of a malignant cell forms the basis of certain LB tests that rely on the demonstration of aneuploidy to detect CTCs or CACs (cytogenetically abnormal cells [24, 25, 33, 34]. Genetic mutations arising in CTCs can be characterized by polymerase chain reaction (PCR) or next generation sequencing (NGS) on a single cell basis as well as by *fluorescence–in-situ-hybridization* (FISH) and immunohistochemistry. [23, 25, 35–37].

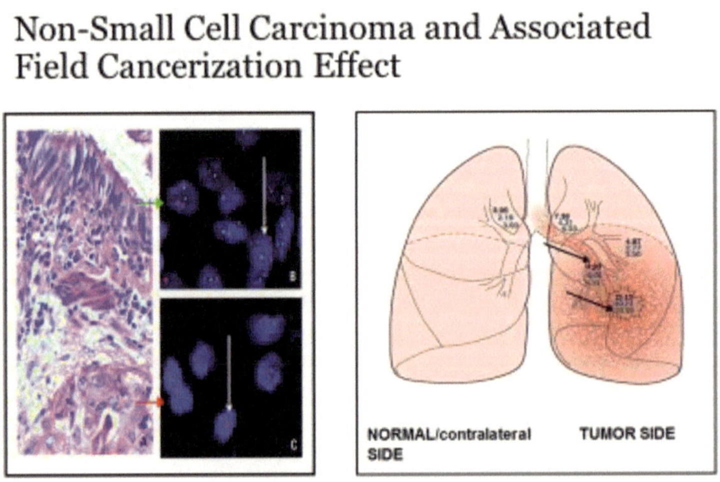

Figure 3.
Left hand panel: A. section of histologically normal ciliated bronchial epithelial cells, overlying adenocarcinoma of bronchial origin. B. Microdissection of bronchial epithelial cells adjacent to NSCLC and hybridized by FISH showed deletion of gene for surfactant protein a (SP-A) in adjacent bronchial epithelial cells, with fewer green signals (SP-A) versus red signals (centromeric 10). C. Tumor cells (white arrow) show 3 signals of centromeric 10 versus 2 signals of 10q22.3 (SP-A) (green) consistent with deletion of 10q22.3 (SP-A). (adapted from Jiang et al. [32]). Right hand panel: Composite diagram of 110 cases of NSCLC demonstrating field cancerization effect of left lung following hybridization of lung sections from tumor, bronchus adjacent to tumor, proximal bronchus on side of tumor, and normal lung on contralateral side for 3 different DNA FISH probes at 3p, and 10q) expressed as percentage deletion. The highest percentages of deletion occur in the main tumor mass, however there is evidence of increased deletion of 3p and 10q throughout the lung parenchyma and in the proximal ipsilateral main bronchus (shaded areas), compared to the contralateral side. (SPORE grant, lung cancer, the University of Texas, M.D. Anderson cancer center).

Before entering the blood stream, CTCs are required to undergo epithelial mesenchymal transition (EMT) in order to traverse the endothelial lining of small blood vessels and capillaries [37]. The CTCs have a much larger diameter than the diameter of a capillary and need to become deformable. This process requires CTC transformation involving micro- RNAs that can interfere with the translation of proteins by messenger RNA and facilitate the adhesion of the CTCs to the endothelium and subsequent migration into the blood stream [38]. The number of CTCs are extremely rare and are estimated at one CTC per $1x10^{-6}$ -10^{-7}. The half- life of CTCs in the blood is very short and estimated to be less than 2.5 hours [39].

7. Circulating tumor DNA (ctDNA) and cell free tumor DNA (cfDNA)

Studies have shown that tumor-specific biomarkers exist in the blood. These biomarkers represent tumor-derived elements from cancer cells undergoing apoptosis and death while traversing the blood stream. These biomarkers include circulating tumor DNA (ctDNA) which are fragments of DNA derived from

Comparison	CTCs	cfDNA
Origin	Intact cells	Necrotic apoptotic cells, exosomes
Definition	Tumor cells derived from primary and metastases	Fragmented DNA in circulation, includes DNA from normal dying cells, ctDNA, cfNucleic acids
Capture and Analysis Methods	Enrichment via gradient density, immunomagnetic or microfluidic based via antigen dependent methods, filtration(ISET), CellSearch detection, FISH for chromosomal abnormalities or translocations and fusions *(ALK,ROS1, MET)*	Enrichment: plasma collection Detection: PCR- or sequencing based, droplet pcr, digital pcr, Next Generation Sequencing (NGS)
Advantages	Extensive downstream analysis (DNA, RNA, protein) Cell culture via capture of viable single cells for *in vitro* or *in vivo* animal studies; NGS sequencing for mutations or copy number variations, FDA approved for prognosis and detection in stage IV breast, Colorectal and prostate cancers, Cell Search™ System. OncoDx iFISH for ARv7 Possibility to monitor expression of checkpoint inhibitors, PD-L1, PD-1 to guide immunotherapy Slide based methods such as for FISH (ref Katz), or IHC (Epic Science) can be archived	Easy to isolate from whole blood Long term storage for subsequent analysis High sensitivity read out Clinically validated for EGFR mutations in NSCLC, comprehensive genomic profiling for additional genetic mutations (Guardant 360, Foundation Medicine for comprehensive genomic profiling and tumor mutation burden (TMB), and microsatellite instability).
Disadvantages	Low cell numbers Labor intensive as both detection and enrichment steps may require highly sensitive and often expensive instrumentation Lack of uniformity of platforms to capture CTCs	Not sensitive enough for detection of early stage cancers Limited downstream analysis (DNA only) regarding cell culture, PDl1 assessment Only feasible in a high tumor burden setting

Modified from [43].

Table 1.
Comparison of circulating tumor cells (CTCs) and cell free DNA (cfDNA).

malignant cells which reside in a background of cell-free DNA (cfDNA). The DNA describes DNA that is freely circulating in the blood stream, but is not necessarily of tumor origin; cell free nucleic acid (cfNAs)includes DNA and RNA derived from cfDNA, cell free RNA (cfRNA),miRNA and exosomes [25]. Circulating tumor DNA fragments (ctDNA) result from activation of nucleases in apoptotic cells and increase in response to rapid cell turnover. The burden of ctDNA is proportional to the total tumor burden throughout the body as well as the metabolic tumor volume as measured by Positron Emission Tomography (PET-CT) [40]. ctDNA is cleared by the kidneys, liver and the spleen [41] and is easier to enrich from whole blood than CTCs, but until recently, before the advent of NGS for LB, its widespread use was limited by the need-to-know which mutations to target by PCR [42]. A comparison of CTCs versus ctDNA is presented in **Table 1**.

8. EGFR mutations detected by LB

In 2016, the U.S. Food and Drug Administration (FDA) approved the first test in LB for ctDNA, the Cobas® test (Roche, USA), which was a companion diagnostic test for the use of targeted therapy, for detecting the presence of common EGFR mutations (exon 19 deletions and the L858R point mutation), which are discovered in up to 16% of Western patients and in 50% of Asian patients with NSCLC [28]. The use of tyrosine kinase inhibitors (TKIs) in NSCLC, such as a first line TKI, like Erlotinib, is guided by the presence of alterations in EGFR with notably better response of patients harboring EGFR exon 19 deletions compared to point mutations in EGFR exon 21, whereas patients who have developed the T790M mutation after receiving first and second generation TKI's will have an improved PFS response to the third-generation EGFR TKI, Osimertinib. [44]. Resistance to TKI's may be intrinsic or acquired, with the latter occurring as an acquisition of an additional genetic mutation to a target therapy such as EGFR or through secondary mutations such as gene amplifications in other genes such as Her2neu or MET, or changes in tumor histology [28]. Thus, one disadvantage of LB compared to tissue biopsy for monitoring advanced disease, is the inability to detect transformation of NSCLC to a small cell lung cancer phenotype, which would necessitate different chemotherapy that would include etoposide and a platinum drug such as carboplatin or even the addition of an immunotherapy drug such as Atezolizumab (Tecentriq) that targets PD-L1 [28].

9. LB for detection of actionable mutations in addition to EGFR

By using a comprehensive multi-genome test panel, as opposed to a single targeted PCR test, a LB test may reveal several different mutations that may be amenable to targeted therapies. Serial blood monitoring may in addition, reveal newer actionable mutations. The use of NGS to look for actionable genes or biomarkers in formalin fixed paraffin embedded tissue sections in cancer patients with advanced disease, has been successfully applied in order to institute targeted therapies, and has resulted in improved clinical outcomes [45]. However, it has been shown that "undergenotyping" or incomplete testing for all guideline recommended biomarkers continues to be a challenge in the treatment of patients with metastatic NSCLC [27].

Studies have also shown that the results of mutational profiles from LB ctDNA in advanced or metastatic NSCLC can be very similar to that obtained in FFPE tissue from primary tumor or metastatic sites [27]. A large prospective study of comprehensive ctDNA genotype analysis (Guardant360®) in patients with metastatic NSCLC compared to standard-of-care physician requested tissue genotyping, demonstrated that guide-line recommended biomarkers were significantly more likely to be discovered using the ctDNA LB test compared to tissue genotyping [27]. There are eight guideline recommendedbiomarkers and include *EGFR* mutations, *ALK* fusions, *ROS* fusions, *BRAF* V600E mutations, *RET* fusions, *MET* amplification and *MET* exon 14 skipping variants, and *ERBB2 (HER2)* mutations. There was >98% concordance for FDA –approved therapy targets (*EGFR, ALK, ROS1*, and *BRAF*) between tissue and cfDNA. In addition, there was a faster mean turnaround time in obtaining results of cfDNA compared to tissue (9 versus 15 days). Significantly, addition of the LB test in addition to tissue genotyping, increased the detection of actionable mutations, including those with negative, or not assessed or insufficient tissue results.

There are differences between the mutational profiles in ever-smoker versus never smokers in NSCLC, as well as differences in demographically different populations. As an example, 93% of 904 never smokers with lung adenocarcinomas in East-Asian populations using surgically resected frozen tumor tissue were shown to harbor an actionable mutation that could be exploited as a therapeutic target as compared to 31.2% of 1770 patients (779 current or former smokers) with NSCLC [46]. In this latter study, comprising 2674 patients, the incidence of METex 14 skipping was 1.3% in NSCLC and 1.9% in non-smokers with adenocarcinoma. By comparison, a NGS LB study of 6,034 Western patients with advanced NSCLC, reported METex14 skipping in 3.6% of all patients, demonstrating that this actionable mutation can be successfully detected by LB, with a genomic profile very similar to the aforementioned data obtained on tissue biopsy [47].

In another NGS study a hybrid-capture based 508-gene panel (Oseq-NT) was used, that included 119 patients with advanced EGFR –TKI-naïve NSCLC and 15 EGFR –TKI-resistant patients. In this study, somatic cfDNA mutations by NGS, were detected in 82.8% of patients. Actionable genetic mutations were detected as 27.7%, predominantly EGFR mutations, including the EGFR T790M mutation as well as BRAF mutations, MET mutation and gene fusions for EML4-ALK and KIF5B-RET [48]. In August 2020, the first NGS companion diagnostic test, the Guardant360® CDx test, that used LB to identify patients with specific types of mutations of EGFR in metastatic NSCLC was granted FDA approved [49]. This test uses a more sensitive and specific digital sequencing method compared to standard NGS assays, in 20 ml of blood, combined with high throughput tumor profiling or large panel genetic sequencing to simultaneously detect mutations in 55 tumor genes.

At the time of this writing, the FDA approval is only valid for targeted therapy in relation to EGFR. If other somatic mutations are detected by this EGFR assay, patients may then be referred to appropriate clinical trials where suitable targeted therapies are being used. There are 73 genes listed on the Guardant Health website for point mutations, indels, amplifications and fusions. These include amongst other genes, *ALK, BRAF, TP53, MET, NOTCH1, EGFR, ERBB2(Her2), CDK6, FGFR1, NTRK.* For a full description the reader is referred to the website (http://www.guardanthealth.com/). A second similar test called Foundation One Liquid CDx®, (Roche, Switzerland), received expanded approval in late October 2020 by the FDA for additional targeted drugs, known as companion diagnostics [50]. This test covers single gene alterations in more than 300 cancer -related genes, as well as multi-gene signatures such as micro-satellite instability and tumor mutational burden (TMB). TMB may be used as a predictive biomarker for delivering immune check point inhibitors and refers to the totality of somatic, and coding base substitutions or mutations, and short insertions or deletions per tumor genome, which may result in high numbers of tumor neo-antigens, and increase the likelihood of immune recognition by the immune system.

10. Clonal hematopoiesis

The development of somatic mutations in DNA as a result of the aging process can affect certain stem cells most commonly in blood and bone marrow, and less frequently in other tissues, such as the skin, colon and esophagus. In the blood, random somatic mutations in genes (*DNMT3A, TET2,* and *ASXL1*) involved in epigenetic regulation may confer relative "fitness" on certain hematopoietic stem cells, which permits unregulated proliferation of a process known as clonal hematopoiesis (CH). This results in clonal expansion of these cells [51, 52]. CH is highly prevalent in the elderly, with between 10 and 20% of individuals over the age of seventy, harboring a clone of appreciable size. Because break- down of peripheral blood cells, including CH, comprises a large component of cfDNA, CH, which may also contain somatic DNA mutations, may be a source of "biological background noise" that can lead to false positive plasma genotyping. This has been reported in patients with advanced EGFR-mutant NSCLC where mutations in *KRAS, JAK2 V617F* and *TP53* were detected and confirmed as derived from CH and not tumor [53]. To overcome the possibility of false-positive genotyping due to CH in patients with NSCLC, paired peripheral blood cell and plasma genotyping may need to be performed, so that inappropriate therapy can be avoided.

11. CfDNA for early detection of cancer

In spite of the spectacular success in applying precision therapy via LB to patients with advanced NSCLC, in early stage LC, the presence of very low amounts of mutated tumor DNA fragments in plasma, makes it difficult to be able to detect actionable genetic mutations in the pool of cell-free DNA (cfDNA). In 2019, the FDA granted break-through Device Designation to Cancer SEEK™, which was developed for early detection of eight common-cancer types, and combines multiplexed PCR detection of over 1000 mutations identified from numerous cancer samples in cfDNA, together with a panel of validated serum protein biomarkers [54, 55] including cancer-antigen 125(CA-125), carcinoembryonic antigen (CEA), cancer antigen 19–9(CA 19–9), prolactin(PRL), hepatocyte growth factor (HGF), osteopontin (OPN), myeloperoxidase (MPO) and tissue inhibitor of metallo-proteinases 1(TIMP-1) The median sensitivity to detect the different types of cancers was 70%, ranging from 98% in ovarian cancers to 33% in breast and lung cancers [54]. While this assay has very high specificity, it has low sensitivity to detect early stage 1 lung and breast cancers. In addition, because the assay is limited in its capacity to determine in which organ the cancer is present, it may be necessary to institute additional expensive screening tests such as LDCT scan, or other endoscopic or ultrasound tests, in order to discover the organ of origin of the cancer [56] which may call into question, the actual clinical value and expense of this screening test.

In recent years, large multi-center prospective clinical screening trials involving thousands of patients using cfDNA have been conducted, such as the Circulating Cell Free Genome Atlas (CCGA) study to determine if genome-wide cfDNA sequencing in conjunction with machine learning can accurately detect and determine the tissue of origin of a large number of cancer types [54] for early cancer screening purposes. An off-shoot of this study, whole genome bisulfite screening (WGBS) has examined methylation patterns of cell-free DNA fragments using a vast targeted methylation panel based on the The Cancer Genome Atlas (TCGA) in a large variety of cancer patients versus non-cancer controls and was able to identify with high specificity, but with lower sensitivity, especially for the less advanced stage cancers, the presence of cancer as well as the tissue of origin (GRAIL) several years in advance of the manifestation of the tumor [55–57]. Studies are in progress employing computational biology and machine learning in prospective studies in large cohorts of healthy individuals for early detection of clinically actionable information from vast amounts of cell free nucleic acids (cfNAs) both DNA and RNA, released into the blood stream through high intensity sequencing. The goal is to discover unique genetic signatures indicative of early cancer.

12. Composition of blood cells and numbers of CTCs

CTCs are extremely rare events in the peripheral blood stream, with actual numbers depending on the platform used to evaluate the numbers of CTCs. For example, using a label-dependent method that relied on immuno-magnetic beads conjugated to an antibody to EpCAM, (CellSearch®) between 2 CTCs/ml of blood for early stage breast cancer, to >5 CTCs/ml of blood, could be detected in patients with advanced stage breast cancer [58, 59]. These rare cells are surrounded by up to several hundred million lymphocytes and neutrophils per ml of blood. On the other hand, using a label-free method to enumerate cytogenetically abnormal cells (CACs) by 2-color FISH, patients with NSCLC of all stages had significantly higher numbers of CACs than did controls. Depending on the DNA probe used, mean numbers of CACs ranged from $7.23 \pm 1.32/\mu l$ for deletions of surfactant protein A gene at 10q22.3 to $45.52 \pm 7.49/\mu l$ for deletions of EIF1B, eukaryotic translation initiation factor, a gene located on 3p22.1 [34]. The numbers of CACs detected for patients with NSCLC were far higher than the CTCs reported in NSCLC for the Cell Search Instrument [34] and could be accounted for by the definition of CACs as a single deletion of a genetic probe compared to the internal control DNA probe, as well as the label-free method of enumeration, in which all CACs irrespective of immunophenotype, and including cancer stem cells, malignant EMT cells and malignant epithelial cells, were counted.

In early stage LC, the vast majority of CACs are CK -/CD45- /EpCAM- and may express EMT or stem cell markers [25] hence the discrepancy between the FISH method and the Cell Search method [34]. In addition to single CTCs, clusters of cells may break off from the primary tumor and travel in clusters through the blood stream. CTC clusters may form "tumor micro-emboli "(TMI) consisting of up to 50 cells (**Figure 7**), that may demonstrate more aggressive properties than single CTCs, as they may be surrounded platelets, lymphocytes, neutrophils [60], similar to the cellular components that comprise the microenvironment seen in tumors, which may be protect TMI from destruction while circulating in the peripheral blood. TMI together with CTCs have also been detected in LB from patients with early breast cancer.

13. Concept of lineage plasticity

For malignant epithelial cells to metastasize, it is postulated that they need to adopt an epithelial to mesenchymal transition (EMT) phenotype and undergo lineage plasticity by changing their genotypic and phenotypic characteristics. During the shift from an epithelial to a mesenchymal state, the adhesion molecules expressed by the cell are modified, allowing it to adopt a migratory and invasive behavior. EMT is induced by specific transcription factors such as Snail, Zeb and Twist, and miRNA's which together with epigenetic and post translational regulators, mediate the process of EMT. EMT is involved in wound healing, embryogenesis and cancer metastases. Most importantly, EMT has been shown to trigger the dissociation of cancer cells from the primary epithelial tumor mass and enable these cells to disseminate as CTCs into the blood stream. In a label- free study of peripheral blood mononuclear cells (PBMCs), it was demonstrated by FISH that there were higher numbers of CACs in patients with lung cancer and breast cancer across all stages than had previously been reported by other methods [25, 59, 61, 62]. This included label-dependent bead-based antibody capture systems for EpCAM, in which captured cells, that are CK+/ CD45- and stain for DAPI are defined as CTCs [58]. Notably, the FISH assay identified far higher numbers of CACs in patients in both early and advanced NSCLC compared to the low numbers of CTCs reported by EpCAM immune-antibody-cell capture methods including the CTC –chip [63]. It was also demonstrated by IHC for stem cell markers (ALDH1), mesenchymal markers (SNAIL) and CK combined with FISH, using a method known as FICTION, [64] that the CACs that were previously identified based solely on genetic abnormalities [34] actually represented diverse cohorts of pluri-potential CTCs including malignant stem cells and cells which had undergone EMT with loss of epithelial markers [25]. Further evidence for lineage plasticity and phenotypic switching was obtained by serial monitoring of blood for CTCs both before, and at several time points after, resection of LC [25]. In early stage LC the vast majority of CACs are negative for epithelial and lymphoid markers (CK-/CD45-), most likely representing EMT cells and stem cells. At later time points or as LC becomes more advanced, more CACs that are CD45+/CK+ or CK+/ CD45- are identified [25]. The not infrequent finding of genetically abnormal circulating cells co-expressing CD45+/CK+, or CK -/CD45- contradicts the classic definition of a CTC as defined by the FDA approved CellSearch® test [58]. This observation may account for the higher sensitivity of an antigen-independent gene-based test. It has also been shown that only a minority of CTCs with stem cell properties are able to survive and initiate metastases [65].

Figures 4 and **5** depict a 43-year-old patient with stage IB, poorly differentiated squamous carcinoma, showed CACs of all lineages(lineage plasticity). a CD45–/ CK+ cell showing 3 red (10q22.3) and 3 green (Cep10) signals. b CD45+/CK– cell with 2 green (Cep10) and 3 red (10q22.3) signals. c CD45–/ALDH1+ stem cell with

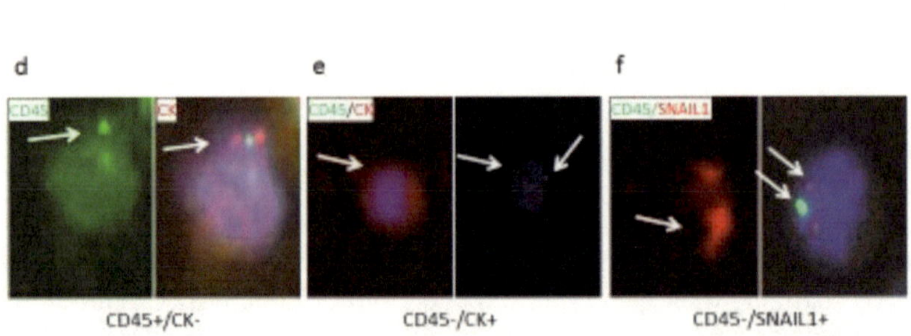

Figure 4.
Demonstrating lineage plasticity in CACs (by combined immunofluorescence and FISH (FICTION)).

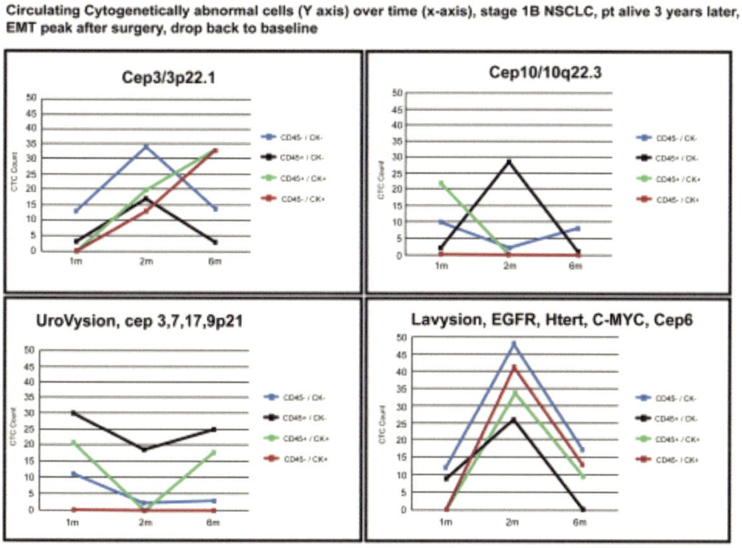

Figure 5.
*Histogram of CACs from the same patient as in **Figure 4**. FICTION method for CD45 and CK, combined with DNA probes for Cep3/3p22.1, Cep10/10q22.3, UroVysion Cep3,7,17, 9p21.3, and LAVysion, EGFR, TERT, C-MYC, and Cep6,showed increase of double-negative CTCs at 2 months in Cep3/3p22.1 abnormal cells and increase of CD45+/CK–CTCs in Cep10/10q22.3 abnormal cells, and increase of all CTC lineages in EGFR, C-MYC, and Cep6 abnormal cells at 2 months, followed by a marked decrease in all CTCs at 6 months [25]. Note that "CAC peaks" as shown in 3/4 of the above diagrams,occurred at two months post surgery, and returned to baseline at 6 months in patients with a good prognosis.*

2 red (10q22.3) and 1 green (Cep10) signal. d CD45+/CK– cell with 2 red (10q22.3) and 1 green (Cep10) signal. e CD45–/CK+ cell with 2 red (10q22.3) and 1 green (Cep10) signal. f EMT cell with 2 red (10q22.3) and 1 green (Cep10) signal. White arrows indicate the location of FISH signals [25]. **Figure 5** is derived from the same patient and demonstrates CACs from baseline before surgery to 6 months following surgery, with a return of CACs to baseline, following a peak in CACs observed at 2 months post surgery (**Figures 4**).

The significance of the EMT phenotype in initiating metastases was demonstrated by studies of CTC derived xenografts (CDX) from patients with advanced NSCLC, which demonstrated a mesenchymal phenotype [28, 66].

14. Methods for isolation of CTCs from blood

Different platforms have been developed to isolate CTCs. These can be divided into affinity, label or antigen dependent methods or affinity- or antigen-independent or label-free methods (**Figure 6**).

Affinity or label dependent devices include the CellSearch® System and the Mag –sweeper, as well as the CTC chip, because all rely on magnetic particles, beads, or posts, coated with antibodies to EpCAM that capture CTCs secondary to the expression of EpCAM on their surface membranes (**Figure 6a,b**).

Label free methods can isolate CTCs based on their physical properties and include:

a. CTC separation via density gradient centrifugation, which enables enrichment of CTCs [67] followed by *fluorescence in situ hybridization* (FISH) to identify cytogenetically abnormal cells (Sanmed Multiplex 4 color FISH test) (**Figure 6e**) [24] or immunocytochemistry for different biomarkers expressed on cancer cells such as Her2neu, estrogen receptors (ER) or cytokeratin's.

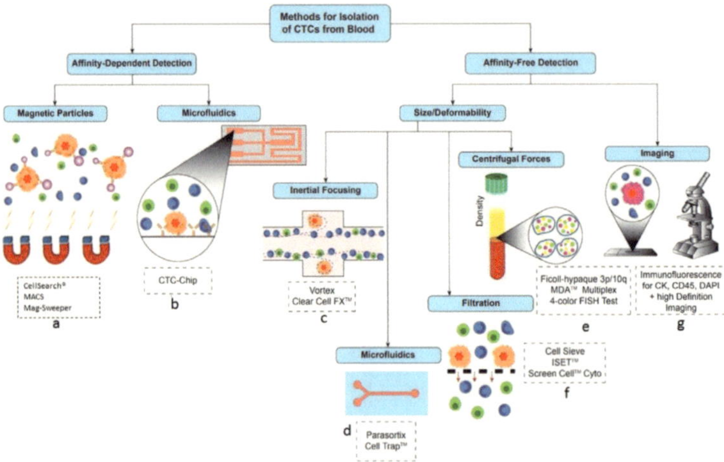

Figure 6.
Diagram depicting methods for isolation and detection of CTCs using either a) affinity –dependent detection devices usually employing magnetic particles, beads or posts coated with EpCAM such as a) CellSearch®, MACS or mag-sweeper or b) CTC chip or B) affinity-free detection devices relying on physical properties of CTCs such as larger size or deformability compared to other blood cells using c) inertial focusing or d) trapping of cells when passed through a Parasortix® filtration cassette or e) enriched on a Ficoll–Hypaque gradient due to specific gravity and centrifugal forces and characterized based on genetic abnormalities by FISH such as the Sanmed™ multiplex 4-color FISH test or f) trapped on filtration membranes that only permit passage of white blood cells with a pore size smaller than CTCs such as cell-sieve, ISET™, screen cell™ Cyto and g) total cell capture coupled with red blood cell lysis and immunocytochemistry or FISH together with high resolution imaging for cell morphology for detection of CTCs, such as the Epic or Tethis SBS platforms.

b. Microfluidic devices that use physical properties of the larger less deformable CTCs that allows inertial focusing to detect CTCs (Vortex Clear Cell FX™) (**Figure 6c**) and include a micro cavity array system that traps CTCs into 10,000 cavities arranged in a 100x100 array with each cavity fabricated to have a diameter of 8–9 μm [68].

c. A microfluidic device that traps cells (Parsortix™ Cell Trap) (**Figure 6d**) [1].

d. Various filtration devices that use membranes or screens with small pores that allow the WBCs to flow through but trap single CTCs and clusters of CTCs based on the larger size of the CTCs on the surface (Cell Sieve, ISET™, Screen Cell™Cyto) (**Figure 6f**) [1].

e. Imaging methods that promote total tumor cells capture by minimal sample manipulation examining all nucleated cells in the blood by immunofluorescence (IF) for different antigens and tumor markers such as CK, ER, AR, Her2, or CD45 or FISH for aneuploidy and high-definition imaging for cell morphology (such as the EPIC™ test or Tethis SBS Platform) (**Figure 6g**) [1, 69, 70].

15. Antigen dependent devices or methods

15.1 Immunomagnetic devices

The CellSearch® (Menarini-Silicon Biosystems, San Diego, CA) method relies on ferrofluid based immunomagnetic separation of EpCAM expression to isolate epithelial cells [58, 59, 71] which are confirmed as CTCs by staining positive for high expression of cytokeratin's CK8, 18 and 19, and absence of expression of CD45, a lymphoid marker. Thereafter the cell, is stained with DAPI (4, 6-diaminidino-2-phenylidole) a nuclear stain. The requirements tor this test are 7.5 ml of whole blood, collected in special CellSave tubes (**Figure 1**). Most CTCs will go through epithelial–mesenchymal transition (EMT) when they extravasate into the bloodstream, resulting in a loss or down regulation of EpCAM expression and are therefore poorly detected by this isolation method [60, 62, 71]. Loss of EpCAM is particularly notable in early stage NSCLC. In spite of the loss of epithelial marker expression in the CTC population, CellSearch® is the only CTC test that was approved in 2004 by the US Food & Drug Administration for clinical use for patients with metastatic breast, colorectal and prostate cancer, as well as prediction of survival in advanced NSCLC [58]. Since then, this test has been used in many studies with reliable and reproducible results [72–74]. CellSearch® has shown prognostic significance in detecting CTCs in most breast cancer subtypes, with a cut-off of ≤2 being a marker for long time survival [75] while ≥5 CTCs was associated with a decrease in 5 year survival. This device in its conventional set up, has drawbacks regarding sensitivity for capturing the whole dynamic range of plasticity that CTCs may demonstrate as it may not detect many cells that have lost or down regulated their EpCAM expression. Thus, numerous studies of solid tumors have reported zero or only 1–2 CTCs that can be recovered by the Cell Search instrument as currently configured [59, 71]. There are also certain solid tumors such as NSCLC, pancreatic cancer and triple –negative breast cancer, where the predominant component of CTCs are of the EMT type and hence, would not be detected by CellSearch® [25, 59].

15.2 Microfluidic chips

Microfluidic chips allow for cells to be captured, immobilized and then washed out, after which they can be subjected to molecular assays. Blood flows through 78,000 micro posts placed at very narrow intervals, forcing cells to move along narrow channels and enhancing their opportunities for contact with posts coated with EpCAM (**Figure 6b**), thus CTCs expressing EpCAM, become immobilized and attach to the walls of the chip resulting in the negative depletion of white blood cells (WBCs) which lack expression of EpCAM. Other chips may use antibodies such as anti-CD45 or anti CD66 for negative depletion resulting in retention of WBCs and elution of CTCs. The advantages of the CTC-chip compared to the CellSearch® instrument is the higher yield of CTC capture (median 50 CTCs per milliliter), as well as on-chip lysis which permits extraction of DNA and RNA for molecular analysis [63].

15.3 Bead based subtraction-enrichment strategies

Positive immunomagnetic bead-based CTC enrichment methods may rely on epithelial antigens such as EpCAM for capture and/or intra-cellular tumor cell antigens such as cytokeratin for detection, however, CTCs undergoing epithelial-mesenchymal transition, may be missed [76–79]. To avoid this failure, negative selection approaches exist for unbiased CTC enrichment [80]. Negative immunomagnetic selection uses a cocktail of antibodies against hematopoietic antigens such as CD2, CD14, CD16, CD19, CD45, CD61, CD66b and Glycophorin A, to enrich for CTCs, by removing contaminating white blood cells and platelets. An example of such an assay is the RosetteSep™ (STEMCELL Technologies). Antibody labeled WBCs can also be removed by AutoMACS Separator (Miltenyi Biotec). A major disadvantage of negative selection approaches is the lower CTC purity as compared to the positive selection approaches; however negative selection approaches show promise for identifying more CTCs for downstream analyses. Both epithelial and mesenchymal cancer cells could be enriched from patient samples [76, 79–82].

15.4 Magsweeper

MagSweeper technology is an automated immunomagnetic cell separator that uses a magnetic arm to collect cells coated with anti-EpCAM antibodies [79]. This EpCAM based isolation method can capture high-purity cells from metastatic cancer patients, but adsorption of background cells to the capturing device or the entrapment within the large magnetic particles used for labeling rare cells in large volume could lead to nonspecific contamination. However, MagSweeper is not commercially available, which might require further analysis to validate the effectiveness of the test [83].

15.5 CellCollector

The CellCollector is a modification of a medical device for use in vivo. It uses a wire with an antibody against EpCAM that is attached to the surface and is inserted through a cannula straight into patients' bloodstream and left exposed to a high volume of blood for 30 minutes to collect CTCs [84]. This device has been used successfully ex vivo to quantitate the number of CTCs in 15ml of blood from patients with prostate cancer [85]. In spite of the complicated in vivo application procedure, Luecke et al. [86] reported that the CellCollector can capture a higher volume of CTCs compared with the CellSearch method (73% vs. 29%) in 62 lung cancer patients. Further studies with larger samples will be required to demonstrate the efficiency of this technology.

16. Antigen independent platforms

16.1 Enrichment free platforms or "No Cell Left Behind"

Following red cell lysis of a whole blood sample, CTCs are captured by analyzing all nucleated cells present so that the final result is fully representative of the entire cell population in the blood sample except for the red blood cells. (Epic Science, San Diego, CA) [69, 87]. This test attempts to identify CTCs defined as: a) CK+/CD45- with abnormal morphology; b) CK - /CD45- with abnormal morphology, which may be cancer stem cells or cells undergoing EMT; c) Apoptotic CTCs, which are the abnormal cells described in a and b, but with nuclear fragmentation and d) CTC clusters, 2 or more individual cells bound together. Cells are stained with a cocktail of cytokeratin, CD45 and DAPI and then analyzed at high resolution by digital pathology methods for numerous nuclear, nucleolar and cytoplasmic features. Machine learning algorithms then quantify CTC subtypes into different categories. Cells of interest are confirmed by a trained operator as to whether they represent CTCs. This platform is also used for nuclear localization of AR-V7 in CTCs from patients with metastatic prostate cancer, which if positive, is indicative of resistance to androgen –targeted therapy, suggesting alternative therapies such as chemotherapy or other therapies [87].

A similar approach has been used for detection of CTCs and in early breast cancer using of IF for estrogen receptors and CK/and or Her2 and morphology in bright field. In combination with proprietary slides to enhance cell retention (Tethis,

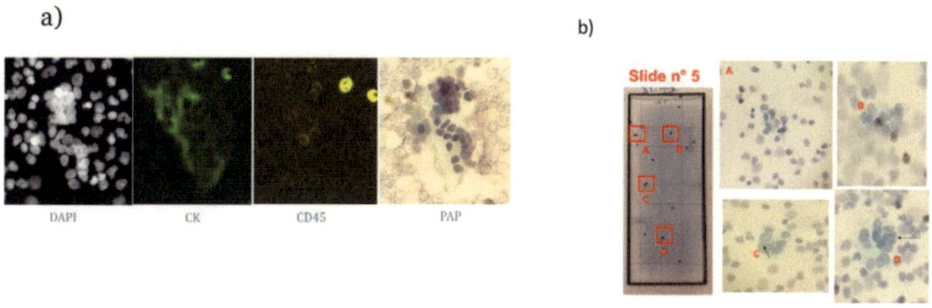

Figure 7.
CTC clusters in early breast cancer (a) 40x magnification of a CTC cluster stained with DAPI, and immunostained with CK and CD45, and stained with Papanicolau; (b) bright field analysis of a whole slide showing different CTC clusters (Papanicolau staining).

Milan, Italy), this method allows gently and quick white blood cell adhesion as a monolayer with no selection, avoiding shear stress or manipulation associated with enrichment methods and thereafter examining the whole repertoire of nucleated cells [69] (**Figure 7**) thus leaving the architecture of CTCs in the peripheral blood intact. This method, which has been automated and standardized in its pre-analytical phase of sample preparation on slides, has shown high sensitivity and specificity in single CTCs and also CTCs cluster detection in a pilot study of early breast cancer [69]: identification of CTC clusters in early breast cancer is a novel finding that will deserve further confirmation in larger clinical trials. The presence of CTC clusters in metastatic settings has been clearly associated with a more aggressive tumor phenotype [70]: identification of such biomarkers in early settings could open new perspectives for the evaluation of their prognostic relevance and consequent therapeutic decision in early breast cancer.

16.2 *Fluorescence-in-situ hybridization* or FISH-based assays

A novel way to look at the genotype of individual cells is to perform interphase FISH (iFISH) using DNA probes that may be localized to locus specific, centromeric or telomeric sites on the chromosomes. iFISH can identify if cells are diploid (normal) or aneuploid (malignant) based on the gains and/or loss of chromosomes. Panels of probes may be custom made and designed specifically to detect certain types of cancers, such as the Sanmed ™ test for LC, in which cDNA subtraction hybridization using DNA extracted from resected NSCLC specimens versus normal lung tissue was used to discover universally deleted genes [88]. The latest automated fluorescence technology using pseudo -confocal microscopy, permits up to 6 different DNA probes to be quantitated simultaneously in a single nucleus using different color fluorescent tags [89] thus allowing an opportunity for up to 6 different genetic markers to be analyzed on a per cell basis (Bioview, Rehovoth, Is.) and creating opportunities to devise novel biomarkers customized to different subtypes of cancers.

To maximize the enumeration of CTCs by FISH, a gradient centrifugation process is used, which causes the neutrophils and RBCs to precipitate at the bottom of the tube, while cells with abundant cytoplasm, such as CTCs, peripheral blood mononuclear cells (PBMCs) including monocytes and lymphocytes, band at the buffy coat due to the effect of specific gravity [24, 25, 67] (**Figure 8**). For chromosomal abnormality enumeration, thousands of purified cells from the buffy coat are subjected to iFISH, with multiple DNA probes labeled with different fluorescent tags [24] in order to identify nuclei containing gains or polysomies, and/or deletions of different targeted genes. These cells are also known as cytogenetically abnormal cells or CACs. Preparations are scanned on an automated fluorescent microscope

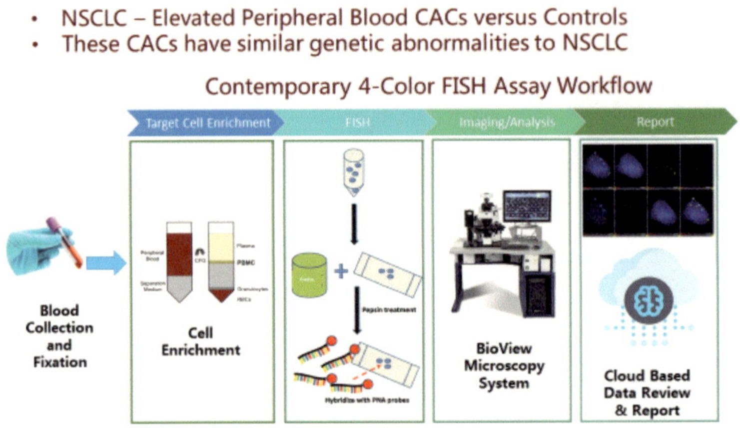

Figure 8.
The workflow of CAC enumeration, from left to right, collection of 10 ml of peripheral blood, enrichment of peripheral blood mononuclear cells, hybridization of FISH probes, fluorescence image acquisition and analysis followed by cloud based data review and report [90].

with multiple filter wheels of different wavelengths to detect different color signals (e.g., Bioview Duet Instrument Rehovoth™, Il). This instrument can be programmed to count cells of a certain size and to exclude cells the size of a lymphocyte or smaller cells. At the end of each scan, a pie chart is produced, according to a predetermined classification of signals. Digitization of cells subjected to FISH, can be performed fairly rapidly, however manual evaluation by a qualified technologist, of genetically abnormal cells, is mandatory, but can be time-consuming. Using strict criteria, only cells with intact nuclei that demonstrate good hybridization signals of all probes are analyzed (**Figure 8**).

In a 4-color FISH test such as the Sanmed™ test, the goal of the analysis is to find unequivocal aneuploid CTCs as defined by polysomy of 2 or > signals of different nucleic acid probes per nucleus. This criterion is the same one that is recommended for a similar 4-color FISH test, the Urovysion™ FISH test (Vysis, Abbott Labs, Chicago, Il) for the diagnosis of urothelial carcinoma in urine specimens in patients to rule out bladder cancer [91]. A threshold for calling a specimen positive or negative is established based on the lowest number of CTCs present in cancer patients with histologically confirmed primary cancers as compared to the highest number of CTCs present in a matched control population. The optimal threshold is the one that most accurately predicts the presence of cancer [24].

Recently, Katz et al. [24] used a 4-color FISH assay to evaluate cytogenetic abnormalities of 3p22.1 and 10q22.3 in 207 patients, including 100 control subjects, who were at risk of developing NSCLC, based on risk factors for LC as well as suspicious LDCT findings, using ≥3 CTCs as a threshold for malignancy, and successfully identified patients at stage I and II NSCLC with a high degree of accuracy (**Figure 9**, **Table 2**).

CTCs were identified as a complete cell with a nucleus larger than a lymphocyte nucleus that contained polysomy of at least 2 of 4 FISH probes per nucleus. Strikingly, the accuracy of this method to detect early-stage LC was significantly higher than other published EpCAM based technologies, most likely due to the high sensitivity of the 4-color probe cocktail that is used to detect cytogenetically abnormal circulating cells and is not dependent on EpCAM expression [24, 71, 95].

An environmental study that employed the 4-color FISH assay showed an 89.47% sensitivity and an 85.00% specificity to detect LC in 89 Chinese bus drivers who had indeterminate lung nodules on LDCT following chronic and consistent exposure to occupational pollutants [92]. Similarly, Liu et al. in a prospective

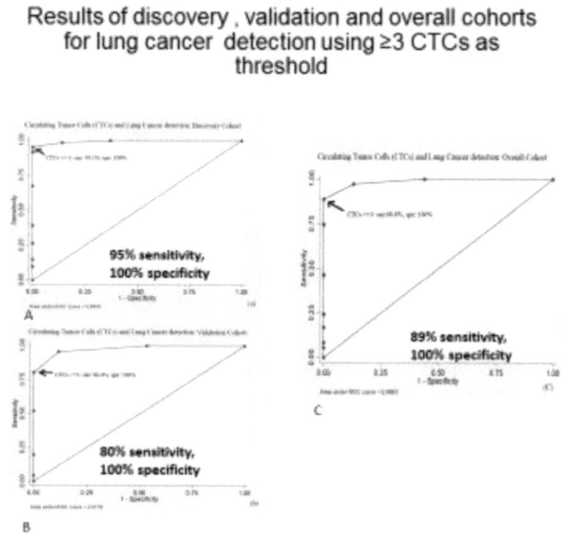

Figure 9.
High degree of sensitivity and specificity demonstrated in 3 separate cohorts comprising patients with predominantly early stage cancer and controls using a threshold of ≥3 CTCs to determine the presence of malignancy, A) discovery cohort, first 118 B) validation cohort, subsequent 89 and C) overall cohort, 207 patients (107 patients and 100 controls) [24].

Population	Type of nodules	Lung cancer stages	Sensitivity	Specificity	References
Chinese Bus Drivers, n = 89	Non-specific	Stage I	89.47%	85%	[92]
Chinese, n = 339	Solid, mGGN and PGGN	StageI	Solid nodules 63.0% mGGN 73.0% pGGN 66.7%	Non-specific	[90]
Chinese, n = 125	5–10 millimeters	StageI	70.4%	86.4%	[93]
Chinese, n = 534	Non-specific	Non-specific	Non-specific	Non-specific	[94]
Americans, n = 207, includes 100 control subjects (white = 72%, African Americans = 8%, Hispanic =1%, Asian = 19%)	Non-specific	Stage I = 55, stage II = 10, stage III = 18, stage IV = 17 Stage not ascertained = 7	88.8%	100%	[24]

Abbreviations: mGGNs, mixed ground glass nodules, pGGNs, mixed ground-glass nodules.

Table 2.
Performance of 4 color FISH test in LDCT detected lung nodules for identification of lung cancer in different populations [24, 90, 92–94].

case–control study involving 339 participants, indicated that the 4 color FISH test yielded 67.2 sensitivity% and 80.8% specificity in stage I NSCLC patients, including those with solid nodules (38.7%), mixed ground-glass nodules (mGGn) (31.9%)

and pure ground-glass nodules (pGGn) (28.4%) [90] detected by LDCT. In addition, in this study the discriminatory capability between CACs and traditional tumor serum biomarkers such as CEA, TPSA, NSE, CA19–9 and CYFRA21-1 was compared to the results of the 4 color FISH assay and showed that the sensitivity of the CAC assay was significantly higher for small nodules and ground glass nodules when compared to the serum biomarkers [90].

In a different study, 125 individuals with newly discovered pulmonary nodules 5–10 millimeters in diameter by LDCT, underwent LB for the 4 color FISH test prior to surgery, followed by histopathological examination of the resected nodules. Here, in spite of the extremely small size of the nodules, the FISH test demonstrated a 70.4% sensitivity and an 86.4% specificity for the diagnosis of LC [93]. The advantages of using this assay were demonstrated in yet another study that collected lung LDCT images of 534 patients with pulmonary nodules and invited experienced physician to score the patients' lung cancer risk and to compare the risk score to that

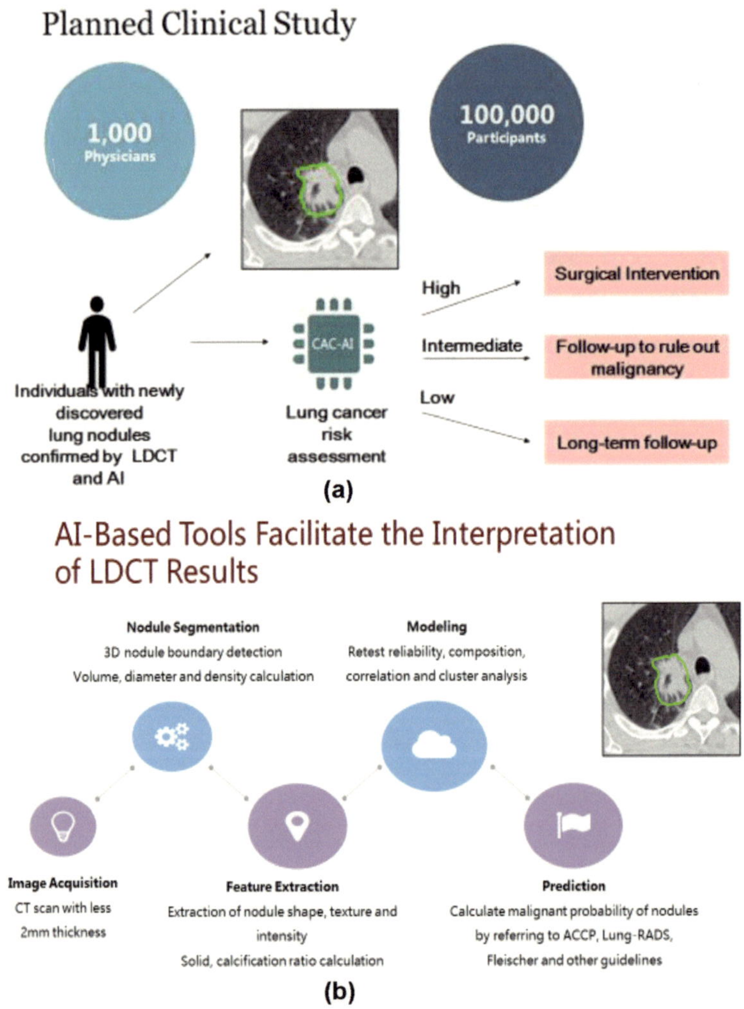

Figure 10.
(a) Overview of proposed clinical study to test robustness of AI assisted LDCT of lung nodules combined with evaluation of Sanmed test by AI in order to evaluate whether a pulmonary nodule is low, intermediate or high risk for cancer, with follow up recommendations. (b) Overview of AI based tools, include nodule segmentation, feature extraction, modeling and prediction based on established radiology guidelines, such as lung-RADS and the Fleischner society, in order to improve and standardize interpretation of lung nodules. Bueno et al. [96].

calculated by Artificial Intelligence with deep learning. In all 11 cases where both physicians and AI incorrectly predicted the lung cancer risk factor, the results of the 4- color FISH test was consistent with the results of the histopathological examinations [94]. When LDCT image analysis is insufficient to make a clinical decision, the 4 -color FISH test may be a valuable complementary tool for individuals with indeterminate LDCT results.

Based on initial studies, it appears that the multiplex–FISH LB assay is robust and has the potential to be scaled up for widespread use. Reproducible results with an acceptable degree of clinical utility were obtained on numerous blood samples from different geographic locations, in which pre-analytical values were kept constant, regarding the volume of blood (10 mL collected in K2EDTA vacuum tubes), as well as methods of fixation and stabilization of blood samples for up to 96 hours at room temperature, before being processed in a centralized certified laboratory according to standard operating procedures. The multiplex- FISH CTC assay is currently being tested in a prospective study comprising large cohorts of at-risk subjects, in combination with computerized scanning of LDCT detected indeterminate lung nodules in order to confirm that the FISH assay, in conjunction with the artificial intelligence (AI) interpretation of the lung nodule may have an important and synergistic role to play in early LC detection (**Figure 10a** and **b**).

16.3 FISH quantitation by artificial intelligence (AI)

A drawback of the different FISH assays has been the length of time taken to manually evaluate and accurately enumerate fluorescent signals due to overlapping cells and/or other technical difficulties such as splitting of signals, resulting in inaccurate counting and overcalling of CTCs and distinguishing CTCs from debris and leukocytes [94, 97]. However, the development of machine learning algorithms in implementing the CTC counting procedure has been able to make the process far more efficient and accurate. Machine learning(ML) algorithms that function in advancing cell image analysis can automatically input layers with a geometric relationship, as well as precisely capture the rows and columns of images; thus ML can rapidly recognize CTCs with extra intra-nuclear structures compared to normal cells, in order to reduce the artificial errors and improve the precision of

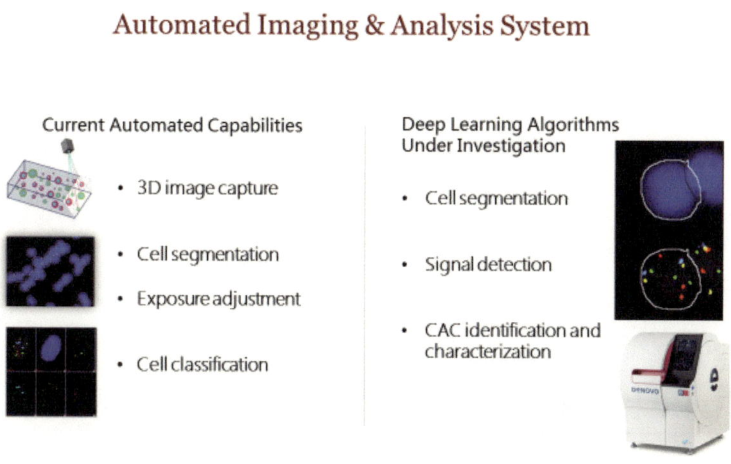

Figure 11.
Diagram of instrumentation (De novo®, BioView, Rehovoth, is) currently in use (left hand panel) for automated imaging comprising 3D image capture, cell segmentation, exposure adjustment and cell classification. Right hand panel depicts deep learning algorithms to improve classification of cells including cell segmentation, signal detection and CAC identification and characterization.

CTC identification [98, 99]. For example, the BioView platform automates image collection and is able to utilize an algorithm for identifying CTCs according to cell size, cell shape, nucleus to cytoplasm ratios, and occurrence of biomarkers identified by target features, and can automatically select CTCS from other cells in peripheral blood in a timely manner and has been widely applied in many FISH based CTC enrichment processes [100, 101] (**Figure 11**). In another AI study involving analysis of the 4-color FISH LB assay, FISH probes were segmented using 3D-Unets, which enabled a significant reduction in false –positive enumeration of polysomies obtained during traditional computer vision microscopy, while retaining all verified CTCs, greatly improving the efficiency of the scoring pathologists and the accuracy of the test [102].

16.4 Filtration methods

16.4.1 Filtration devices

CTCs may be isolated by the size of epithelial cells (ISET) (Rarecells Diagnostics, Paris, France) [103, 104] via a blood filtration approach which enriches 10 ml of peripheral blood collected in buffered EDTA and kept at room temperature. The membrane used is made of polycarbonate and allows cells <8 microns to pass through, while the larger epithelial and mononuclear white blood cells remain on top (**Figure 6f**). Half of the membrane can be used for morphology via a May Grunewald Giemsa stain, and the second half can be used for immunocytochemistry using a pan-cytokeratin antibody and an anti-vimentin antibody applied to the filters. Malignant cells are identified cytologically according to usual characteristic nuclear and cytoplasmic features. Another similar platform is the CellSieve method that uses microfilters and a pressure monitored filtration pump from Creative MicroTech, Inc., Rockville, MD (**Figure 12**). Another filtration device similar to that has enhanced cell recovery for in vivo quantitation of rare CTCs via multiphoton intravital flow cytometry [105]. Successful size- based isolation of CTCs has been described using a microcavity array system that traps CTCs into 10,000 cavities arranged in a 100x100 array with each cavity fabricated to have a diameter of 8–9 μm [68]. This method was shown to be superior to CellSearch in detecting CTCs from patients with NSCLC and small cell lung cancer. Filtration devices have been successfully and

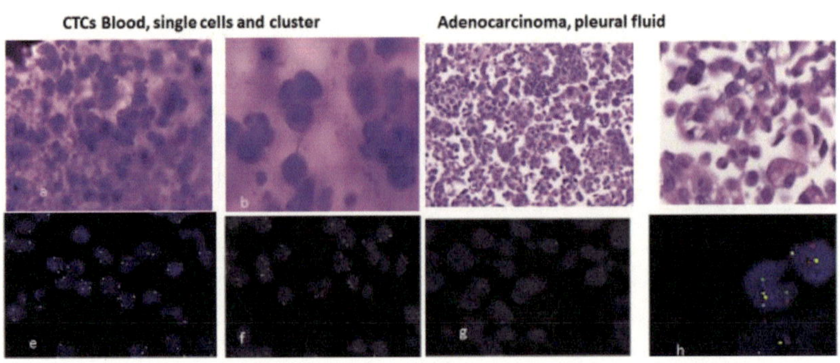

Figure 12.
Filter preparation, screen cell, of CTCs derived from a patient with stage IV adenocarcinoma of lung showing numerous CTCs, both single and in clusters a) diff- Quik 20X b) diff -Quik 40X, c) same patient, clusters of adenocarcinoma, morphologically resembling CTCs, in pleural fluid, hematoxylin and eosin 10X, d) 40X, e) CTCs multiplex 4 color FISH (3, 3p, 10, 10q) demonstrating aneuploidy 400X, f) EML-ALK translocation, CTCs X400, g)pleural fluid X400, h) multiplex 4 color FISH (3, 3p, 10, 10q), pleural fluid X600.

DOI: http://dx.doi.org/10.5772/intechopen.97631

extensively used [103], to detect CTCs, both for screening for lung cancer in high risk COPD patients, as well as in patients with established diagnosis of LC [71]. In a large study of patients with and without COPD, investigators noted that 5/168 patients with COPD or 3%, all of whom had negative spiral CT scans, manifested CTCs one to 4 years before the appearance of indeterminate lung nodules. All nodules proved to be early stage lung cancer on surgical resection [104]. The CTCs were isolated by the ISET filtration method and were stained with both epithelial and mesenchymal markers. In a side-by-side comparison of 40 patients with advanced NSCLC, predominantly stage IV, using the filtration-based size exclusion technology ISET (Rarecell Diagnostics), investigators detected higher numbers of CTCs including epithelial marker- negative cells in 32/40 or 80% of patients as compared to CellSearch where only 9/40 or 23% of patients were found to have CTCs In addition circulating tumor microemboli (CTM) were detected by filtration but were not detectable by CellSearch [71]. Immunohistochemistry stains on cells isolated by ISET showed variable expression of EGFR, CK and Ki67, however EpCAM expression was not detected. Despite the initial promising results of ISET capability for identifying high risk individuals that could develop LC, in a recent multicenter study, CTC detection using ISET was shown not to be suitable for lung cancer screening. In this study, factors limiting the widespread use of ISET for screening for LC, included pre-analytical factors, such as use of different blood collection tubes such as EDTA (ethylenediaminetetra-acetic acid) or Streck BCT (Streck, Omaha Nebraska) tubes, and imprecise standardization of the filtration method, by different operators [30]. It was subsequently concluded that in order to define a robust CTC test, suitable for real world consumption, large multi-center trials with large numbers of patients, using uniform pre-analytical conditions and identical technical analysis is essential [30].

One notable disadvantage of the filtration methods is that there exist subpopulations of CTCs whose size is smaller or in the same size range as WBCs (around 5 microns) and therefore would be eliminated during the filtration process. This feature may contribute to a lower sensitivity of CTC detection compared to other methods for enrichment of CTCs that do not rely on filtration [81].

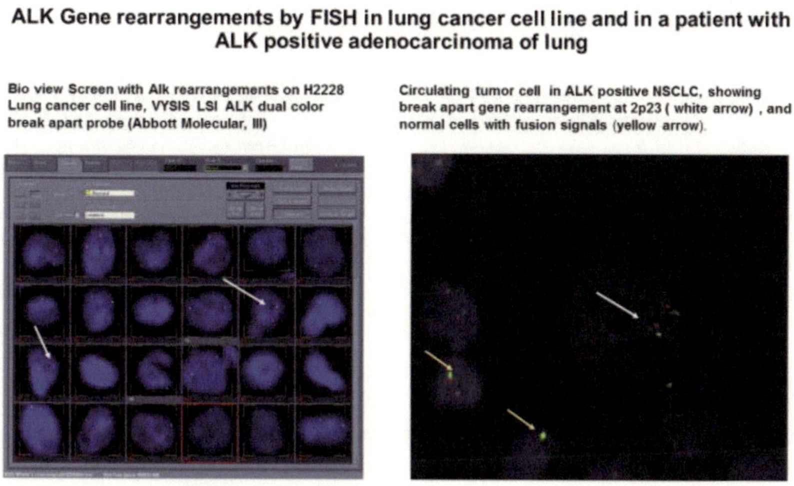

Figure 13.
Left hand panel, showing ALK gene rearrangements (white arrows) in H2228 lung cancer cell line, Vysis ALK break apart FISH probe kit (Abbott, molecular diagnostics, Des Plaines, IL). Right hand panel showing CTCs demonstrating ALK break apart gene rearrangements (white arrow) in CTC and normal cells with fusion signal seen as closely opposed green and red signals (yellow arrows), BioView duet™, scanning system, Rehovot, is.

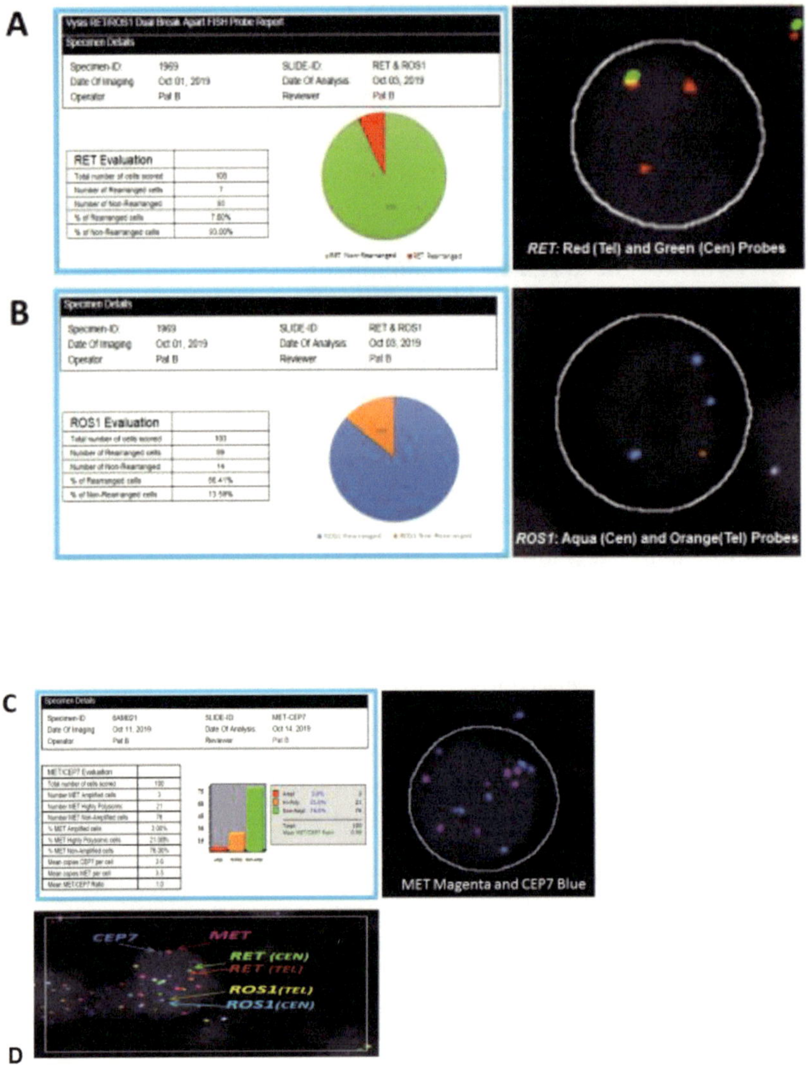

Figure 14.

(A) Multiplex fast FISH assay for detecting ROS1, RET and MET aberrations in FFPE non-small cell lung cancer specimens using Bio View Duet™ scanning system for automated slide imaging and digital analysis of 6-color probe assay. Examples of case reports and representative images of cells positive for RET, ROS1 and MET aberration a) RET break apart probes labeled with Spectrum Green (5′ RET Cen) and Spectrum Red (3′ RET Tel) and captured with corresponding filters. b) ROS1 break apart probes labeled with SpectrumAqua (3' ROS1 Cen) and SpectrumGold (5' ROS1 Tel, pseudocolored in Orange) and captured with appropriate filters rearrangement probe. c) MET gene copy number probe labeled with Alexa 647 (pseudocolored in Magenta) and centromeric probe CEP7 labeled with Alexa 750 (Blue) and captured with appropriate filters. d) Combined image of the multiplex FISH assay with probe mix contained 6 differentially labeled fluorescent probes: 3' ROS1, 5' ROS1, 3' RET, 5' RET, MET and CEP7. (B) Figures supplied courtesy of Dr. Irina Sokolova, Tatyana Grushko and Katerina Pestova, Abbott, Molecular Diagnostics, Des Plains, IL [89].

16.5 Specific chromosomal abnormalities to detect CTCs

A method known as FICTION which combines IFISH and IHC may be used to simultaneously analyze the genotype and phenotype of a single CTC and can be used to study phenotypic and genotypic changes in the same cell [25, 64] The anaplastic lymphoma kinase (*ALK*) fusion gene is a driver gene for non-small cell lung cancer (NSCLC) [106]. *ALK*-positive NSCLC has been considered as a molecular subtype of NSCLC that provides unique clinicopathological characteristics of cancer diagnosis and prognosis [106, 107]. Initially, researchers found that the *EML4-ALK* fusion gene exists in NSCLC patients by PCR and proteomics methods. However, due to the variation of fusion partners of ALK fusion genes, as well as the possibilities of unknown fusion partners, the FISH method with specific probes is an accepted and essential FDA approved companion diagnostic method performed on FFPE sections of NSCLC [108]. Currently, FISH has been considered as the gold standard of detecting ALK rearrangements [107, 109] using the Abbot Vysis *ALK* Break Apart FISH Probe Kit. The kit is designed with the 3′ and 5′ probes labeled by red and green signals; once abnormalities of *ALK* have occurred, deletion or splitting of the signals will be detected [110]. The limitation of the FISH based *ALK* test includes high cost and the utilization of specialized equipment [110, 111]. Studies have demonstrated CTCs containing the *ALK-EMLK1* gene rearrangements in patients with NSCLC [108–112] (see **Figure 13**) as well as in *ex vivo* cultures of CTCs from patients with NSCLC [113].

An enriched cell preparation can be used to detect oncogene fusions due to chromosomal translocations or inversions in lung cancer such as *ALK-EML1, ROS-1* or amplifications of oncogenes such as *Her2neu* or *EGFR*. Recently a novel FISH assay was described that can simultaneously detect *ROS1, RET*, and *MET* chromosomal aberrations in cells of NSCLC on FFPE tissue. This assay has the potential to be used on CTCs [89] (**Figure 14a–d**).

17. PDL-1/PD-1 on CTCs

In recent years the development of tumor immunotherapy drugs, especially immune checkpoint inhibitors (ICIs) targeting the programmed death protein (PD-1)/ programmed death ligand 1(PD-L1) has changed the paradigm in the treatment of malignant tumors and has shown superiority in terms of therapeutic effect and quality of life compared with traditional chemotherapy

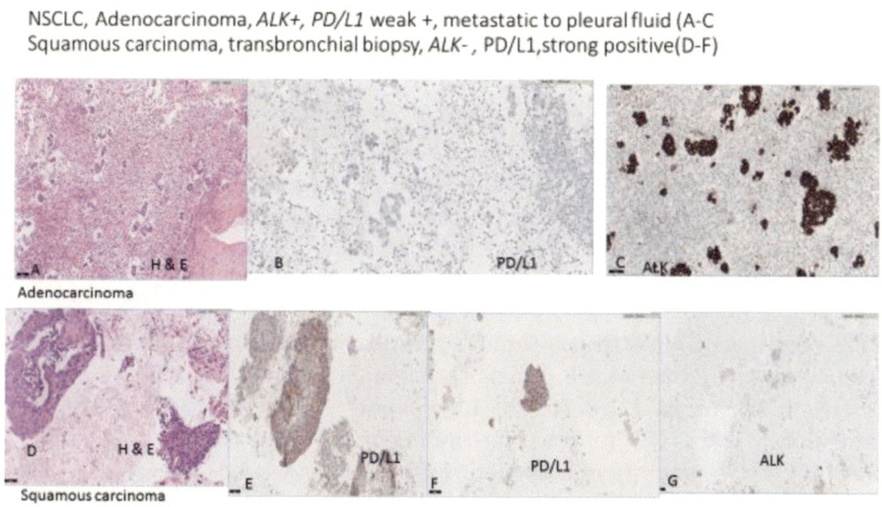

Figure 15.
Top panel: Example of metastatic adenocarcinoma of lung in pleural fluid in a patient with advanced lung cancer, A) papillary and acinar fragments of adenocarcinoma (H&EX20); B) PD/L1 IHC clone 22c3(pharm dx, Dako, CA) showed weak membranous expression, overall score < 50%; C) ALK IHC, clone D5F3 showed strong expression consistent with a positive test. Bottom panel: D) squamous carcinoma lung, moderately differentiated, transbronchial biopsy, H&E X40, E) and F) PD/L1 IHC22C3 shows strong positive membranous staining in >90% of malignant cells, G) Alk IHC, clone D5F3, showed negative expression consistent with a negative result.

[114–118]. Single-agent immune checkpoint inhibitors are now standard of care for advanced non-small cell lung cancer (NSCLC), and emerging data show that combining these agents with established chemotherapy further improves progression free survival and overall survival. The Phase III KEYNOTE-189 and IMPower-130 trial showed significantly improved survival using this strategy for non-squamous NSCLC, and the phase III KEYNOTE-407 trial showed similar results in squamous disease [119].

PD-L1 is a type 1 transmembrane protein with an extra-cellular N-terminal domain which inhibits or blocks the immune response by interacting with the PD-1 receptor which is expressed on activated T- and B-cells, and macrophages. Anti-PD-L1/PD-1 antibodies can reactive the immune system to eradicate tumors by blocking checkpoint proteins from binding with their partner proteins. PD-L1 expression may inform the use of checkpoint inhibitor combination therapy, while overall tumor mutation burden is also an emerging biomarker for ICIs. Antibodies that have FDA approval for NSCLC are two that block PD-1, namely Nivolumab (Opdivo, Bristol-Myers Squibb) approved for third line approval and Pembrolizumab (Keytruda, MSD SHARP and DOHME GMBH), which has approval for first- and second line-treatment, and one antibody blocking PD-L1, namely Atezolizumab (Tecentriq, Roche) for third line–treatment settings.

Immunohistochemistry (IHC) on tumor tissue, using the recommended FDA approved IHC-companion diagnostic for PD-L1, Ventana PD-L1 SP142 assay (Ventana Medical Systems, Tucson, AZ, USA) and PD-L1 IHC 22C3 PharmDx (Dako, North America, Santa Barbara, CA, USA) is the gold standard (**Figure 15**) and is widely adopted in PD-L1 detection.

17.1 Limitations of PD-1/PD-L1 inhibitors

1. Before or throughout therapy with PD-1/PD-L1 inhibitors, variations of PD-L1 expression in cancer cells might occur, causing different sensitivity to PD-1/PD-L1 blockade, which might be missed by a single biopsy.

2. In the tissue microenvironment, cells like lymphocytes and macrophages, also express PD-L1.

3. Patients who receive immunotherapy are often in an advanced stage when tumors develop and evolve, and the PD-L1 expression in the primary tumor may have also changed dynamically. Some of the patients at these stages might not be able to tolerate the side effects caused by invasive tissue biopsy [114–117].

CTCs originate from different tumor sites and thus, better reflect the tumor heterogeneity compared to tissue biopsies. They could therefore be potentially useful as a non-invasive method to detect PD-L1 expression in NSCLC patients [114–120]. In 2016, Schehr et al. [121] reported the finding of PD-L1-positive (PD-L1+) CTCs in NSCLC via in-house immunomagnetic enrichment system. However, other than cells expressing EpCAM, the study also mentioned the co-isolation of CD11b+, CD45-low, and cytokeratin-positive (CK+)- cells that expressed PD-L1, that could be mislabeled as CTCs, thus stressing the importance of proper identification of CTCs to avoid false positive events. Recently, Wang et al. [122] mentioned the dynamic changes of PD-L1 expression by CTCs 13 non-metastatic NSCLC patients. CTCs were in all 13 samples, PD-L1+ CTCs were detected in 66.7% of the sample. A recent study from 106 NSCLC patients, showed a 93% concordance between PD-L1 status in CTCs and tumor tissue, indicating the potential of a CTC test in determining response to ICIs [120].

Another recent study used a novel SE-iFISH (subtraction enrichment interphase FISH) strategy to examine the presence of PD-L1 on aneuploid CTCs and aneuploid circulating tumor endothelial cells (CTECs) to evaluate if their presence could be used as a surrogate biomarker to evaluate the efficiency of second-line anti-PD-1 (Nivolumab) immunotherapy. This study demonstrated that significant numbers of PD-L1+ aneuploid CTCs and CTECs could be detected in histopathologic hPD-L1-patients. In contrast to decreased PD-L1+ CTCs, the number of multiploid PD-L1+ CTECs (≥tetrasomy 8) undergoing post-therapeutic karyotype shifting increased in patients along with tumor progression following anti-PD-1 treatment and was associated with a significantly shorter PFS compared to those without PD-L1+ CTECs [123].

Many issues of PD-1/PD-L1 expression still need to be validated, including ensuring that the clones of antibody cocktail used for staining are standardized and equivalent in performance to the antibody clones included in the IHC kits that have received regulatory approval as companion diagnostics, as well as the threshold used to call a test PD-L1 positive, and whether the effect of the therapeutic use of anti-PDL1 antibodies interferes with the binding of diagnostic PD-L1 antibodies on CTCs [124]. Currently there are over 400 listed clinical trials for LC patients using ICI's alone or in combination with traditional chemotherapies [124]. Thus, if the CTC test, can be standardized, it will be of tremendous value as a complementary diagnostic tool for real time monitoring of PD-L1 expression for advanced lung cancer patients.

18. Conclusion

LB has evolved as a transformative technology for cancer diagnosis. Enormous strides have been made in recent years by the scientific and oncology communities to expand upon the tremendous value contained in a LB specimen. These readily obtained samples provide a real time window into the presence of cancer cells, the molecular evolution of the underlying tumor and its metastatic cascade and represent a far more feasible method for the longitudinal monitoring of the cancer patients as compared to direct tissue biopsy. Currently CTCs and ctDNA may be used in screening for early stage LC, as a diagnostic test to discriminate between a benign or malignant nodule on LDCT scan, as a decision –making tool or companion diagnostic for instituting targeted therapy for different genetic mutations, for detecting the presence of minimum- residual disease and as a monitoring tool for detecting response to immune-check point inhibitors. There are however still discrepancies in how to harness the power of CTCs, especially in the area immune-check point inhibitors, where standardization of CTC capture and companion PD-L1 antibodies, together with inter-laboratory standardization in interpretation of these tests, will be mandatory. Another key objective of future research will be the ability to establish mouse models from CTCs to monitor the epigenetic, and genetic profiling, functional and signaling pathways of malignant cells in response to different therapies. In order for LB for LC to become well accepted as a reliable source for actionable therapy large scale studies involving consortia of academic institutions and public/private partnerships are needed to establish reliable platforms for capturing and detecting CTCs and ctDNA that validate pre-existing discovery studies. Notwithstanding these caveats, it is apparent that LB is becoming an indispensable weapon in the battle against cancer.

Acknowledgements

The authors gratefully acknowledge the following people who have contributed to this book chapter: Ms. Sharon Mehl for assisting with the editing and references, Dr. Robert Mattaliano, Sanmed Diagnostics Inc. for permission to use **Figures 1a, 8, 10a, b,** and **11** adapted from his presentation on Liquid Biopsy at the Tricon Molecular Medicine Meeting, San Francisco, February 2021 as well as for editing and reviewing the manuscript, Dr. Irina Sokolova, Vysis, Abbott Molecular, Chicago, Il for supplying the multiplexed 6 color FISH figures and Dr. Efrat Ofek, of Sheba Hospital, Tel Hashomer, Tel Aviv University, Israel for supplying pleural fluid and transbronchial biopsy specimens (**Figure 14**), and Ms. Camilla Avivi of Sheba Hospital, Tel Hashomer, Tel Aviv University for her expert immunocytochemical staining.

The authors have obtained permission from Karger Publishers, License number 5001350625847, Feb 03,2021 to reproduce 3 figures and one table from Liquid Biopsy: Recent Advances in the Detection of Circulating Tumor Cells and Their Clinical Applications, authored by Katz Ruth L., Zaidi Tanweer M., Ni Xiaohui, Copyright © 2020, © 2020 S. Karger AG, Basel, Vol 25, license date Feb 03, 2021.

The authors have obtained permission from John Wiley and Sons, License number 5020371212886, to use licensed content from Cancer Cytopathology, Apr 22,2020, vol 128, entitled: Identification of circulating tumor cells using 4-color fluorescence in situ hybridization: Validation of a noninvasive aid for ruling out lung cancer in patients with low- dose computed tomography-detected lung nodules., authored by Ruth L. Katz, Tanweer M. Zaidi, Deep Pujara, et al., **Figures 2a, c–e,** and **3**.

Funding

- The study was supported in part by LunglifeAI (Thousand Oaks, CA, USA), Thermo Fisher Scientific, and a SPORE grant for lung cancer, and Sanmed Biotech, Zhuhai, China.

- National Cancer Institute. Grant Numbers: CA123208, CA55769; Division of Cancer Prevention, National Cancer Institute. Grant Number: K07CA093592; NIH SPORE GRANT. Grant Number: P50CA70907

- The study was supported partially by Program for Guangdong and Zhuhai Introducing Innovative and Entrepreneurial Teams (Fund No. 2019ZT08Y297/ZH01110405170017PWC); Program for Zhuhai Industrial Core and Key Technology Research (Fund No. ZH22044702190132HJL).

Conflict of interest

Dr. Ruth Katz is a consultant for Sanmed Bio, and on the scientific board of Lung life AI, Dr. Xin Ye and Ms. Xiaozheng Yang are employed by Sanmed Bio, Zhuhai, China. Dr. Katz is also an inventor of the Mutiplex LB FISH Test, licensed by MD Anderson Cancer Center to Lunglife AI, and sublicensed to Sanmed Biotech Ltd., Zhuhai, China as the Sanmed test for CACs. Dr. Katz was an employee of MD Anderson Cancer center from 1976 to 2018, during which time she developed the Mutiplex LB FISH Test. Dr. Katz and MD Anderson Cancer center, may in the future, be beneficiaries of royalties from this test,

She holds the following patents:

UTMDACC, Katz RL, Feng J: Detection and diagnosis of smoking-related cancers, United States, 12/761,134/UTSC: 658USC2, 4/15/2010, issued.

- UTMDACC, Katz RL: Circulating tumor and tumor stem cell.

  Detection using genomic specific probes, United States, UTFC.

  P1234WO, 12/10/2015, pending.

  Chinese Application No. 201580075104.1 based on PCT/US2015/065057 and U.S. Provisional Application No. 62/090,167; Entitled "CIRCULATING TUMOR AND TUMOR STEM CELL DETECTION USING GENOMIC SPECIFIC PROBES" by Ruth Katz.

  In the Name of Board of Regents, The University of Texas System Our Ref. UTFC.P1234CN; Your Ref. MDA14–035.

- The four-color FISH test described within this chapter is licensed to LunglifeAI (Los Angeles, CA, USA) and sublicensed to San Med Bio (Zhuhai, China) and Livzhon Pharma, China.

Dr. Roberta Carbone is a Tethis employee and holds equity and/or stock options: she holds a patent on the SBS technology (Method for immobilizing biological samples for analytical and diagnostic purposes, WO2019021150A1).

Author details

Xin Ye[1], Xiao Zheng Yang[1], Roberta Carbone[2], Iris Barshack[3] and Ruth L. Katz[3]*

1 Sanmed Biotech Ltd., Zhuhai, China

2 Tethis S.p.A., Milan, Italy

3 Chaim Sheba Hospital, Tel Aviv University, Ramat Gan, Israel

*Address all correspondence to: ruarik18@gmail.com

References

[1] Habli Z, Al Chama W, Saab R et al *Circulating tumor cell detection technologies and clinical utility: challenges and opportunities.* Cancers et al. 2020,12, 1930 doi.10.3390/cancers12071930

[2] Bray F, Ferlay J, Soerjomataram I, et el. *Global cancer statistics 2018: GLOBOCAN estimates of incidence and mortality worldwide for 36 cancers in 185 countries*. CA. Cancer J Clin. 2018. doi:10.3322/caac.21492

[3] Torre LA, Bray F, Siegel RL et al, *Global cancer statistics*, 2012. CA Cancer J Clin. 2015. doi:10.3322/caac.21262

[4] Cao M, Chen W. *Epidemiology of lung cancer in China*, Thorac Cancer. 2019. doi:10.1111/1759-7714.12916

[5] de Groot PM, Wu CC, Carter BW. *The epidemiology of lung cancer*. Transl Lung Cancer Res. 2018. doi:10.21037/tlcr.2018.05.06

[6] Birring SS, Peake MD. *Symptoms and the early diagnosis of lung cancer.* Thorax. 2005.doi:10.1136/thx.2004.032698

[7] Henschke CI, Yankelevitz DF, Libby DM, et al. *Survival of patients with stage I lung cancer detected on CT screening.* N Engl J Med. 2006. doi:10.1056/NEJMoa060476

[8] Lu T, Yang X, Huang Y, et al. *Trends in the incidence, treatment, and survival of patients with lung cancer in the last four decades*. Cancer Manag Res. 2019. doi:10.2147/CMAR.S187317

[9] Henschke CI, McCauley DI, Yankelevitz DF, et al. *Early Lung Cancer Action Project: Overall design and findings from baseline screening.* Lancet. 1999. doi:10.1016/S0140-6736(99)06093-6

[10] Kaneko M, Eguchi K, Ohmatsu H, et al. *Peripheral lung cancer: Screening and detection with low-dose spinal CT versus radiography*. Radiology. 1996. doi:10.1148/radiology.201.3.8939234

[11] Henschke CI, Naidich DP, Yankelevitz DF, et al. *Early Lung Cancer Action Project: Initial findings on repeat screening.* Cancer. 2001. doi:10.1002/1097-0142(20010701) 92:1<153:AID-CNCR1303>3.0.CO;2-S

[12] *Reduced Lung-Cancer Mortality with Low-Dose Computed Tomographic Screening*. N Engl J Med.2011. doi:10.1056/nejmoa1102873

[13] de Koning HJ, van der Aalst CM, de Jong PA, et al. *Reduced Lung-Cancer Mortality with Volume CT Screening in a Randomized Trial*. N Engl J Med. 2020. doi:10.1056/nejmoa1911793

[14] Huang KL, Wang SY, Lu WC, et al. *Effects of low-dose computed tomography on lung cancer screening: A systematic review, meta-analysis, and trial sequential analysis*. BMC Pulm Med 2019. doi:10.1186/s12890-019-0883-x

[15] American Cancer Society. *Lung Cancer Early Detection, Diagnosis, and Staging*. New York, NY Springer. 2019.

[16] National Comprehensive Cancer Network. *NCCN guidelines for patients lung cancer*. Natl Compr Cancer Netw 2018.

[17] Jaklitsch MT, Jacobson FL, Austin JHM, et al. *The American Association for Thoracic Surgery guidelines for lung cancer screening using low-dose computed tomography scans for lung cancer survivors and other high-risk groups.* J Thorac Cardiovasc Surg 2012. doi:10.1016/j.jtcvs.2012.05.060

[18] Gould MK, Tang T, Liu ILA, et al. *Recent trends in the identification of incidental pulmonary nodules.* Am .J

Respir Crit Care Med. 2015. doi:10.1164/rccm.201505-0990OC

[19] Tanner NT, Aggarwal J, Gould MK, et al. *Management of pulmonary nodules by community pulmonologists a multicentre observational study.* Chest. 2015. doi:10.1378/chest.15-0630

[20] Lokhandwala T, Bittoni MA, Dann RA, et al. *Costs of Diagnostic Assessment for lung cancer: a Medicare claims analysis.* Clin Lung Cancer. 2017. doi: 10.1016/j.cllc.2016.07.006

[21] Mascalchi M, Sali L. *Lung cancer screening with low dose CT and radiation harm-from prediction models to cancer incidence data.* Ann Transl Med 2017;5(17). doi:10.21037/atm.2017.06.41

[22] Wisnivesky JP, Henschke CI, Yankelevitz DF. *Diagnostic percutaneous transthoracic needle biopsy does not affect survival in stage I lung cancer*. Am J Respir Crit Care Med. 2006. doi:10.1164/rccm.200602-160OC

[23] Evangelista L, Panunzio A, Scagliori E et al *Ground glass pulmonary nodules: their significance in oncology patients and the role of computer tomography and 18F–fluorodeoxyglucose positron emission tomography*. Eur J Hybrid Imaging. 2018. doi:10.1186/s41824-017-0021-z

[24] Katz RL, Zaidi TM, Pujara D, et al. *Identification of circulating tumor cells using 4-color fluorescence in situ hybridization: Validation of a non-invasive aid for ruling out lung cancer in patients with low-dose computed tomography–detected lung nodules*. Cancer Cytopathol. 2020;128(8):553-562.

[25] Katz RL, Zaidi TM, Xiaohui N, Liquid Biopsy: Recent advances in the detection of circulating tumor cells and their clinical applications. Bui MM, Pantanowitz (eds): Modern Techniques in Cytopathology. Monogr Clin Cytol Basel, Karger, 2020, vol 25, pp43-66 (DOI: 10.1159/000455780)

[26] Liu M.C., Oxnard G.R., Klein E.A., et al *Sensitive and specific multi-cancer detection and localization using methylation signatures in cell-free DNA*, Elsevier enhanced. Annals of Oncology, volume 31, Issue 6, 2020, 745-759

[27] Leigh1, N.B., Page R.D., Raymond V.M. et al. *Clinical utility of comprehensive cell-free DNA analysis to identify genomic biomarkers in patients with newly diagnosed metastatic non-small cell lung cancer*. Clinical Cancer Res. AACR journals.org April 15, 2019 doi: 10.1158/1078-0432.CCR-19-0624

[28] Pawlikowska P, Faugeroux V, Oulhen et al *Circulating tumor cells (CTCs) for the non-invasive monitoring and personalization of non-small cell lung cancer (NSCLC) therapies*. J Thoracic Dis 2019;11(Suppl 1): S45-S56. doi:10.21037/jtd.2018.12.80

[29] Marquette CH, Boutros J, Benzaquen J, Ferreira M, Pastre J, Pison C, Padovani B, Bettayeb F, Fallet V, Guibert N, Basille D, Ilie M, Hofman V, Hofman P; AIR project Study Group. Circulating tumour cells as a potential biomarker for lung cancer screening: a prospective cohort study. Lancet Respir Med. 2020 Jul;8(7):709-716. doi: 10.1016/S2213-2600(20)30081-3. Erratum in: Lancet Respir Med. 2020 Dec;8(12): e94. PMID: 32649919.

[30] Paul Hofman, *Liquid biopsy for lung cancer screening: usefulness of circulating tumor cells and other circulating biomarkers,* September 8,2020, Cancer Cytopathology September 8,2020, DOI: 10.1002/cncy.22367,

[31] Akhoundova D, Martinez J M, Musmann L.E., et al, *The role of the liquid biopsy in decision-making for patients with non-small cell lung cancer* J Clin. Med.2020,9, 3674; doi:10.3390/jcm9113674

[32] Jiang F Jiang, F, Caraway NP, Zhang H-Z, et al. Surfactant protein A gene

deletion and prognostics for patients with stage I non-small cell lung cancer DOI: 101158/1078-0432 CCR-04-2087 Published August 2005.

[33] Freitas, MO.; Gartner, J.; Rangel-Pozzo, A et al. *Genomic instability in circulating tumor cells.* Cancers 2020, *12*, 3001.

[34] Katz RL, He W, Khanna A, et al. *Genetically abnormal circulating cells in lung cancer patients: antigen-independent fluorescence in situ hybridization- based case-control study.* Clin Cancer Res.doi: 10.1158/1078-0432.CCR-09-3358

[35] Zong C, Lu S, Chapman AR, Xie XS. *Genome-wide detection of single-nucleotide and copy-number variations of a single human cell*. Science (New York, NY) 2012;338:1622-6.

[36] Chen C, Xing D, Tan L, et al. *Single-cell whole-genome analyses by linear amplification via transposon insertion (LIANTI).* Science (New York, NY) 2017;356:189-94.

[37] Agashe R and Kurzrock R, *Circulating tumor cells: from the laboratory to the cancer clinic*. Cancer 2020, 12, 2361: doi: 10.3390/cancers 12092361

[38] Oliveto S, Mancino M, Manfrini, N et al. *Role of microRNAs in translation regulation and cancer.* World .J. Biol. Chem 2017, 8, 45-46

[39] Arechederra M, Avila MA, Berasain C, *Liquid biopsy for cancer management: a revolutionary but still limited new tool for precision medicine.* Advances in Laboratory Medicine, April 2020 https: doi.org/10.1515/ almed-2020-0009

[40] Chang, S, Hur J Y, Choi, Yoon-La, Chang HL, Kim, WS. *Current status and future perspectives of liquid biopsy in non-small cell lung cancer, Journal of Pathology and Translational Medicine* 2020: 54; 204-212.https//doi. org/10.4132/jptm.2020.02.27

[41] Hussain H, Melnikova VO, Kosko K, et al, *Monitoring daily dynamics of early tumor response to targeted therapy by detecting circulating tumor DNA in urine.* Clin Cancer Res 2017;23;4716-23)

[42] Zhou C, Cheng Y, et al *Detection of EGFR T790M in Asia Pacific patients across 3 platforms,* Ann Oncol. 2017. From Current Status and future perspectives of LB in NSCLC.

[43] Circulating Tumor Cells and Cell Free DNA Workshop, Int. J. Mol.Sci. 2016, 17, 1505; doi:10.3390/ijms17091505

[44] Predictive and prognostic biomarkers © S. Karger Publishers Ltd 2020 64 Fast Facts

[45] Mehta A, Smreti V, Sanjeev, KS, et al. *Biomarker testing for advanced lungcancer by next-generation sequencing; a valid method to achieve a comprehensive glimpse at mutational landscape*. Applied Cancer Research, doi.org/10.1186/ s4124-020-00089-8

[46] Zheng, D, Wang, R, Ting, Y, et al. *Met exon 14 skipping defines a unique molecular class of non-small cell lung cancer*. Oncotarget. 2016 Jul 5; 7(27):41691-41702. doi: 10.18632/ oncotarget.9541

[47] Le X, Heymach JV. *New verse for a familiar song: Small molecule inhibitors for MET exon 14 skipping non-small cell lung cancer.* Oncologist, 2020;25(10):822-825,doi: 10.1634/ theoncologist.2020-0760.Epub 2020 Aug 27. PMID:33400286:PMCID: PMC7543381

[48] Hou H, Yang X, Zhang X, et al, *Discovery of targetable genetic alterations in advanced non-small cell lung cancer using a next generation sequencing –based circulating tumor DNA assay.* Sci Rep 2017;7;14605)

[49] *FDA approves first liquid biopsy next generation sequencing companion diagnostic test*. https://www.fda.gov/news-events/press-announcements 11/11/2020)

[50] *Foundation Medicine liquid biopsy gets FDA approval for multiple companion diagnostic indications, companion diagnostic indications.* Precision Oncology News October 20202828

[51] Steensma, DP et al, *Clonal hematopoiesis as a model for premalignant changes during aging.* Exp Hematol,2020. PMID: 31838005.Review.

[52] Jaiswal, S and Ebert, B.L. *Clonal hematopoiesis in human aging and disease.* Science 366,586 (2019) 1 November 2019

[53] Yuebi Hu, Bryan C. Ulrich, Julianna Supplee, et al.*False –Positive Plasma Genotyping Due to Clonal Hematopoiesis.* Clinical Cancer research, September 2018, Volume 24, Issue 18 DOI: 10.1158/1078-0432.CCR-18-0143 P

[54] Cohen, Joshua et al, Detection and localization of surgically resectable cancers with a multi-analyte blood test. Science 23 Feb 2018, vol 359,Issue 6378,pp.926-930,DOI.10. 1126/science.aar3247.

[55] Liu, MC, Oxnard, GR, Klein, EA, *Sensitive and specific multi-cancer detection and localization using methylation signatures in cell-free DNA*. Annals of Oncology, vlume 31, issue 6, 2020

[56] Young, Christmas, Hopkins, Editorial, J Thoracic Dis. Clin Cancer Res.(18) September 15, 2018 Editorial, *Multi-analyte assays and early detection of common cancers*, J Thor Dis 2018;10 (Suppl.18): S2165-S2167

[57] Lei Fu, K, Zhou, Wenyu et al. *Applying Circulating DNA methylation in the diagnosis of lung cancer.* Precision Clinical Medicine 2019)

[58] Miller MC, Doyle G V., Terstappen LWMM. *Significance of Circulating Tumor Cells Detected by the CellSearch System in Patients with Metastatic Breast Colorectal and Prostate Cancer.* J Oncol. 2010. doi:10.1155/2010/617421

[59] Zhang L, Ridgway LD, Wetzel MD, et al. *The identification and Characterization of breast cancer CTCs competent for brain metastasis.* Science translational medicine 2013;5:180ra48. .2013;5:180ra48.

[60] Hou JM, Krebs MG, *Lancashire L, et al. Clinical significance and molecular characteristics of circulating tumor cells and circulating tumor microemboli in patients with small-cell lung cancer*.J Clin Oncol. 2012doi:10.1200/JCO.2010.33.3716

[61] Wang L, Balasubramanian P, Chen AP et al. *Promise and limits of the CellSearch platform for evaluating pharmacodynamics in circulating tumor cells.* Semin Oncol. 2016. doi:10.1053/j.seminoncol.2016.06.004

[62] Truini A, Alama A, Dal-Bello MG, et al. *Clinical applications of circulating tumor cells in lung cancer patients by CellSearch system*. Front Oncol. 2014. doi:10.3389/fonc.2014.00242

[63] Maheswaran S, Haber DA. *Circulating tumor cells: a window into cancer biology and metastasis*. Current Opinion in Genetics Development. 2010; 20:96-99.

[64] Jiang F, Katz RL. *Use of interphase fluorescence in situ hybridization as a powerful diagnostic tool in cytology*. Diagnostic molecular pathology: American journal of surgical pathology, Part B 2002;11:47-57.

[65] Nieto,A, Huang, R, Jackson, R, et al EMT Cell; 2016;166;21-4. http://dx.doi.org/10.1016/j.cell.2016.06.028

[66] Hodgkinson CL, Morrow CJ, Li Y, et al. *Tumorigenicity and genetic profiling of circulating tumor cells in small-cell lung cancer*. Nature medicine

[67] Katz RL, Lukeman JM. *The comparative diagnostic accuracy of cancer-cell detection obtained with Ficoll-Hypaque gradient separation and standard centrifugation technics on body-cavity fluids*. Am J Clin Pathol 1980; 74:18-24.

[68] Hosokawa,M,Kemnotsu, H, Yasuhiro,K et al (2013) Size based isolation of circulating tumor cellsin lung cancer patients using a micro-cavitary array system. PLos ONE 8(6):e67466, doi: 10.1371/Journal. Pone.0067466

[69] Ilona Krol et al. Detection of Clustered Circulating Tumor Cells in Early Breast Cancer, BJC 2021, in press.

[70] Aceto N, Bardia A, Miyamoto DT, Donaldson MC, Wittner BS, Spencer JA, Yu M, Pely A, Engstrom A, Zhu H, Brannigan BW, Kapur R, Stott SL, Shioda T, Ramaswamy S, Ting DT, Lin CP, Toner M, Haber DA, Maheswaran S. Circulating tumor cell clusters are oligoclonal precursors of breast cancer metastasis. Cell. 2014 Aug 28;158(5):1110-1122. doi: 10.1016/j. cell.2014.07.013. PMID: 25171411; PMCID: PMC4149753.

[71] Krebs MG, Hou JM, Sloane R, et al. *Analysis of circulating tumor cells in patients with non-small cell lung cancer using epithelial marker-dependent and -independent approaches*. J Thorac Oncol.2012;7(2):306-315. doi:10.1097/ JTO.0b013e31823c5c16

[72] Pantel K, Speicher MR. *The biology of circulating tumor cells*. Oncogene. 2016. doi:10.1038/onc.2015.192

[73] Pantel K, Brakenhoff RH. *Dissecting the metastatic cascade*. Nat Rev Cancer. 2004. doi:10.1038/nrc1370

[74] Eslami-S Z, Cortés-Hernández LE, Alix-Panabières C. *Epithelial cell adhesion molecule:an anchor to isolate clinically relevant circulating tumor cells*. Cells. 2020. doi:10.3390/cells9081836

[75] Christofanilli M, Budd GT, Ellis MJ et al, *Circulating tumor cells, disease progression, and survival in metastatic breast cancer.* N Eng J Med 2004; 351:781-791.

[76] Mikolajczyk SD, Millar LS, Tsinberg P, et al. *Detection of EpCAM-Negative and Cytokeratin-Negative Circulating Tumor Cells in Peripheral Blood.* Journal of oncology 2011;2011:252361.

[77] Grover PK, Cummins AG, Price TJ, et al. *Circulating tumour cells: the evolving concept and the inadequacy of their enrichment by EpCAM-based methodology for basic and clinical cancer research.* Annals of oncology: official journal of the European Society for Medical Oncology 2014;25:1506-1516.

[78] Gabriel MT, Calleja LR, Chalopin A, et al. *Circulating Tumor Cells: A Review of Non-EpCAM-Based Approaches for Cell Enrichment and Isolation*. Clinical chemistry 2016;62:571-581.

[79] Liu Z, Fusi A, Klopocki E, et al. *Negative enrichment by immunomagnetic nanobeads for unbiased characterization of circulating tumor cells from peripheral blood of cancer patients.* Journal of translational medicine 2011;9:70.

[80] Lapin M, Tjensvoll K, Oltedal S, et al. *MINDEC-An Enhanced Negative Depletion Strategy for Circulating Tumour Cell Enrichment.* Scientific reports 2016;6:28929.

[81] Ge F, Zhang H, Wang DD et al. *Enhanced detection and comprehensive in situ phenotypic characterization of circulating and disseminated heteroploid epithelial and glioma tumor* cells. Oncotarget.2015:6(29):27049-27064 doi:10.18632/oncotarget.4819)

[82] Millner LM, Linder MW, Valdes R. *Circulating tumor cells: A review of present methods and the need to identify heterogeneous phenotypes.* Ann Clin Lab Sci. 2013.

[83] Talasaz AH, Powell AA, Huber DE, et al. *Isolating highly enriched populations of circulating epithelial cells and other rare cells from blood using a magnetic sweeper device.* Proc Natl Acad Sci U S A. 2009. doi:10.1073/pnas.0813188106

[84] Man Y, Wang Q, Kemmner W. *Currently Used Markers for CTC Isolation - Advantages, Limitations and Impact on Cancer Prognosis.* J Clin Exp Pathol. 2011. doi:10.4172/2161-0681.1000102

[85] Theil G, Fischer K, Weber E, et al. *The use of a new CellCollector to isolate circulating tumor cells from the blood of patients with different stages of prostate cancer and clinical outcomes - A proof-of-concept study.* PLoS One. 2016. doi:10.1371/journal.pone.0158354

[86] Luecke K, Gasiorowski L, Herold S, et al. *Characterization in lung cancer patients.* J Clin Oncol. 2015. doi:10.1200/jco.2015.33.15_suppl.e22035

[87] Scher HI, Graf RP, Schreiber NA, et al. *Phenotypic Heterogeneity of Circulating Tumor Cells Informs Clinical Decisions between AR Signaling Inhibitors and Taxanes in Metastatic Prostate Cancer*. Cancer Res 2017;77:5687-5698.

[88] Jiang F, Yin Z, Caraway NP et al. *Genomic profiles in stage I primary non small cell lung cancer using comparative genomic hybridization analysis of cDNA microarrays.* Neoplasia 2004;6: 623-635.

[89] Sokolova,I, Bedroske PB, Grushko T, et al. *Multiplex fast FISH assay for detecting ROS1, RET and MET aberrations in FFPE specimens using BioView image analysis.,* Abbott Molecular, Des Plaines, Il. Poster #4256, AACR 2020

[90] Liu WR, Zhang B, Chen C, et al. *Detection of circulating genetically abnormal cells in peripheral blood for early diagnosis of non-small cell lung cancer.* Thorac Cancer. *2020.* doi: 10.1111/1759-7714.13654

[91] Halling KC, King W, Sokolova A, et al. *Assessing the value of reflex fluorescence in situ hybridization testing in the diagnosis of bladder cancer when routine urine cytological examination is equivocal.* J Urol. 2000; 164: 1768-1775

[92] Chen BS. *Integrating circulating genetically abnormal cells to early lung cancer screening in Chinese bus drivers.* Poster presented at: The IASLC North America Conference on Lung Cancer; Oct 16-17; Online

[93] Sun JY. *Clinical utility of circulating genetically abnormal cells in differential diagnosis of benign from malignant pulmonary nodules sized between 5-10mm*. Poster presented at: The IASLC Liquid Biopsy; Oct 2-3; Online

[94] Xu T. *Artificial intelligence for differential diagnosis between benign and malignant pulmonary nodules: a real-world, multicenter, diagnostic study.* Poster presented at: The American Society of Clinical Oncology annual meeting; May 29-31; online

[95] Zhu Y, Lowe ACY. *Multiplexed fluorescence in situ hybridization–based detection of circulating tumor cells: A novel liquid-based technology to facilitate accurate and early identification of non–small cell lung cancer patients.* Cancer Cytopathol. 2020;128(8):518-519. doi:10.1002/cncy.22277

[96] Bueno,J,Landeras,M,Chung, JH, Updated Fleischner Society Guidelines for Managing Incidental Pulmonary Nodules: Common Questions and Challenging Scenarios.RadioGraphics 2018; 38:1337-1350 https://doi.org/10.1148/rg.2018180017

[97] Stoecklein NH, Fischer JC, Niederacher D et al. *LWMM. Challenges for CTC-based liquid biopsies: Low CTC frequency and diagnostic leukapheresis as a potential solution*. Expert Rev Mol Diagn. 2016. doi:10.1586/14737159.2016.1123095

[98] Karabacak NM, Spuhler PS, Fachin F, et al. *Microfluidic, marker-free isolation of circulating tumor cells from blood samples.* Nat Protoc. 2014. doi:10.1038/nprot.2014.044

[99] He B, Lu Q, Lang J, et al. *A new method for CTC Images Recognition based on machine learning.* Front Bioeng Biotechnol. 2020;8(August):1-10. doi:10.3389/fbioe.2020.00897

[100] Asante DB, Calapre L, Ziman M et al. *Liquid biopsy in ovarian cancer using circulating tumor DNA and cells: Ready for prime time?* Cancer Lett. 2020.

[101] Raillon C, Che J, Thill S, et al. *Toward microfluidics label-free isolation and enumeration of circulating tumor cells from blood samples*. Cytom Part A. 2019;95(10):1085-1095. doi:10.1002/cyto.a.23868

[102] Savadikar C, Tahvillian S, Baden L, et al, *towards designing accurate FISH probe detection using 3D U-Nets on microscopic blood cell images.* CoDS, COMAD 2020, January 5-7, Hyderabad, India.

[103] Tang CM, Zhu P, Li S et al. *Filtration and Analysis of Circulating Cancer Associated Cells from the Blood of Cancer Patients.* Methods in molecular biology (Clifton, NJ) 2017;1572:511-24.

[104] Ilie M, Hofman V, Long-Mira E, et al. *"Sentinel" circulating tumor cells allow early diagnosis of lung cancer in patients with chronic obstructive pulmonary disease*. PloS one 2014;9:e111597.

[105] He W, Wang H, Hartmann LC et al. *In vivo quantitation of rare circulating tumor cells by multiphoton intravital flow cytometry*. Proc Natl Acad Sci U S A. 2007. doi:10.1073/pnas.0703875104

[106] Straughan M Azoury DC Shukla S. *Anaplastic lymphoma kinase inhibitors in non-small cell lung cancer*. Curr Drug Targets. 2016. doi:10.2174/1573399811666150615144336

[107] Villalobos P, Wistuba II. *Lung cancer biomarkers*. Hematol Oncol Clin North Am. 2017. doi:10.1016/j.hoc.2016.08.006

[108] Kim H, Chung JH. *Overview of clinicopathologic features of ALK-rearranged lung adenocarcinoma and current diagnostic testing for ALK rearrangement*. Transl Lung Cancer Res. 2015. doi:10.3978/j.issn.2218-6751.2014.12.02

[109] Heuckmann JM, Pauwels P, Thunnissen E. *Comprehensive Hybrid Capture–Based Next-Generation Sequencing Identifies a Double ALK Gene Fusion in a Patient Previously Identified to Be False-Negative by FISH*. J Thorac Oncol. 2017. doi:10.1016/j.jtho.2016.11.2229

[110] Pailler E, Adam J, Barthélémy A, et al. *Detection of circulating tumor cells harboring a unique ALK rearrangement in ALK-positive non–small-cell lung cancer.* J Clin Oncol. 2013. doi:10.1200/JCO.2012.44.5932

[111] Hu L, Ru K, Zhang L, et al. *Fluorescence in situ hybridization (FISH): An increasingly demanded tool for biomarker research and personalized medicine.* Biomark Res. 2014;2(1):1-13. doi:10.1186/2050-7771-2-3

[112] Sholl LM, Aisner DL, Varella-Garcia M, et al. *Multi-institutional oncogenic driver mutation analysis in lung adenocarcinoma: The lung cancer mutation consortium experience*. J Thorac Oncol. 2015. doi:10.1097/JTO.0000000000000516

[113] Kapeleris, J, Kulasinghe, A, Warkianai, ME et al *Ex vivo culture of Circulating tumor cells derived from non-small cell lung cancer* Trans Lung Cancer Res 2020; 9 (5):1795-1809 1Httpdx.doi.org/10.21037/tlcr-20-521

[114] Ilie, M.; Szafer-Glusman, E.; Hofman, V. et al. *Detection of pd-l1 in Circulating tumor cells and white blood cells from patients with advanced non-small-cell lung cancer.* Ann. Oncol. Off. J. Eur. Soc. Med. Oncol. 2018, *29*, 193-199

[115] Ribas A, Wolchok JD. *Cancer immunotherapy using checkpoint blockade.* Science *(80-)*. 2018. doi:10.1126/science.aar4060

[116] Alsaab HO, Sau S, Alzhrani R, et al. *PD-1 and PD-L1 checkpoint signaling inhibition for cancer immunotherapy: mechanism, combinations, and clinical outcome.* Front Pharmacol. 2017. doi:10.3389/fphar.2017.00561

[117] Lowery MA, Oreilly EM. *New approaches to the treatment of pancreatic cancer: From tumor-directed therapy to immunotherapy*. BioDrugs. 2011. doi:10.2165/11592470-000000000-00000

[118] Bastien JP, Minguy A, Dave V, et al. *Cellular therapy approaches harnessing the power of the immune system for personalized cancer treatment*. Semin Immunol. 2019. doi:10.1016/j.smim.2019.101306

[119] .Melosky B, Juergens R, Hirsh V, et al. *Amplifying Outcomes: Checkpoint Inhibitor Combinations in First-Line Non-Small Cell Lung Cancer*. Oncologist. 2020;25(1):64-77. doi:10.1634/theoncologist.2019-0027

[120] Janning M, Kobus F, Babayan A, et al. *Determination of PD-L1 expression in circulating tumor cells of NSCLC patients and correlation with response to PD-1/PD-L1 inhibitors*. Cancers (Basel). 2019;11(6):1-16. doi:10.3390/cancers11060835

[121] Schehr JL, Schultz ZD, Warrick JW, et al. *High specificity in circulating tumor cell identification is required for accurate evaluation of programmed death-ligand 1.* PLoS One. 2016. doi:10.1371/journal.pone.0159397

[122] Wang Y, Kim TH, Fouladdel S, et al. *PD-L1 Expression in Circulating Tumor Cells Increases during Radio(chemo)therapy and Indicates Poor Prognosis in Non-small Cell Lung Cancer*. Sci Rep. 2019.

[123] L. Zhang, X. Zhang, Y. Liu, T. Zhang, Z. Wang, M. Gu, Y. Li, D.D. Wang, W. Li, P.P. Lin (2020) *PD-L1+ aneuploid circulating tumor endothelial cells (CTECs) exhibit resistance to the checkpoint blockade immuno therapy in advanced NSCLC patients.* Cancer Lett 469:355-366 https://d oi.org/10.1016/J.CANLET.2019.10.041
Published: 2020-01

[124] Kloten,V, Lampignano, R, Krahn, T et al. *Circulating Tumor cell PD-L1 Expression as biomarker for therapeutic efficacy of immune checkpoint inhibition in NSCLC,* Cells,2019,8,809;doi:10.3390/cells8080809

Chapter 9

Current Advances in Clinical Application of Liquid Biopsy

Shawn Baldacchino

Abstract

Liquid biopsy solutions are available for niche clinical applications. The patient benefits of such solutions are evident: ease of sampling, acceptable and repeatable. To date a number of solutions have received regulatory approval with more comprehensive, multi-cancer companion diagnostic approaches receiving approval in late 2020. Given these breakthrough advances and the ongoing clinical studies in early detection of cancer, the liquid biopsy field is making strides in technology. While circulating tumour DNA (ctDNA) solutions are quickly penetrating the market, strides in circulating tumour cells (CTC) and extracellular vesicles (EV) technologies is unlocking their potential for liquid biopsy. ctDNA solutions are paving the way towards clinical translation into the distinct applications across the cancer continuum. This chapter presents a detailed review of current approved liquid biopsy tests and provides a summary of advanced-stage prospective technologies within the context of distinctive clinical applications.

Keywords: circulating tumour cells, CTC, extracellular vesicles, EV, cfDNA, ctDNA, methylation, liquid biopsy, cancer screening, precision medicine, companion diagnostics

1. Introduction

Precision medicine is driven by discoveries in cancer biology that enable targeted therapy against specific oncogenic molecular targets. Using small selective inhibitory molecules or monoclonal antibodies, therapies aim to effectively target tumour cells with minor effects on normal cells [1]. Targeted therapies significantly contribute to improved cancer survival, however the results have not been commensurate with expectations [2]. Tumours accumulate mutations, many of which are passenger or dispensable aberrations that can be bypassed to confer resistance. Malignant cells interact and exploit their immediate and distant microenvironment. Tumours exhibit clonal evolution that results in heterogeneity [3, 4]. Cancer is a cell disorder characterised not only by its genetics but transcriptomic, proteomic expression patterns and cellular interactions. This is driving an integrative approach to cancer diagnosis and therapeutic options [5–7].

Until recently, precision medicine was limited to the solid tissue space but is now becoming established in the liquid biopsy field with several approved solutions (**Tables 1** and **2**). The broad term, liquid biopsy, alludes to a test or series of tests that can provide information comparable and potentially beyond the limits of the tissue biopsy harnessing body fluid constituents. Body fluids investigated for liquid biopsy applications are comprehensive including but not limited to blood,

Single Cancer Indication						
Test (Manufacturer)	Technology	Biomarker	Cancer Type	Approval	Application	Sample
CellSearch® (Menarini Silocon Biosystems)	CTC immuno-isolation and detection by immune-fluorescence	CTC with CD45-, EpCAM+ and (CK8, 18 and/or 19)	Metastatic Breast, Colorectal, Prostate	FDA / CE-IVD	Prognostic	Blood
Cobas® EGFR mutation test V2 (Roche)	PCR	EGFR	NSCLC	FDA	CDx	Plasma
Therascreen (Qiagen)	PCR	• PIK3CA	• Breast	FDA / CE-IVD	CDx	Blood
		• KRAS	• CRC			
		• BRAF	• CRC			
		• EGFR	• NSCLC			
		• FGFR	• Urothelial			
Target Selector™ (Biocept) [8]	Switch-Blocker, qPCR, NGS	EGFR	NSCLC	CE-IVD	CDx	Blood / FFPE
OncoBEAM (Sysmex)	Digital PCR	KRAS & NRAS	mCRC	CE-IVD	CDx	Plasma
Idylla (Biocartis)	PCR	• KRAS	• mCRC	CE-IVD	CDx	Plasma
		• NRAS, BRAF	• mCRC			
HCCBlood Test (Epigenomics AG) [9]	Bisulfite converted DNA & PCR	SEPT9 methylation	HCC (patients with liver cirrhosis)	CE-IVD	Diagnostic aid	Plasma
Epi proColon® (Epigenomics AG) [10, 11]	Bisulfite converted DNA & PCR	SEPT9 methylation	CRC	FDA / CE-IVD	Ancillary Screening	Plasma
COLOGUARD (ExactSciences) [12]	QuARTS & Immunoassay	BMP3 & NDRG4 methylation, KRAS, ACTB Haemoglobin	CRC or advanced adenoma	FDA	Ancillary screening	Stool
IntPlex® (DiaDx) [13, 14]	PCR	• BRAF	• mCRC	CE-IVD	CDx	Plasma
		• EFGR	• mCRC			

Single Cancer Indication						
Xpert® Bladder Cancer Detection Xpert® Bladder Cancer Monitor (Cepheid) [15]	RT-PCR	UPK1B, IGF2, CRH, ANXA10, ABL1	Bladder (patients with haematuria) NMIBC	CE-IVD	Diagnostic aid Surveillance for recurrence	Urine
UroVysion (Abbott) [16]	FISH	Aneuploidy 3,7,17 and loss of 9p21 (p16)	Bladder (patients with haematuria)	FDA / CE-IVD	Diagnostic aid	Urine
Uromonitor (Uromonitor)	PCR	FGFR3 and TERT PCR	NMIBC (patients with haematuria)	CE-IVD	Diagnostic aid, Surveillance for recurrence	Urine
Epicheck (Nucleix) [17]	Methylation-sensitive restriction Enzyme digestion, PCR	15 DNA methylation markers	Bladder	CE-IVD	Surveillance for recurrence	Urine

Table provides a general overview and may not be exhaustive [CDx: Companion diagnostic; mCRC: metastatic colorectal carcinoma; CTC: Circulating tumour cells; ddPCR: droplet digital Polymerase chain reaction; FDA: Food & Drug Administration; FISH: Fluorescent in situ hybridisation; HCC: Hepatocellular carcinoma; CE-IVD: In vitro Diagnostic device certification; NMIBC: Non-muscle invasive bladder cancer; NSCLC: Non-small cell lung carcinoma; PCR: Polymerase chain reaction; QuARTS: Quantitative allele-specific real-time target and signal amplification; RT-PCR: reverse transcription PCR] [18, 19].

Table 1.
Overview of current approved (FDA/IVD) ctDNA liquid biopsy solutions for single cancer indications.

Pan-Cancer / Multi-cancer Indication						
Test (Manufacturer)	**Technology**	**Biomarker**	**Cancer Type**	**Approval**	**Application**	**Sample**
FoundationOne Liquid CDx (FoundationOne) [20]	NGS (324 genes)	• ALK, EGFR	• NSCLC	FDA	CDx	Plasma
		• BRCA1/2	• Ovarian			
		• BRCA1/2 & ATM	• Prostate			
		• PIK3CA	• Breast			
Guardant360 (Guardant Health) [21, 22]	NGS (73 genes)	• Tumour mutation profiling	• Any solid tumour	FDA	CDx	Plasma
		• EGFR	• NSCLC			

Table provides a general overview and may not be exhaustive. [CDx: Companion diagnostic; mCRC: metastatic colorectal carcinoma; FDA: Food & Drug Administration; NGS: Next-generation sequencing; NSCLC: Non-small cell lung carcinoma] [18, 19].

Table 2.
Overview of current approved (FDA/IVD) ctDNA liquid biopsy solutions indicated for use with 2 or more solid cancers.

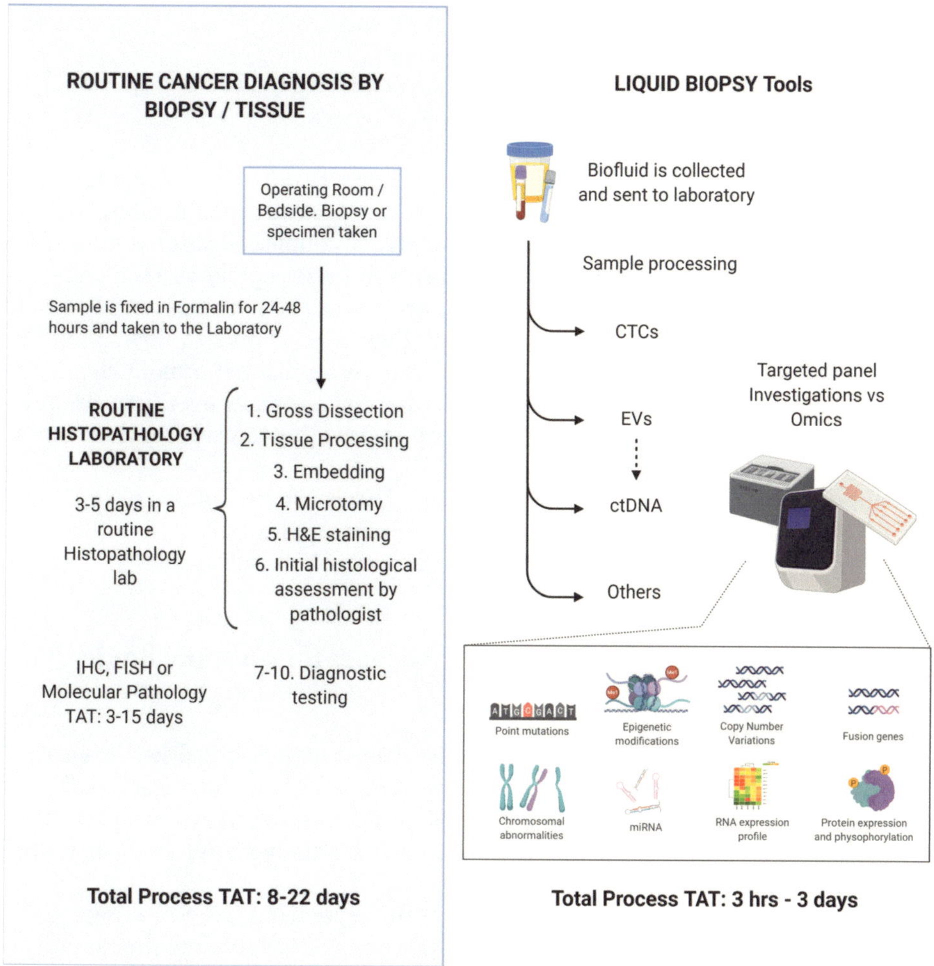

Figure 1.
Comparison of workflows of emerging liquid biopsy tools with routine cancer diagnostics by tissue biopsy. Liquid biopsy solutions remain complimentary to the clinical standard of care. [CTC: Circulating tumour cells; EVs: Extracellular vesicles; ctDNA: Circulating tumour DNA; FISH: Fluorescent in situ hybridisation; H&E: Haematoxylin and eosin; IHC: Immunohistochemistry; TAT: Turn-around time; created with BioRender.com].

urine [16], cerebrospinal fluid [23], stool [24], breast milk [25], saliva/sputum, oesophageal brushing, Pap smears/brushing [26], tears [27], pleural effusion [28] and ascitic fluid [29].

Liquid biopsy testing may encompass investigations of circulating tumour DNA (ctDNA) or cell-free DNA (cfDNA) and RNA (ctRNA), circulating tumour cells (CTCs), tumour-derived extracellular vesicles (EVs) and tumour-educated platelets [30]. Rapidly advancing technologies for immunoprofiling of leukocytes and T-cell receptor (TCR) profiling also present a potential liquid biopsy tool with a particular role in metastatic cancer patients for immunotherapy [31, 32].

The potential applications of liquid biopsy are numerous and throughout the cancer journey:

1. Cancer detection for screening or earlier detection [33, 34],

2. Diagnosis / Prognosis/Predictive (Companion Diagnostics, CDx) [30],

3. Therapeutic response monitoring (Detection of resistance mechanisms) [35, 36],

4. Minimal Residual Disease detection [37],

5. Post-remission surveillance to predict/detect relapse, metastases and clonal evolution [37, 38].

The main advantages of a liquid biopsy assay relate to the ease of sampling. Collecting the sample is generally not invasive and repeatable enabling longitudinal monitoring. The risk of complications and pain from sample collection is minimal presenting a very acceptable procedure that beckons better uptake as a screening procedure. Liquid biopsy methods are less laborious than tissue biopsy methods and can be analysed in a much shorter time-frame (**Figure 1**). Moreover, liquid biopsies offer an overall snapshot of the tumour which represents distinct tumour clones, mitigating tumour region selection bias [30]. Monitoring cancer over time also provides insight on the temporal heterogeneity, a potential tool to study mechanisms of response and resistance [32, 39].

Following is a review of the advances of liquid biopsy in the context of the current state of tissue molecular pathology for clinical application. A brief illustration of future prospects is also described based on ongoing clinical studies.

2. Molecular pathology: overcoming challenges for solid and liquid biopsy

Challenges to comprehensively characterise cancer in the clinical setting exist, relating to pre-analytical (sample collection & processing), analytical and post-analytical factors. Molecular pathology of solid cancer on formalin-fixed paraffin embedded (FFPE) tissue presents technical challenges arising from tissue fixation and processing but also sample availability.

A study evaluating factors for next-generation sequencing (NGS) testing failure showed that on average 22.5% of cases do not meet quality requirements. Insufficient tissue or insufficient DNA accounted for 62% and 29% of failures with 6% failing at library preparation [40]. The study highlights increased failure from fine needle aspirates and biopsy specimens with a low failure rate in excisional specimens (1.7%) [41]. Whole genome sequencing approaches show non-uniform coverage in FFPE DNA samples resulting in sub-optimal somatic copy number alteration detection. Nonetheless clinically actionable variants are generally detected [42]. Sensitive NGS applications require good quality DNA to achieve adequate assay performance and coverage. Recent developments in DNA extraction methods and optimisation improve assay performance [42, 43]. In fact NGS solutions have been achieving regulatory approval such like Oncomine Dx (ThermoFisher Scientific) for targeted therapies in non-small cell lung carcinoma (NSCLC) [44]; Praxis (Illumina) characterising 56 KRAS/NRAS mutations for colorectal cancer companion diagnostics (CDx); Memorial Sloan Kettering-Integrated Mutation Profiling of Actionable Cancer Targets (MSK-IMPACT), the first U.S. Food & Drug Administration (FDA) approved tissue profiling test that detecting aberrations across 341 cancer genes for solid cancer tissue diagnostics but not prescriptive for any specific therapeutic product [45]; and FoundationOne CDx which is the first FDA-approved broad CDx test that is clinically and analytically validated for all solid tumours for therapeutic indication and has a success rate of >95% on FFPE [46].

Targeted gene panels or single gene polymerase chain reaction (PCR) assays are more easily translated to clinical application given their very specific intended use. Recent advances can mitigate the effects of DNA fragmentation and PCR inhibition [47]. Technical challenges are greater for detection of RNA signatures due to high degree of RNA fragmentation and introduced technical bias [48]. A study assessing the performance of PCR on RNA derived from FFPE reports that only 50% (37/74) of samples were informative. RNA profiling on FFPE samples requires alternative technologies that can robustly detect degraded RNA with reduced technical bias [49–51].

Liquid biopsy options involve far less sample processing and better sample quality. Nonetheless tumour signatures are generally rare, similar to finding 'the needle in a haystack', and assays require high sensitivity to avoid false negative results. In the search for a sensitive, specific and reliable method, liquid biopsy technologies are becoming more diverse and complex [52–54]. Moreover, pre-analytical considerations are critical to ensure high sensitivity and reproducible performance. These requirements vary depending on the analysed liquid biopsy component. Expert recommendations for minimal requirements for clinical cfDNA testing have been published to emphasise the need for standardisation of the test processes [55].

3. Current state of liquid biopsy application

3.1 Liquid biopsy for companion diagnostics

A particular study of previously untreated metastatic non-small cell lung carcinoma (NSCLC) shows that cfDNA technologies have the potential to detect guideline-recommended biomarkers with a higher sensitivity compared to standard of care tissue genotyping methodology [22]. Currently, ctDNA assays are being recommended for use in lung patients with progression of secondary clinical resistance and in some clinical settings where tissue is limited or insufficient for molecular testing. ctDNA assays are not recommended for the diagnosis of primary lung tumours [56]. ctDNA liquid biopsy solutions are currently approved as additional tools to the standard of care and when results are negative, tissue testing is recommended when available. Lung cancer tissue is not easily available and sampling implies potential serious complications such as pneumothorax, haemorrhage and respiratory failure. Only 50% of cases in the MarkER Identification Trial (MERIT) trial had sufficient sample for the planned molecular analyses [40]. This presents a clinical need for liquid biopsy to potentially identify a route for targeted treatment.

Advanced-stage technologies within the liquid biopsy field harness ctDNA. These approaches mainly focus on hallmark mutations or other changes in the DNA (methylation). The first FDA approved ctDNA liquid biopsy was the cobas® EGFR mutation test V2 (Roche) as a companion diagnostic [57]. This was followed by several other targeted panel companion diagnostics (**Table 1**). The main available plasma liquid biopsy solutions detect mutations in clinically actionable biomarkers that predict response to specific targeted therapies. The main biomarkers detected are EGFR, FGFR, KRAS, NRAS, BRAF and PIK3CA.

Selected diagnostic panels are useful as companion diagnostics for clinical trials and patient selection for specific targeted therapeutics. Nonetheless, established targets would then be integrated into larger diagnostic panels that provide a comprehensive and exhaustive approach to cancer diagnostics. Recently the FDA approved the first two NGS-based liquid biopsy solutions: Guardant360 (August, 2020) and FoundationOne CDx (November 2020) (**Table 2**). Unlike PCR-based targeted panels, large NGS panel tests interrogate a large-set of genes generating more clinically useful information but present a challenge to validate and regulate [58]. Similar to tissue-based NGS approaches, generated clinical information assists the definition of a spectrum of potential therapeutic options to identify a sequence of treatments to achieve optimised response [59]. In contrast, to tissue biopsy molecular analysis, liquid biopsy solutions are expected to generate a collective picture of cancer heterogenous clones enabling a comprehensive therapeutic approach which may be key to avoid clonal residual disease or recurrence [60].

A recent study evaluated the post-progression ctDNA (Guardant360 assay) with matched multiple lesion biopsies to assess heterogeneity during acquired resistance [61]. This study reveals distinct mutational profiles across metastatic lesions of gastrointestinal origin. The majority of private alterations across lesions could be detected by cfDNA. In another study, combined analysis of solid (192 genes) and liquid biopsies (27 genes) (OncoSTRAT&GO™, OncoDNA, Gosselies, Belgium), only found 40% of variants to be shared between the solid and liquid biopsy, with 51% of variants being exclusive to tissue and 9% to blood [62]. The liquid exclusive variants increased to 14% after a year from tissue sampling reflecting temporal heterogeneity [62]. The disparity in mutation calling may be a result of distinct shedding rates across tumour stage and types or sensitivity of the ctDNA assay. Although further studies are needed, such studies suggest that liquid biopsy can complement tissue molecular pathology to improve the detection of clinically actionable aberrations to overcome spatial and temporal heterogeneity especially in late-stage disease.

3.2 Liquid biopsy for cancer detection

Similar to CDx assays, current solutions for primary cancer diagnosis are either ancillary solutions or to be used when the routine screening/diagnostic test is not an option. Thus, liquid biopsy approaches are currently another tool that assist and improve the overall performance of cancer detection. Approved liquid biopsy solutions for bladder cancer screening and colorectal cancer screening are available (**Table 1**) to support current screening methods. Evidently, when standard of care investigations are not available, liquid biopsy can provide means of detection. For instance, Epi proColon® (Epigenomics) is available only to patients who are unwilling or unable to be screened by recommended methods. This can potentially improve screening uptake with current colorectal cancer screening uptake reported between 53 and 61% [63–65]. The more acceptable, repeatable advantages of liquid biopsy enable multi-line testing or triage testing to select patients for further investigation, similar to the faecal immunochemical testing (FIT) to the colonoscopy procedure. Cologuard (ExactSciences) offers an approved stool molecular test for the detection of colorectal cancer with a reported increased sensitivity for detecting any stage CRC (92%) and 42% sensitivity for advanced precancerous lesions [12]. Specific cases presenting positive Cologuard test and negative follow-up colonoscopy raised concerns for lack of recommendations for patient management in these scenarios [66].

A first-line or triage test should be cost-effective, especially for screening purposes, to achieve a net cost–benefit. A recent health technology assessment evaluates EGFR T790M resistance mutation testing in patients with advanced NSCLC can lead to fewer tissue biopsies although a follow-up confirmatory tissue biopsy is required when liquid biopsy tests negative [67]. EGFR T790M mutation detection from urine has also been shown to be feasible for NSCLC patients to reduce biopsy procedures and mitigate biopsy related complications [68].

In a similar approach, the ExoDx Prostate test (ExosomeDx, a Bio-Techne brand), can be used to assess cancer risk in patients with elevated prostate specific antigen (PSA) to assist the decision to proceed or defer a prostate biopsy. ExoDx is the first exosome-based (RNA biomarkers) liquid biopsy solution to receive a Breakthrough Device Designation by the U.S. FDA [69]. Prostate cancer screening by PSA has highlighted the risks of over diagnosis and over treatment accompanied by a lack of tangible benefit [70, 71]. This created a need to better inform clinical decisions to follow-up with invasive diagnostic procedures and treatment and accentuates the need for sensitive tests that are also highly specific. Specific clinical applications require performance parameters that balance risk of non-detection with overtreatment depending on the backbone standard of care tests.

3.3 Liquid biopsy for prognosis and therapy intervention

CellSearch® (Menarini Silicon Biosystems), a CTC detection system, was the first liquid biopsy approach to be approved by FDA in 2004. The CellSearch technology immunomagnetically captures CTCs from whole blood, that express the Epithelial cell adhesion molecule (EpCAM) and enumerates CTCs with the profile of CD45 negative and cytokeratin 8, 18, and/or 19 positive [72]. The CellSearch system provides prognostic information for patients with metastatic breast, prostate or colorectal cancer. A major limitation of this method is the reliance on the EpCAM marker. CTCs have been described to be heterogeneous and not all CTCs express EpCAM. Such methods are restrictive to the epithelial phenotype and have intrinsic selection bias [73]. Label-free CTC enrichment solutions, such as Parsortix® (ANGLE) and ClearCell® FX1 system (Biolidics) are European CE marked as *in vitro* diagnostic device (CE-IVD) solutions for CTC enrichment but require downstream analysis to derive clinically relevant information. Moreover, isolated CTC remain viable and can potentially be cultured and studied further although finding optimal conditions for culturing CTC subtypes is challenging [74]. CTC enrichment by size discrimination shows a reduced recovery rate (~60%) for smaller sized cell lines (SKBR3) [75] presenting with a selective enrichment and failing to detect a subset of cells similarly to immunoisolation methods. CTC enrichment by depletion of leukocytes also results in reduced recovery [76]. Current advances in flow cytometry resolution and imaging may enable the suppression of pre-enrichment to enable a quick and efficient detection of CTC [77–79]. These approaches have a definite role in therapeutic monitoring, identifying treatment response and early resistance and are ready for clinical studies [80, 81].

ctDNA abundance, mutation count and a KEAP1, KRAS, MET signature predict overall survival in advanced NSCLC patients (N = 949). Interestingly, patients with at least one ctDNA clearance during the course of treatment had a significantly better progression-free survival and overall survival than patients with consistent ctDNA levels throughout treatment [82]. The prognosis and predictive potential of ctDNA is yet to be translated into practical clinical assays. While the potential role of EV in cancer prognosis has been shown [83], further studies are required to define EV isolation and prognostic correlations in larger patient cohorts.

4. Current outlook for early cancer detection

5-year survival rates for patients diagnosed with stage I and stage IV cancer respectively are 98% and 26% for breast cancer, 92% to 10% for colorectal cancer and 57% to 3% for lung cancer [84]. Earlier diagnosis would greatly improve cancer survivability but is currently a great challenge. Detecting cancer early is a cornerstone of the UK's NHS Long term plan. There have been numerous efforts to achieve early cancer screening, through public awareness (Be Clear on Cancer and Detect Cancer Early campaigns), introducing new screening tests (Bowel screening) and targeted lung health checks (following the NELSON trial) and many more.

Complex approaches, by GRAIL [85], Thrive's CancerSEEK [86], FoundationMedicine, Base Genomics, Freenome aim to expand the potential of early diagnosis from blood. Grail's Galleri, Thrive's CancerSEEK and Natera's Signatera have achieved FDA Breakthrough device status while in the trial stage. Early diagnosis remains a challenge with sensitivity being a critical factor. Achieving early diagnosis in the blood using ctDNA is more complex, mainly because there is a huge amount of "normal" DNA circulating in the blood. The smaller the cancer the smaller and less detectible the cancer signature is in the blood. As any cancer grows, it sheds more DNA, more cellular debris and more cancer cells into the bloodstream which eventually leads to the cancer spreading to distant organs. Although the ctDNA shedding rate can vary among patients, a mathematical model can predict tumour size by assessing haploid genome equivalents per plasma volume (correlation: $R^2 = 0.32$; $P = 2.6x10–^{16}$) [87]. The smaller the tumour, the higher the probability of a false negative result for a particular actionable mutation.

Till date there is no FDA-approved solution for early cancer detection from blood with targeted panel solutions available as ancillary diagnostics from stools for colorectal cancer (ColoGuard & Epi ProColon) and from urine for bladder cancer (Xpert Bladder Cancer detection & Uromonitor). Interestingly, a blood test detecting Septin 9 (SEPT9) methylation to aid the detection of hepatocellular carcinoma (HCC) in patients with cirrhosis, has been CE-IVD marked (HCCBloodTest by Epigenomics) [9].

Following are some illustrative examples of ongoing clinical studies investigating the application of liquid biopsy for multi-cancer detection.

4.1 CancerSEEK, PapSEEK, UroSEEK

A series of liquid biopsy tests for early diagnosis have been developed at the Johns Hopkins University: CancerSEEK, PapSEEK and UroSEEK.

CancerSEEK measures 8 protein biomarkers by immunoassays and mutations on 16 genes by PCR and sequencing in blood samples to detect and localise the cancer. A study of eight cancer types (colorectal, ovary, pancreas, breast, upper gastrointestinal tract, lung and liver) resulted in a median sensitivity of 70%, ranging from 33% in breast and 98% in ovarian cancer. Across stages of the disease the test was 43%, 73% and 78% sensitive respectively [86]. In a following prospective, interventional study (DETECT-A) CancerSEEK was coupled with positron emission tomography– computed tomography (PET-CT) for cancer detection. During this trial, the blood test sensitivity for all cancer types was 27.1% and specificity of 98.9%. Of note, 108 participants out of 10,006 in this study had a positive blood test without cancer, most of who (101) were followed up by PET-CT and 38 also had a subsequent procedure to rule out cancer [34]. This highlights the importance of the high specificity levels required for potential screening tests and clearly defined second-line testing with a good consideration of the risk of overtreatment.

PapSEEK was developed for Pap brush samples or Tao brush samples and detects aneuploidy and somatic mutations on 18 genes by multiplex-PCR (AKT1, APC, BRAF, CDKN2A, CTNNB1, EGFR, FBXW7, FGFR2, KRAS, MAPK1, NRAS, PIK3CA, PIK3R1, POLE, PPP2R1A, PTEN, RNF43, and TP53). 81% endometrial cancer and 29% ovarian cancer were detected by PapSEEK on Pap brush samples which increased to 93% and 45% respectively when intrauterine samples were collected using a Tao brush. False positive rate was 1.4% for Pap brush samples which improved to >99% specificity when using the Tao brush [88].

UroSEEK detects mutations within 11 genes (FGFR3, TP53, CDKN2A, ERBB2, HRAS, KRAS, PIK3CA, MET, VHL, MLL, TERT promoter) as well as aneuploidy. In an early detection cohort UroSEEK was 83% sensitive and 93% specific while in the surveillance cohort sensitivity was 71% and specificity 80% which was a significant improvement compared to cytology alone [89].

4.2 Galleri

Recently, the UK's National Health Service (NHS) has taken bold steps and will be partnering with GRAIL to confirm Galleri's clinical and economic performance in the NHS system [90]. The study will investigate the effectiveness of the Galleri test on 140,000 asymptomatic, healthy patients and 25,000 participants showing signs and symptoms of cancer. The Galleri test is a genome-wide test interrogating methylation patterns in plasma samples, optimised during the The Circulating Cell-free Genome Atlas Study (CCGA). Methylation patterns, measured by whole genome-bisulfite sequencing, were found to perform better than whole genome and targeted (507genes) sequencing for the detection of cancer [85]. A further study to evaluate the performance of the optimised method, included 6,689 participants with more than 50 cancer types which were approximately equally distributed across stage of the disease (I- IV). The test achieved 99.3% specificity and 55.2% sensitivity across all cancers in the validation sets. Sensitivity improved when detecting more advanced cancer, reporting a detection of 39% of Stage I cancer, 69% of Stage II cancer and 83–92% sensitivity in Stage III & IV cancer. Cancer detection performance varied across different cancer types [85].

Such clinical studies represent landmark studies that paving the way for clinical service to initiate the introduction of liquid biopsy technologies for cancer screening.

5. Potential for EVs and integrative solutions

Tumour derived extracellular vesicles (EV) show great potential for liquid biopsy. EVs carry protein, DNA, RNA and small-RNA cargo shielding it from degradation [33, 91]. The cargoes carried by EVs represents a molecular fingerprint of the cell of origin [30]. A study comparing cfDNA and EV DNA in pleural effusion for EGFR testing by qPCR, shows an improved detection rate when using EV DNA (72.2% vs. 61.1%) [28]. Moreover, research has described that 90% of prostate cancer ctDNA is found in large EVs [92]. EVs are released in abundant quantities presenting an intriguing solution for increase detection sensitivity [30]. TearExo® is a potential solution detecting EV diagnostic and prognostic markers from tears for diagnosis of breast cancer [27].

Despite these advantages, implementation of EVs into clinical cancer diagnostics is hampered by challenges and lack of standardisation in the isolation methods and analytical sensitivity [93]. With improved and standardised technologies and focused efforts, tumour EVs can potentially be used to selectively pick out tumour-derived DNA from a background of normal DNA enhancing ctDNA technology sensitivity but also enable analysis of DNA, RNA and protein from the same sample, potentially for yet earlier detection.

Several challenges remain to be elucidated. EV populations are diverse and the functions and contents of EVs across their size distribution is not well known. The shedding rates across different tumour types or disease states are cannot be assessed without a standardised and accurate method for sizing and specific size isolation. Several concerted efforts are leading the way to technical standardisation to robustly understand the role of EVs [93, 94].

Solutions that integrate multi-modal testing are budding, such as Epic Sciences' Comprehensive cancer profiling that performs CTC, ctDNA and immune-cell analysis from a single blood draw relying characterising protein, morphology and genomics. CancerSEEK integrates protein markers with ctDNA analysis. Such approaches may be key to unlock the full potential of liquid biopsies but present technical, workflow and interpretation challenges [95].

6. Conclusion

Liquid biopsy is currently a clinically useful tool for assisting companion diagnostics, cancer screening programmes and surveillance. There is an evident prevalence of ctDNA solutions which are already available for the companion diagnostic space and are expected to be accessing the earlier diagnostic space soon following clear delineation of the clinical value and applications. CTC solutions, the first approved liquid biopsy tool for clinical use, have a role in defining cancer prognosis and therapeutic monitoring for timely and effective therapeutic decisions. The clinical value and approach remain to be defined by further clinical studies and translation into practical, clinically applicable solutions.

The full potential of EVs is being uncovered with concerted efforts to establish rigour and standardisation driving reproducible research. Apart from the role of EVs for therapeutic applications, EVs show great potential for early diagnosis of cancer, therapeutic monitoring and post-therapeutic surveillance. Versatile and open technologies could facilitate integrated solutions to maximise the potential of liquid biopsy. Nonetheless, translation to the clinical setting will require practical solutions with clearly defined clinical applications.

Promising data is emerging across potential applications for liquid biopsy with multi-cancer early detection solutions expected in the near future.

Author details

Shawn Baldacchino
Applied Biotech Ltd, Cambridge, UK

*Address all correspondence to: shawn.baldacchino@appliedbiotechltd.com; shawn.baldacchino@gmail.com

References

[1] Falzone L, Salomone S, Libra M. Evolution of cancer pharmacological treatments at the turn of the third millennium. Front Pharmacol. 2018;9(November 2018):1300.

[2] Tu SM, Bilen MA, Tannir NM. Personalised cancer care: promises and challenges of targeted therapy. J R Soc Med. 2016;109(3):98-105.

[3] Bremnes RM, Dønnem T, Al-Saad S, Al-Shibli K, Andersen S, Sirera R, et al. The role of tumor stroma in cancer progression and prognosis: Emphasis on carcinoma-associated fibroblasts and non-small cell lung cancer. J Thorac Oncol [Internet]. 2011;6(1):209-17. Available from: http://dx.doi.org/10.1097/JTO.0b013e3181f8a1bd

[4] Liu Q, Zhang H, Jiang X, Qian C, Liu Z, Luo D. Factors involved in cancer metastasis: a better understanding to "seed and soil" hypothesis. Mol Cancer [Internet]. 2017 Dec;16(1):176. Available from: http://www.ncbi.nlm.nih.gov/pubmed/29197379

[5] Lopez JS, Banerji U. Combine and conquer: Challenges for targeted therapy combinations in early phase trials. Nat Rev Clin Oncol. 2017;14(1):57-66.

[6] Green S. Cancer beyond genetics: On the practical implications of downward causation [Internet]. 2019. Available from: http://philsci-archive.pitt.edu/16297/

[7] Sandoval GJ, Hahn WC. Going beyond genetics to discover cancer targets. Genome Biol. 2017;18(1):17-9.

[8] Poole JC, Wu SF, Lu TT, Vibat CRT, Pham A, Samuelsz E, et al. Analytical validation of the Target Selector ctDNA platform featuring single copy detection sensitivity for clinically actionable EGFR, BRAF, and KRAS mutations. PLoS One. 2019;14(10):1-22.

[9] Oussalah A, Rischer S, Bensenane M, Conroy G, Filhine-Tresarrieu P, Debard R, et al. Plasma mSEPT9: A Novel Circulating Cell-free DNA-Based Epigenetic Biomarker to Diagnose Hepatocellular Carcinoma. EBioMedicine [Internet]. 2018;30:138-47. Available from: https://doi.org/10.1016/j.ebiom.2018.03.029

[10] Warren JD, Xiong W, Bunker AM, Vaughn CP, Furtado L V., Roberts WL, et al. Septin 9 methylated DNA is a sensitive and specific blood test for colorectal cancer. BMC Med [Internet]. 2011;9(1):133. Available from: https://doi.org/10.1186/1741-7015-9-133

[11] Lamb YN, Dhillon S. Epi proColon® 2.0 CE: A Blood-Based Screening Test for Colorectal Cancer. Mol Diagnosis Ther. 2017;21(2):225-32.

[12] Imperiale TF, Ransohoff DF, Itzkowitz SH, Levin TR, Lavin P, Lidgard GP, et al. Multitarget Stool DNA Testing for Colorectal-Cancer Screening. N Engl J Med. 2014;370(14):1287-97.

[13] Thierry AR. A targeted Q-PCR-based method for point mutation testing by analyzing circulating DNA for cancer management care. Methods Mol Biol. 2016;1392:1-16.

[14] DiaDx | Liquid Biopsy For Personalized Medecine In Oncology [Internet]. [cited 2021 Jan 12]. Available from: https://diadx.com/

[15] Pichler R, Fritz J, Tulchiner G, Klinglmair G, Soleiman A, Horninger W, et al. Increased accuracy of a novel mRNA-based urine test for bladder cancer surveillance. BJU Int [Internet]. 2018 Jan 1 [cited 2021 Jan 12];121(1):29-37. Available from: http://doi.wiley.com/10.1111/bju.14019

[16] Batista R, Vinagre N, Meireles S, Vinagre J, Prazeres H, Leão R, et al.

Biomarkers for bladder cancer diagnosis and surveillance: A comprehensive review. Diagnostics. 2020;10(1):1-19.

[17] Witjes JA, Morote J, Cornel EB, Gakis G, van Valenberg FJP, Lozano F, et al. Performance of the Bladder EpiCheck™ Methylation Test for Patients Under Surveillance for Non–muscle-invasive Bladder Cancer: Results of a Multicenter, Prospective, Blinded Clinical Trial. Eur Urol Oncol [Internet]. 2018;1(4):307-13. Available from: https://doi.org/10.1016/j.euo.2018.06.011

[18] De Richter P. Conquering Complexity : The Coming Revolution in Oncology Biomarker Testing [Internet]. 2017 [cited 2021 Jan 10]. Available from: https://www.ipsos.com/sites/default/files/2017-06/Ipsos_Healthcare_Conquering_Complexity_June_2017.pdf

[19] List of Cleared or Approved Companion Diagnostic Devices (In Vitro and Imaging Tools) | FDA [Internet]. [cited 2021 Jan 11]. Available from: https://www.fda.gov/medical-devices/vitro-diagnostics/list-cleared-or-approved-companion-diagnostic-devices-vitro-and-imaging-tools

[20] FDA approves liquid biopsy NGS companion diagnostic test for multiple cancers and biomarkers | FDA [Internet]. [cited 2021 Jan 11]. Available from: https://www.fda.gov/drugs/fda-approves-liquid-biopsy-ngs-companion-diagnostic-test-multiple-cancers-and-biomarkers

[21] FDA Approves First Liquid Biopsy Next-Generation Sequencing Companion Diagnostic Test | FDA [Internet]. [cited 2021 Jan 11]. Available from: https://www.fda.gov/news-events/press-announcements/fda-approves-first-liquid-biopsy-next-generation-sequencing-companion-diagnostic-test

[22] Leighl NB, Page RD, Raymond VM, Daniel DB, Divers SG, Reckamp KL, et al. Clinical Utility of Comprehensive Cell-free DNA Analysis to Identify Genomic Biomarkers in Patients with Newly Diagnosed Metastatic Non–small Cell Lung Cancer. Clin Cancer Res. 2019;25(15):4691-700.

[23] De Mattos-Arruda L, Mayor R, Ng CKY, Weigelt B, Martínez-Ricarte F, Torrejon D, et al. Cerebrospinal fluid-derived circulating tumour DNA better represents the genomic alterations of brain tumours than plasma. Nat Commun. 2015;6:1-6.

[24] Robertson DJ, Imperiale TF. Stool Testing for Colorectal Cancer Screening. Gastroenterology [Internet]. 2015;149(5):1286-93. Available from: http://www.sciencedirect.com/science/article/pii/S0016508515007726

[25] Halvaei S, Daryani S, Eslami-S Z, Samadi T, Jafarbeik-Iravani N, Bakhshayesh TO, et al. Exosomes in Cancer Liquid Biopsy: A Focus on Breast Cancer. Vol. 10, Molecular Therapy - Nucleic Acids. 2018. p. 131-41.

[26] Wan JCM, Massie C, Garcia-Corbacho J, Mouliere F, Brenton JD, Caldas C, et al. Liquid biopsies come of age: Towards implementation of circulating tumour DNA. Nat Rev Cancer. 2017;17(4):223-38.

[27] Takeuchi T, Mori K, Sunayama H, Takano E, Kitayama Y, Shimizu T, et al. Antibody-Conjugated Signaling Nanocavities Fabricated by Dynamic Molding for Detecting Cancers Using Small Extracellular Vesicle Markers from Tears. J Am Chem Soc. 2020;142(14):6617-24.

[28] Lee JS, Hur JY, Kim IA, Kim HJ, Choi CM, Lee JC, et al. Liquid biopsy using the supernatant of a pleural effusion for EGFR genotyping in pulmonary adenocarcinoma patients: A comparison between cell-free DNA and extracellular vesicle-derived DNA. BMC Cancer. 2018;18(1):1-8.

[29] Villatoro S, Mayo-de-Las-Casas C, Jordana-Ariza N, Viteri-Ramírez S, Garzón-Ibañez M, Moya-Horno I, et al. Prospective detection of mutations in cerebrospinal fluid, pleural effusion, and ascites of advanced cancer patients to guide treatment decisions. Mol Oncol [Internet]. 2019/10/11. 2019 Dec;13(12):2633-45. Available from: https://pubmed.ncbi.nlm.nih.gov/31529604

[30] De Rubis G, Rajeev Krishnan S, Bebawy M. Liquid Biopsies in Cancer Diagnosis, Monitoring, and Prognosis. Trends Pharmacol Sci [Internet]. 2019;40(3):172-86. Available from: https://doi.org/10.1016/j.tips.2019.01.006

[31] Hofman P, Heeke S, Alix-Panabières C, Pantel K. Liquid biopsy in the era of immuno-oncology: Is it ready for prime-time use for cancer patients? Ann Oncol. 2019;30(9):1448-59.

[32] Russano M, Napolitano A, Ribelli G, Iuliani M, Simonetti S, Citarella F, et al. Liquid biopsy and tumor heterogeneity in metastatic solid tumors: The potentiality of blood samples. J Exp Clin Cancer Res. 2020;39(1):1-13.

[33] Brock G, Castellanos-Rizaldos E, Hu L, Coticchia C, Skog J. Liquid biopsy for cancer screening, patient stratification and monitoring. Transl Cancer Res. 2015;4(3):280-90.

[34] Lennon AM, Buchanan AH, Kinde I, Warren A, Honushefsky A, Cohain AT, et al. Feasibility of blood testing combined with PET-CT to screen for cancer and guide intervention. Science. 2020;369(6499):eabb9601.

[35] Pasini L, Ulivi P. Liquid Biopsy for the Detection of Resistance Mechanisms in NSCLC: Comparison of Different Blood Biomarkers. J Clin Med. 2019;8(7):998.

[36] Ulz P, Heitzer E, Geigl JB, Speicher MR. Patient monitoring through liquid biopsies using circulating tumor DNA. Int J Cancer. 2017;141(5):887-96.

[37] Pantel K, Alix-Panabières C. Liquid biopsy and minimal residual disease — latest advances and implications for cure. Nat Rev Clin Oncol [Internet]. 2019;16(7):409-24. Available from: http://dx.doi.org/10.1038/s41571-019-0187-3

[38] Vacante M, Ciuni R, Basile F, Biondi A. The liquid biopsy in the management of colorectal cancer: An overview. Biomedicines. 2020;8(9):308.

[39] Venesio T, Siravegna G, Bardelli A, Sapino A. Liquid Biopsies for Monitoring Temporal Genomic Heterogeneity in Breast and Colon Cancers. Pathobiology. 2018;85(1-2):146-54.

[40] Reck M, Hermes A, Tan EH, Felip E, Klughammer B, Baselga J. Tissue sampling in lung cancer: A review in light of the MERIT experience. Lung Cancer [Internet]. 2011;74(1):1-6. Available from: http://dx.doi.org/10.1016/j.lungcan.2011.05.002

[41] Al-Kateb H, Nguyen TDT, Steger-May K, Pfeifer JD. Identification of major factors associated with failed clinical molecular oncology testing performed by next generation sequencing (NGS). Mol Oncol. 2015;9(9):1737-43.

[42] Robbe P, Popitsch N, Knight SJL, Antoniou P, Becq J, He M, et al. Clinical whole-genome sequencing from routine formalin-fixed, paraffin-embedded specimens: pilot study for the 100,000 Genomes Project. Genet Med. 2018;20(10):1196-205.

[43] McDonough SJ, Bhagwate A, Sun Z, Wang C, Zschunke M, Gorman JA,

et al. Use of FFPE-Derived DNA in Next Generation Sequencing: DNA extraction methods. PLoS One. 2019;14(4):e0211400.

[44] Nucleic Acid Based Tests | FDA [Internet]. [cited 2021 Jan 10]. Available from: https://www.fda.gov/medical-devices/vitro-diagnostics/nucleic-acid-based-tests

[45] Cheng DT, Mitchell TN, Zehir A, Shah RH, Benayed R, Syed A, et al. Memorial sloan kettering-integrated mutation profiling of actionable cancer targets (MSK-IMPACT): A hybridization capture-based next-generation sequencing clinical assay for solid tumor molecular oncology. J Mol Diagnostics [Internet]. 2015;17(3):251-64. Available from: http://dx.doi.org/10.1016/j.jmoldx.2014.12.006

[46] Takeda M, Takahama T, Sakai K, Shimizu S, Watanabe S, Kawakami H, et al. Clinical Application of the FoundationOne CDx Assay to Therapeutic Decision-Making for Patients with Advanced Solid Tumors. Oncologist [Internet]. 2020 Dec 16;n/a(n/a):1-9. Available from: https://doi.org/10.1002/onco.13639

[47] Dietrich D, Uhl B, Sailer V, Holmes EE, Jung M, Meller S, et al. Improved PCR Performance Using Template DNA from Formalin-Fixed and Paraffin-Embedded Tissues by Overcoming PCR Inhibition. PLoS One. 2013;8(10):1-10.

[48] Minshall N, Git A. Enzyme- and gene-specific biases in reverse transcription of RNA raise concerns for evaluating gene expression. Sci Rep. 2020;10(1):1-7.

[49] Baldacchino S, Saliba C, Scerri J, Scerri C, Grech G. Optimization of a Multiplex RNA-based Expression Assay Using Breast Cancer Archival Material. JoVE [Internet]. 2018;(138):e57148. Available from: https://www.jove.com/t/57148

[50] Knudsen BS, Allen AN, McLerran DF, Vessella RL, Karademos J, Davies JE, et al. Evaluation of the branched-chain DNA assay for measurement of RNA in formalin-fixed tissues. J Mol Diagnostics [Internet]. 2008;10(2):169-76. Available from: http://dx.doi.org/10.2353/jmoldx.2008.070127

[51] Veldman-Jones MH, Brant R, Rooney C, Geh C, Emery H, Harbron CG, et al. Evaluating robustness and sensitivity of the nanostring technologies ncounter platform to enable multiplexed gene expression analysis of clinical samples. Cancer Res. 2015;75(13):2587-93.

[52] Campos CDM, Jackson JM, Witek MA, Soper SA. Molecular Profiling of Liquid Biopsy Samples for Precision Medicine. Cancer J (United States). 2018;24(2):93-103.

[53] Jia Y, Ni Z, Sun HAO, Wang C. Microfluidic Approaches Toward the Isolation and Detection of Exosome Nanovesicles. IEEE Access. 2019;7:45080-98.

[54] Ferreira MM, Ramani VC, Jeffrey SS. Circulating tumor cell technologies. Mol Oncol [Internet]. 2016;10(3):374-94. Available from: http://dx.doi.org/10.1016/j.molonc.2016.01.007

[55] Deans ZC, Butler R, Cheetham M, Dequeker EMC, Fairley JA, Fenizia F, et al. IQN path ASBL report from the first European cfDNA consensus meeting: expert opinion on the minimal requirements for clinical ctDNA testing. Virchows Arch. 2019;474(6):681-9.

[56] Lindeman NI, Cagle PT, Aisner DL, Arcila ME, Beasley MB, Bernicker EH, et al. Updated Molecular Testing Guideline for the Selection of Lung

Cancer Patients for Treatment With Targeted Tyrosine Kinase Inhibitors: Guideline From the College of American Pathologists, the International Association for the Study of Lung Cancer. J Thorac Oncol [Internet]. 2018 Mar;13(3):323-58. Available from: https://doi.org/10.1016/j.jtho.2017.12.001

[57] Kwapisz D. The first liquid biopsy test approved. Is it a new era of mutation testing for non-small cell lung cancer? Ann Transl Med. 2017;5(3):1-7.

[58] U.S. Food and Drug Administration. Optimizing FDA's Regulatory Oversight of Next Generation Sequencing Diagnostic Tests—Preliminary Discussion Paper [Internet]. Vol. 3. 2015. Available from: https://www.fda.gov/media/90403/download

[59] Allegretti M, Fabi A, Buglioni S, Martayan A, Conti L, Pescarmona E, et al. Tearing down the walls: FDA approves next generation sequencing (NGS) assays for actionable cancer genomic aberrations. J Exp Clin Cancer Res. 2018;37(1):1-3.

[60] Walens A, Lin J, Damrauer JS, McKinney B, Lupo R, Newcomb R, et al. Adaptation and selection shape clonal evolution of tumors during residual disease and recurrence. Nat Commun [Internet]. 2020;11(1):1-15. Available from: http://dx.doi.org/10.1038/s41467-020-18730-z

[61] Parikh AR, Leshchiner I, Elagina L, Goyal L, Levovitz C, Siravegna G, et al. Liquid versus tissue biopsy for detecting acquired resistance and tumor heterogeneity in gastrointestinal cancers. Nat Med [Internet]. 2019;25(9):1415-21. Available from: http://dx.doi.org/10.1038/s41591-019-0561-9

[62] Finzel A, Sadik H, Ghitti G, Laes J-F. The combined analysis of solid and liquid biopsies provides additional clinical information to improve patient care. J Cancer Metastasis Treat. 2018;4(5):21.

[63] Jones RM, Devers KJ, Kuzel AJ, Woolf SH. Patient-Reported Barriers to Colorectal Cancer Screening. A Mixed-Methods Analysis. Am J Prev Med. 2010;38(5):508-16.

[64] Fraser CG, Digby J, McDonald PJ, Strachan JA, Carey FA, Steele RJC. Experience with a two-tier reflex gFOBT/FIT strategy in a national bowel screening programme. J Med Screen. 2012;19(1):8-13.

[65] Steele RJ, McDonald PJ, Digby J, Brownlee L, Strachan JA, Libby G, et al. Clinical outcomes using a faecal immunochemical test for haemoglobin as a first-line test in a national programme constrained by colonoscopy capacity. United Eur Gastroenterol J. 2013;1(3):198-205.

[66] Mulat B, Boroda K, Hertan H. 1673 Multitarget Stool DNA Test (Cologuard™): A Double-Edged Sword. Am J Gastroenterol | ACG [Internet]. 2019;114(p S935-S936). Available from: https://journals.lww.com/ajg/Fulltext/2019/10001/1673_Multitarget_Stool_DNA_Test__Cologuard____A.1674.aspx

[67] (Quality) OH. Cell-Free Circulating Tumour DNA Blood Testing to Detect EGFR T790M Mutation in People With Advanced Non-Small Cell Lung Cancer: A Health Technology Assessment. Ont Health Technol Assess Ser [Internet]. 2020 Mar 6;20(5):1-176. Available from: https://pubmed.ncbi.nlm.nih.gov/32206157

[68] Sands J, Li Q, Hornberger J. Urine circulating-tumor DNA (ctDNA) detection of acquired EGFR T790M mutation in non-small-cell lung cancer: An outcomes and total cost-of-care analysis. Lung Cancer [Internet]. 2017;110(November 2016):19-25.

Available from: http://dx.doi.org/10.1016/j.lungcan.2017.05.014

[69] Tutrone R, Donovan MJ, Torkler P, Tadigotla V, McLain T, Noerholm M, et al. Clinical utility of the exosome based ExoDx Prostate(IntelliScore) EPI test in men presenting for initial Biopsy with a PSA 2-10 ng/mL. Prostate Cancer Prostatic Dis [Internet]. 2020;23(4):607-14. Available from: http://dx.doi.org/10.1038/s41391-020-0237-z

[70] Pinsky PF, Prorok PC, Kramer BS. Prostate Cancer Screening — A Perspective on the Current State of the Evidence. N Engl J Med. 2017;376(13): 1285-9.

[71] Ilic D, Neuberger MM, Djulbegovic M, Dahm P. Screening for prostate cancer. Cochrane Database Syst Rev [Internet]. 2013 Jan 31 [cited 2021 Jan 14];2013(1). Available from: https://pubmed.ncbi.nlm.nih.gov/23440794/

[72] Miller MC, Doyle G V., Terstappen LWMM. Significance of Circulating Tumor Cells Detected by the CellSearch System in Patients with Metastatic Breast Colorectal and Prostate Cancer. J Oncol. 2010;2010:1-8.

[73] Wang L, Balasubramanian P, Chen AP, Kummar S, Evrard YA, Kinders RJ. Promise and limits of the CellSearch platform for evaluating pharmacodynamics in circulating tumor cells. Semin Oncol [Internet]. 2016;43(4):464-75. Available from: http://www.ncbi.nlm.nih.gov/pubmed/27663478

[74] Guo T, Wang CS, Wang W, Lu Y. Culture of Circulating Tumor Cells - Holy Grail and Big Challenge. Int J Cancer Clin Res. 2016;3(4):065.

[75] Takahashi Y, Shirai K, Ijiri Y, Morita E, Yoshida T, Iwanaga S, et al. Integrated system for detection and molecular characterization of circulating tumor cells. Patel GK, editor. PLoS One [Internet]. 2020 Aug 13 [cited 2021 Jan 16];15(8):e0237506. Available from: https://dx.plos.org/10.1371/journal.pone.0237506

[76] Xu Y, Liu B, Ding F, Zhou X, Tu P, Yu B, et al. Circulating tumor cell detection: A direct comparison between negative and unbiased enrichment in lung cancer. Oncol Lett. 2017;13(6):4882-6.

[77] Liu Z, Guo W, Zhang D, Pang Y, Shi J, Wan S, et al. Circulating tumor cell detection in hepatocellular carcinoma based on karyoplasmic ratios using imaging flow cytometry. Sci Rep. 2016;6(December):6-15.

[78] Lopresti A, Malergue F, Bertucci F, Liberatoscioli ML, Garnier S, DaCosta Q, et al. Sensitive and easy screening for circulating tumor cells by flow cytometry. JCI Insight. 2019;4(14):1-14.

[79] Dent BM, Ogle LF, O'donnell RL, Hayes N, Malik U, Curtin NJ, et al. High-resolution imaging for the detection and characterisation of circulating tumour cells from patients with oesophageal, hepatocellular, thyroid and ovarian cancers. Int J Cancer. 2016;138(1):206-16.

[80] Krause S, Friedl T, Romashova T, Fasching P, Schneeweiss A, Müller V, et al. Abstract OT1-10-01: DETECT III/IV study trial – The multicenter study program in patients with HER2-negative metastatic breast cancer and circulating tumor cells. In: Cancer Research [Internet]. American Association for Cancer Research (AACR); 2019 [cited 2021 Jan 16]. p. OT1-10-01-OT1-10-01. Available from: https://cancerres.aacrjournals.org/content/79/4_Supplement/OT1-10-01

[81] Stoecklein NH, Fischer JC, Niederacher D, Terstappen LWMM. Challenges for CTC-based liquid biopsies: low CTC frequency and

diagnostic leukapheresis as a potential solution. Expert Rev Mol Diagn [Internet]. 2016 Feb 1;16(2):147-64. Available from: https://doi.org/10.1586/14737159.2016.1123095

[82] Song Y, Hu C, Xie Z, Wu L, Zhu Z, Rao C, et al. Circulating tumor DNA clearance predicts prognosis across treatment regimen in a large real-world longitudinally monitored advanced non-small cell lung cancer cohort. Transl Lung Cancer Res. 2020;9(2):269-79.

[83] Verma M, Lam TK, Hebert E, Divi RL. Extracellular vesicles: Potential applications in cancer diagnosis, prognosis, and epidemiology. BMC Clin Pathol. 2015;15(1):1-9.

[84] ONS. Cancer survival in England - Office for National Statistics [Internet]. Office for national statistics. 2019 [cited 2021 Jan 14]. Available from: https://www.ons.gov.uk/peoplepopulationandcommunity/healthandsocialcare/conditionsanddiseases/datasets/cancersurvivalratescancersurvivalinenglandadultsdiagnosed

[85] Liu MC, Oxnard GR, Klein EA, Swanton C, Seiden M V., Liu MC, et al. Sensitive and specific multi-cancer detection and localization using methylation signatures in cell-free DNA. Ann Oncol. 2020;31(6):745-59.

[86] Cohen JD, Li L, Wang Y, Thoburn C, Afsari B, Danilova L, et al. Detection and localization of surgically resectable cancers with a multi-analyte blood test. Science [Internet]. 2018/01/18. 2018 Feb 23;359(6378):926-30. Available from: https://pubmed.ncbi.nlm.nih.gov/29348365

[87] Avanzini S, Kurtz DM, Chabon JJ, Moding EJ, Hori SS, Gambhir SS, et al. A mathematical model of ctDNA shedding predicts tumor detection size. Sci Adv [Internet]. 2020 Dec 1;6(December):1-10. Available from: http://advances.sciencemag.org/content/6/50/eabc4308.abstract

[88] Wang Y, Li L, Douville C, Cohen JD, Yen TT, Kinde I, et al. Evaluation of liquid from the papanicolaou test and other liquid biopsies for the detection of endometrial and ovarian cancers. Obstet Gynecol Surv. 2018;73(8):463-4.

[89] Springer SU, Chen C-H, Rodriguez Pena MDC, Li L, Douville C, Wang Y, et al. Non-invasive detection of urothelial cancer through the analysis of driver gene mutations and aneuploidy. Elife [Internet]. 2018 Mar 20;7:e32143. Available from: https://doi.org/10.7554/eLife.32143

[90] GRAIL and UK Government to Make Galleri Multi-Cancer Early Detection Blood Test Available to Patients | GRAIL [Internet]. [cited 2021 Jan 15]. Available from: https://grail.com/press-releases/grail-and-uk-government-to-make-galleri-multi-cancer-early-detection-blood-test-available-to-patients/

[91] Fleischhacker M, Schmidt B. Circulating nucleic acids (CNAs) and cancer—A survey. Biochim Biophys Acta - Rev Cancer [Internet]. 2007;1775(1):181-232. Available from: http://www.sciencedirect.com/science/article/pii/S0304419X0600059X

[92] Vagner T, Spinelli C, Minciacchi VR, Balaj L, Zandian M, Conley A, et al. Large extracellular vesicles carry most of the tumour DNA circulating in prostate cancer patient plasma. J Extracell vesicles [Internet]. 2018 Aug 7;7(1):1505403. Available from: https://doi.org/10.1080/20013078.2018.1505403

[93] Théry C, Witwer KW, Aikawa E, Alcaraz MJMJ, Anderson JDJD, Andriantsitohaina R, et al. Minimal information for studies of extracellular vesicles 2018 (MISEV2018): a position statement

of the International Society for Extracellular Vesicles and update of the MISEV2014 guidelines. J Extracell Vesicles. 2018;7(1):1535750.

[94] Geeurickx E, Lippens L, Rappu P, De Geest BG, De Wever O, Hendrix A. Recombinant extracellular vesicles as biological reference material for method development, data normalization and assessment of (pre-)analytical variables. Nat Protoc [Internet]. 2021; Available from: https://doi.org/10.1038/s41596-020-00446-5

[95] Qiu J, Xu J, Zhang K, Gu W, Nie L, Wang G, et al. Refining cancer management using integrated liquid biopsy. Theranostics. 2020;10(5):2374-84.

Section 5

Pathophysiology

Chapter 10

Dopamine: The Amazing Molecule

Mehveş Ece Genç and Emine Nur Özdamar

Abstract

Dopamine (DA) is a neurotransmitter in the central nervous system (CNS) and has been implicated in the pathogenesis of various diseases of motor functions and psychiatric conditions. Dopamine is also the key modulator for motivational behavior and brain reward system and regulates food intake as well. It has some neuroendocrine function too. It is noteworthy that dopamine has so many diverse roles in the CNS. DA has various pathways such as the Nigrostriatal pathway, Mesolimbic pathway, Mesocortical pathway and Tuberohypophyseal pathway. It has D1, D2, D3, D4 and D5 metabotropic receptors and interacts with cholinergic, GABAergic, opioidergic and glutamatergic systems. DA also activates diverse second messengers and pathways. These complicated interactions partly explain its diverse actions. The aim of the present chapter is to summarize data on the contribution of DA in the pathogenesis of many conditions such as Parkinson's disease, Schizophrenia, Attention Deficit Hyperactivity Disorder and addiction.

Keywords: dopamine, Parkinson's disease, Attention deficit hyperactivity disorder, valproic acid

1. Introduction

Dopamine is a neurotransmitter both in the periphery and in the central nervous system. It is synthesized from the amino acid tyrosine. Tyrosine is first hydroxylated by the rate limiting enzyme tyrosine hydroxylase to Levodopa (L-DOPA) and L-DOPA is further converted to Dopamine with the action of L-Amino acid decarboxylase.

2. Dopamine and Parkinson's disease

Parkinson's disease (PD) is a neurodegenerative disorder characterized by progressive loss of dopamine (DA) neurons in substantia nigra pars compacta. According to the epidemiological studies cigarette smoking, coffee, anti-inflammatory agents and high serum uric acid are protective against PD. Teaching staff, medical personnel, people who work in farms, people who are exposed to lead or manganese and people who are deficient of vitamin D have increased risk of getting the disease [1].

There is a prodromal phase in PD before the disease fully develops. Hyposmia and constipation appear first, then depression follows, and finally the motor symptoms become evident such as bradykinesia (slowness of movement), tremor (involuntary shaking, most commonly of the hands) and rigidity (stiff or inflexible muscles), [2]. The cardinal features of PD are summarized in **Figure 1**.

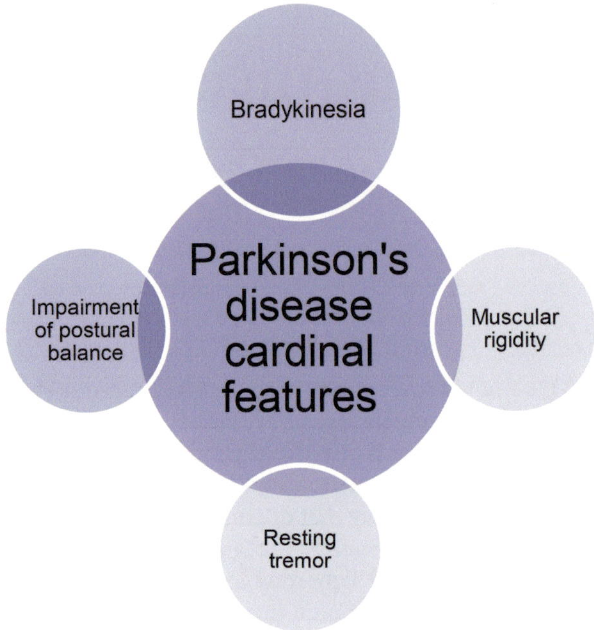

Figure 1.
Cardinal features of Parkinson's disease.

3. Incidence and prevalence of Parkinson's disease

The prevalence and incidence of PD may differ depending on various determinants such as age and gender [3]. A higher incidence of PD were reported in males than females with a ratio ranging between 1.37 to 3.7 [4]. Several studies reported that the prevalence and incidence of PD rises with age [5], with a prevalence rate of 108–257 per 100.000 persons and incidence rate of 11–19 per 100.000 persons [6].

4. Features of Parkinson's disease

Hyposmia is an important feature of Parkinson's disease and might be a significant and valuable sign to take some precautions. As well known olfactory function declines as people age and might have detrimental effects in those people [7].

Dopamine is part of the neuronal system in olfactory system. Gamma Aminobutyric Acid (GABA), Acetylcholine and norepinephrine have been the other transmitters [7].

More recently α-synuclein (α-syn) overexpression in olfactory bulb has been observed and it was related to symptoms and pathology of Parkinson's disease [8]. Scientists developed methods to detect protein aggregation by nasal brushing as a guidance to early diagnosis [9]. Nasal brushing is a non-invasive technique to pick up olfactory epithelium from the olfactory mucosa which is thereafter analyzed by real-time quaking-induced conversion (RT-QuIC) assay. This method has a high sensitiviy (97%) and specificity (100%) for Creutzfeldt–Jakob disease (a neurodegenerative disease) diagnosis [10].

In addition to Parkinson's disease, other neurodegenerative disorders such as Alzheimer's disease and Amyotrophic Lateral Sclerosis are characterized by accumulation of particular proteins in cellular aggregates.

α-Syn is an important molecule of the synapse, under physiologic conditions it regulates synaptic function in its soluble form. In PD patient brains monomers form amyloid-β sheet fibrils that aggregate into Lewy bodies [11]. These presynaptic alterations mediated by accumulation of α-Syn change the size of vesicle pools and function of vesicles, impair neurotransmitter exocytosis, vesicle recycling and neural communication [2].

5. Neuroinflammation and Parkinson's disease

Injury, environmental toxins, endogenous proteins, infection or age cause microglia to become activated and release of inflammatory cytokines such as IL1-β, TNF-α, nitric oxide (NO) and reactive oxygen species (ROS) that cause dopaminergic neuronal deterioration. Damaged neurons further stimulate microglia by α-Syn, ATP and ROS [12]. The events related with neuroinflammation are summarized in **Figure 2**.

Neuroinflammation has been implicated in DA cell loss during Parkinson's disease [13]. In experiments conducted on rats and mice Kurkowska and colleagues have shown that dexamethasone treatment prevented striatal DA depletion and protected DA neurons in substantia nigra (SN) [14].

Aspirin given orally increases the expression of tyrosine hydroxylase in the nigra and upregulates DA in the striatum in both normal and α-syn transgenic mice, indometacin on the other hand, protects neurons in the 1-methyl-4-phenyl-1,2,3,6-tetrahydropyridine (MPTP) model of PD and diminishes microglial activation in the effected area [15, 16].

COX-2 inhibitor celecoxib has also been found to be effective in rats injected with 6-hydroxydopamine (6-OHDA) in the striata, a method that caused retrograde neuronal damage, by reducing DA cell degeneration [17].

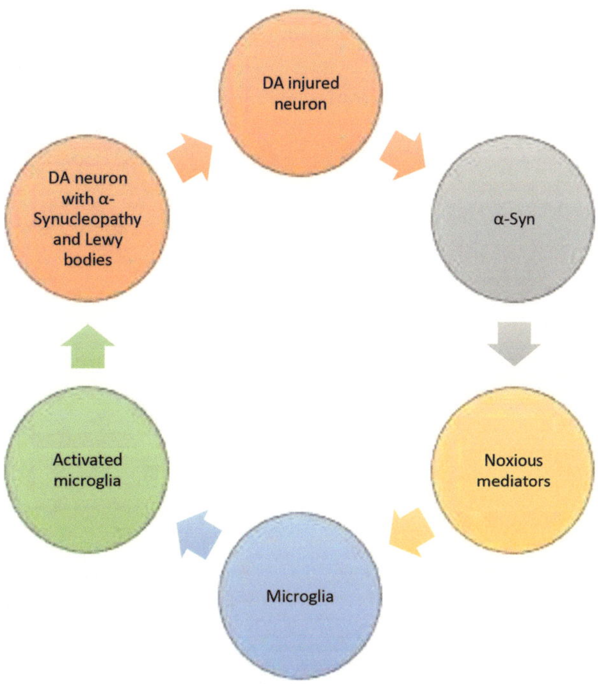

Figure 2.
Stressed DA neurons and release of irritating mediators and producing a vicious cycle [8].

In addition to these drugs, the antiinflammatory cytokine IL-10 and peroxisome proliferator-activated receptor gamma (PPAR-γ) ligand rosiglitazone have been found effective in 6-OHDA rat and MPTP mouse models of PD [18, 19].

However, unlike animal studies there are conflicting results in human reports. While several epidemiologic studies reported that the use of non-steroidal anti-inflammatory drugs (NSAIDs) decrease the risk of PD [20], recent metaanalyses found no association between NSAIDs and the risk of Parkinson's disease [21, 22].

6. Parkinson's disease and valproic acid

Valproic acid (VPA) is an inhibitor of histone deacetylases (HDACs), and has been used in the treatment of epilepsy, migraine, schizophrenia and bipolar

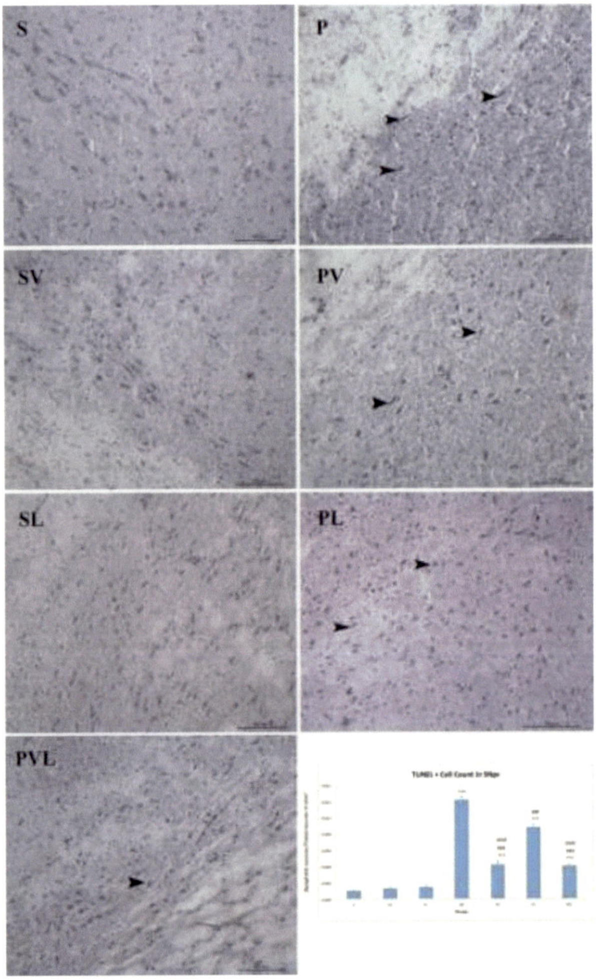

Figure 3.
*Photomicrographs demonstrate TUNEL positive neurons and graph comparing TUNEL positive neurons in right substantia nigra pars compacta. Sham operated (S), sham operated and VPA treated (SV), sham operated and L-DOPA treated (SL), Nigrally 6-OHDA injected (PD), Nigrally 6-OHDA injected and VPA treated (PV), Nigrally 6-OHDA injected and L-DOPA treated (PL), Nigrally 6-OHDA injected and VPA and L-DOPA treated (PVL) groups. Apoptotic neuron (TUNEL positive neuron) is demonstrated with arrow. The magnification is x20. Scale bar represents 100 μm. Nigrally 6-OHDA injected and VPA and L-DOPA treated (PVL) groups. Data are presented as percentage of apoptotic neurons in right substantia nigra pars compacta compared to total neurons in right substantia nigra pars compacta. Data are expressed as mean ± SEM. ***$p < 0.001$ vs. S, SV, SL; ###$p < 0.001$ vs. PD; ΘΘΘ$p<0.001$ v PL.*

disorders [23]. It increases GABA activity, blocks Ca++ and Na + channels and decreases N-methyl-D-aspartate (NMDA) mediated excitation [24, 25].

In a study conducted in our laboratory, VPA was found to be effective in a PD model induced by 6-OHDA injected into the SN of rats. Sham operated animals demonstrated trace amounts of apoptotic neurons, 6-OHDA caused significantly increased amounts of TUNEL positive neurons in susbstantia nigra pars compacta as compared with sham operated groups. Valproic acid treatment significantly diminished the apoptotic neurons in susbstantia nigra pars compacta as compared with 6-OHDA lesioned and saline treated animals. Valproic acid treatment also significantly diminished the apoptotic neurons as compared with 6-OHDA lesioned and levodopa treated animals [26]. The results of the experiment have been illustrated in **Figure 3**.

The neuroprotective effects of VPA could be associated with the glycogen synthase kinase-3 (GSK3) alpha and beta, Akt, ERK and phosphoinositol pathways, tricarboxylic acid cycle, GABA and oxidative phosphorylation (OXPHOS) system [27].

7. Parkinson's disease and therapeutic aids

Parkinson patients are being treated with DA precursor L-DOPA that increases the synthesis of dopamine in the substantia nigra; Catechol-O-methyltransferase (COMT) inhibitors that increase the central uptake of levodopa (entecapone, talcapone), Monoamine oxidase B inhibitors (MAO-B inhibitors) that decrease the metabolism of dopamine (selegiline, rasagiline) and finally D1 and D2 receptor agonists pramipexole and ropinirole.

However, chronic use of dopaminergic medications in the treatment of Parkinson's disease (PD) might cause some motor and non-motor behavioral side effects such as dyskinesias, impulse control disorders (ICDs), (uncontrollable gambling, shopping, binge eating, hypersexuality), punding (aimless, stereotypical repetitive behaviors) and compulsive medication use [28]. The prevalence of ICDs in PD patients using dopamine agonists was reported to range from 2.6% to 34.8% [29]. This brings us to another significant function of dopamine which is IMPULSIVITY.

8. Dopamine and impulsivity

Impulsivity implicates a variety of behaviors that are unsuitable or overly risky, immature, poorly planned, and often results with undesired consequences. Impulsivity is the main symptom of a wide range of psychiatric disorders such as ICDs and drug addiction. Moreover, attention deficit hyperactivity disorder (ADHD) and mania, also contribute to the expression of impulsivity [30]. It is thought that dopamine has an important role in impulsive behavior, based on the therapeutic effects of psychostimulant drugs such as amphetamine and methylphenidate that increase dopaminergic transmission in attention deficit hyperactivity disorder. Namely, there is a paradox regarding why dopamine releasing psychostimulant drugs ameliorate ADHD symptoms, while the drugs that enhance dopamine transmission increase impulsivity, as in the case of medication induced adverse reactions in PD. This discrepancy means that other neurotransmitters also influence impulsivity [31].

The dopamine system and D2 receptors seem to be closely related to impulsive choice. The activation of D2 receptors in the nucleus accumbens region causes an increase in motor impulsivity. There are many studies highlighting the relationship between serotonin, norepinephrine and dopamine dysregulation and impulse control disorders. Particularly, studies with human and animal subjects demonstrated the role of serotonin and dopamine in impulsivity. The importance of serotonin and dopamine interaction in the nucleus accumbens is underlined for impulse control disorders [32, 33].

9. Dopamine and attention deficit hyperactivity disorder

ADHD is one of the most common psychiatric disorders of childhood which is characterized by problems in attention, concentration, mobility and impulse control. Dopamine and noradrenaline levels are low and dysregulated in ADHD and it is thought that symptoms of inattention may indicate dopamine and/or noradrenaline dysfunction in important regions of the cerebral cortex that control cognitive functions [34]. Neuroanatomical regions (cortical-striatal-thalamic-cortical network) that are thought to be important in ADHD are regions known to be the area of dopamine concentration.

Dopamine and norepinephrine are the most well studied neurotransmitters in understanding the etiology of ADHD. These neurotransmitters and their degradation products are found at a lower rate in the cerebrospinal fluid (CSF), blood and urine of children with ADHD. Molecular genetics and neuroimaging studies, as well as therapies with stimulant drugs, have also supported the hypothesis of dopamine dysfunction in ADHD etiology. The fact that methylphenidate, which acts by preventing dopamine reuptake in ADHD pharmacotherapy, has brought the dopaminergic system to the fore in candidate gene studies. Molecular genetic studies have indicated some candidate genes related to the dopamine system, such as D1, D2, D3, D4 and D5 receptors and dopamine transporters (DAT). Among these, the genes that are most emphasized and with positive findings are DRD4 (D4) and DAT1 genes (**Table 1**).

Since stimulant drugs provide increase in extracellular DA by blocking DAT, molecular neuroimaging studies have mostly focused on the DAT [34]. In the meta-analysis of positron emission tomography (PET) and single photon emission computed tomography (SPECT) studies, higher striatal DAT density was reported in patients with ADHD [35].

Receptor	**Enzyme-Transporter**
Dopamin D1 receptor gene (DRD1)	Tyrosine hydroxylase gene (TH)
Dopamin D2 receptor gene (DRD2)	Catechol-O-methyl- transferase gene (COMT)
Dopamin D3 receptor gene (DRD3)	Monoaminoxidase A gene (MAO-A)
Dopamin D4 receptor gene (DRD4)	Dopamine transporter gene (DAT1/SLC6A3)
Dopamin D5 receptor gene (DRD5)	

Table 1.
Candidate genes studied in the dopaminergic pathway.

10. Dopamine and addiction

Addiction is defined as seeking and using substances and chemicals such as alcohol, cannabis, morphine, metamphetamine, nicotine despite their physical and psychological negative effects on individuals. The negative effects are characterized by having trouble in stopping the intake after starting to use and by causing negative emotional states such as dysphoria, anxiety and irritability in case of discontinuation. In addition to addiction, these substances cause changes in the reward system, decision-making, memory and brain structures related to memory.

The mesocorticolimbic system, which is formed by the integration of mesolimbic and mesocortical pathways, is an important part of the reward system and dopamine (DA) is the main neurotransmitter in this system. The addictive substances essentially activate the mesolimbic dopamine pathway. Apart from the mesocorticolimbic system, another dopaminergic pathway, the nigrostriatal pathway also plays a role in addiction development.

There is good evidence that synaptic changes in mesolimbic pathways are involved in food and drug addiction. Namely, drug addiction and obesity are related to decreased striatal dopamine D2 receptor levels [36, 37]. Decreased D2 receptor levels in the striatum was also reported in patients with alcohol dependence [38]. In addition, lower striatal dopamine D2/D3 receptor levels were reported in cocaine and metamphetamine addicted subjects [39].

Even though the drugs that enhance DA activity could be effective for alcohol and/or substance use disorders, contradictory results have been reported by several studies. Hence, there is not enough evidence regarding the use of DA agonists for addiction [40].

11. Dopamine and schizophrenia

The neurotransmitter systems that have been investigated in schizophrenia are dopamine, noradrenaline, serotonin, glutamate and GABA. The most well-studied neurotransmitter in schizophrenia is dopamine. The fact that psychostimulant agents that increase dopamine activity such as amphetamine and cocaine cause schizophrenia-like symptoms in normal individuals and that neuroleptics that block postsynaptic dopamine D2 receptors regress the symptoms of schizophrenia supports the dopamine hypothesis. Overactivation of the dopaminergic neurons in the mesolimbic pathway is thought to play a role in the emergence of delusions and hallucinations, which are positive symptoms of psychosis. Neuroreceptor imaging studies indicated the higher levels of dopamine D2 receptor availability in individuals with schizophrenia [36]. The main mechanism of action of the current antipsychotic drugs is the antagonism of mainly dopaminergic D2 receptors [41].

12. Conclusion

As can be observed easily dopamine is involved in the pathogenesis of many conditions such as Parkinson's disease, Schizophrenia and Attention Deficit Hyperactivity Disorder. It is the key substance for impulsivity and addiction as well.

Author details

Mehveş Ece Genç* and Emine Nur Özdamar
Faculty of Medicine, Department of Medical Pharmacology, Yeditepe University, İstanbul, Turkey

*Address all correspondence to: egenc@yeditepe.edu.tr

References

[1] Seidl SE, Potashkin JA. The promise of neuroprotective agents in Parkinson's disease. Front Neurol. 2011;NOV(November):1-19.

[2] Bridi JC, Hirth F. Mechanisms of alpha-Synuclein Induced Synaptopathy in Parkinson's Disease. Front Neurosci. 2018;12:80.

[3] Ball N, Teo WP, Chandra S, Chapman J. Parkinson's disease and the environment. Front. Neurol 2019; 10: 218.DOI: 10.3389/fneur.2019.00218

[4] Gillies GE, Pienaar IS, Vohra S, Qamhawi Z. Sex differences in Parkinson's disease. Frontiers in Neuroendocrinology 2014;35: 370-384.

[5] Pringsheim T, Jette N, Frolkis A, Steeves TD. The prevalence of Parkinson's disease: a systematic review and meta-analysis. Mov Disord. 2014;29(13):1583-90.

[6] Balestrino R, Schapira AHV. Parkinson disease. Eur J Neurol 2020;27(1):27-42.

[7] Doty RL, Kamath V. The influences of age on olfaction: a review. Front Psychol. 2014;5:20.

[8] Niu H, Shen L, Li T, Ren C, Ding S, Wang L, et al. Alpha-synuclein overexpression in the olfactory bulb initiates prodromal symptoms and pathology of Parkinson ' s disease. 2018;1-17.

[9] Brozzetti L, Sacchetto L, Cecchini MP, Avesani A, Perra D, Bongianni M, et al. Neurodegeneration-Associated Proteins in Human Olfactory Neurons Collected by Nasal Brushing. Front Neurosci. 2020;14.

[10] Behaeghe O, Mangelschots E, De Vil B, Cras B. A systematic review comparing the diagnostic value of 14-3-3 protein in the cerebrospinal fluid, RT-QuIC and RT-QuIC on nasal brushing in sporadic Creutzfeldt–Jakob disease. Acta Neurol Belg 2018;118: 395-403

[11] Lashuel HA, Overk CR, Oueslati A, Masliah E. The many faces of α-synuclein: From structure and toxicity to therapeutic target. Nat Rev Neurosci [Internet]. 2013;14(1):38-48. Available from: http://dx.doi.org/10.1038/nrn3406

[12] Collins LM, Toulouse A, Connor TJ, Nolan YM. Contributions of central and systemic inflammation to the pathophysiology of Parkinson's disease. Neuropharmacology [Internet]. 2012;62[7]:2154-68. Available from: http://dx.doi.org/10.1016/j.neuropharm.2012.01.028

[13] Cebrián C, Sulzer D. Neuroinflammation as a Potential Mechanism Underlying Parkinsons Disease. Parkinsons Dis [Internet]. 2017 Jan 1 [cited 2020 Jan 8];245-79. Available from: https://www.sciencedirect.com/science/article/pii/B9780128037836000080

[14] Kurkowska-Jastrzębska I, Litwin T, Joniec I, Ciesielska A, Przybyłkowski A, Członkowski A, et al. Dexamethasone protects against dopaminergic neurons damage in a mouse model of Parkinson's disease. Int Immunopharmacol [Internet]. 2004;4(10):1307-18. Available from: http://www.sciencedirect.com/science/article/pii/S1567576904001535

[15] Rangasamy SB, Dasarathi S, Pahan P, Jana M, Pahan K. Low-Dose Aspirin Upregulates Tyrosine Hydroxylase and Increases Dopamine Production in Dopaminergic Neurons: Implications for Parkinson's Disease. J Neuroimmune Pharmacol. 2019;14[2]:173-87.

[16] Kurkowska-Jastrzębska I, Babiuch M, Joniec I, Przybyłkowski A, Członkowski A, Członkowska A. Indomethacin protects against neurodegeneration caused by MPTP intoxication in mice. Int Immunopharmacol. 2002;2[8]:1213-8.

[17] Sánchez-Pernaute R, Ferree A, Cooper O, Yu M, Brownell AL, Isacson O. Selective COX-2 inhibition prevents progressive dopamine neuron degeneration in a rat model of Parkinson's disease. J Neuroinflammation. 2004;1:1-11.

[18] Johnston LC, Su X, Maguire-Zeiss K, Horovitz K, Ankoudinova I, Guschin D, et al. Human interleukin-10 gene transfer is protective in a rat model of parkinson's disease. Mol Ther. 2008;16[8]:1392-9.

[19] Schintu N, Frau L, Ibba M, Caboni P, Garau A, Carboni E, et al. PPAR-gamma-mediated neuroprotection in a chronic mouse model of Parkinson's disease. Eur J Neurosci. 2009;29(5):954-63.

[20] Gagne JJ, Power MC. Anti-inflammatory drugs and risk of Parkinson disease A meta-analysis. Neurology 2010; 74: 995-1002.

[21] Poly TN, Islam MR, Yang HC, Jack Li YC. Non-steroidal anti-inflammatory drugs and risk of Parkinson's disease in the elderly population: a meta-analysis. European Journal of Clinical Pharmacology 2019; 75: 99-108.

[22] Alharbi BA, Ghazali JS, Alatwi NA, Alghamdi WM, Alqahtani RM, Alqahtani MM, et al. Non-steroidal anti-inflammatory drugs and Parkinson's disease: a systematic review and metaanalysis. Ann Med Health Sci Res. 2020;10: 1023-1028.

[23] Lai CL, Lu CC, Lin HC, Sung YF, Wu YP, Hong JS, et al. Valproate is protective against 6-OHDA-induced dopaminergic neurodegeneration in rodent midbrain: A potential role of BDNF up-regulation. J Formos Med Assoc [Internet]. 2019;118(1P3):420-8. Available from: https://doi.org/10.1016/j.jfma.2018.06.017

[24] Macdonald RL, Bergey GK. Valproic acid augments GABA-mediated postsynaptic inhibition in cultured mammalian neurons. Brain Res. 1979 Jul;170(3):558-62.

[25] Macdonald RL, Kelly KM. Antiepileptic drug mechanisms of action. Epilepsia. 1995;36 Suppl 2:S2-12.

[26] Dagdelen M, Cumbul A, Uslu U, Gene E. P.1.g.065 Apoptosis in a 6-hydroxydopamine rat model of Parkinson's disease: impact of valproic acid. Eur Neuropsychopharmacol [Internet]. 2014 Oct 1 [cited 2020 Jan 29];24:S241. Available from: https://www.sciencedirect.com/science/article/pii/S0924977X14703761?via%3Dihub

[27] Christian Machado Ximenes J, Crisóstomo Lima Verde E, da Graça Naffah-Mazzacoratti M, Socorro de Barros Viana G. Valproic Acid, a Drug with Multiple Molecular Targets Related to Its Potential Neuroprotective Action. Neurosci Med. 2012;03(01):107-23.

[28] Voon V, Napier C, Frank M, Sgambato-Faure V, Grace AA, Rodriguez-Oroz M, Obeso J, Bezard E, Fernagut PO. Impulse control disorders and dyskinesias in Parkinson's disease: an update. The Lancet Neurology 2017; 16(3): 238-250. DOI: 10.1016/S1474-4422(17)30004-2

[29] Grall-Bronnec M, Victorri-Vigneau C, Donnio Y, Leboucher J, Rousselet M, Thiabaud E, Zreika N, Derkinderen P Challet-Bouju G. Dopamine agonists and impulse control disorders: a complex association. Drug Saf 2018; 41: 19-75. DOI: 10.1007/s40264-017-0590-6

[30] Hollander E, Evers M. New developments in impulsivity. The Lancet 2001; 358(9286): 949-950. DOI: 10.1016/S0140-6736(01)06114-1

[31] Dalley JW, Roiser JP. Dopamine, serotonin and impulsivity. Neuroscience 2012; 215: 42-58. DOI: 10.1016/j.neuroscience.2012.03.065

[32] Arce E, Santisteban C. Impulsivity: a review. Psicothema 2006;18[2]: 213-220.

[33] Winstanley CA, Theobald DEH, Dalley JW, Robbins TW. Interactions between serotonin and dopamine in the control of impulsive choice in rats: therapeutic implications for impulse control disorders. Neuropsychopharmacology 2005; 30: 669-682. DOI: 10.1038/sj.npp.1300610

[34] Del Campo N, Chamberlain SR, Sahakian BJ, Robbins TW. The roles of dopamine and noradrenaline in the pathophysiology and treatment of attention-deficit/hyperactivity disorder. Biol Psychiatry 2011;69:e145–e157. DOI: 10.1016/j.biopsych.2011.02.036

[35] Faraone SV. The pharmacology of amphetamine and methylphenidate: relevance to the neurobiology of attention-deficit/hyperactivity disorder and other psychiatric comorbidities. Neuroscience and Biobehavioral Reviews 2018; 87: 255-270. DOI: 10.1016/j.neubiorev.2018.02.001

[36] Klein MO, Battagello DS, Cardoso AR, Hauser DN, Bittencourt JC, Correa RG. Dopamine: functions, signaling, and association with neurological diseases. Cellular and Molecular Neurobiology 2019; 39: 31-59. DOI: 10.1007/s10571-018-0632-3

[37] Kenny PJ, Voren G, Johnson PM. Dopamine D2 receptors and striatopallidal transmission in addiction and obesity. Curr Opin Neurobiol. 2013; 23(4): 535-538. DOI:10.1016/j.conb.2013.04.012.

[38] Martinez D, Gil R, Slifstein M, Hwang DR, Huang Y, Perez A, Kegeles L, Talbot P Evans S, Krystal J, Laruelle M, Abi-Dargham A. Alcohol dependence is associated with blunted dopamine transmission in the ventral striatum. Biol Psychiatry 2005;58:779-786. DOI: 10.1016/j.biopsych.2005.04.044

[39] Nutt, DJ, Lingford-Hughes A., Erritzoe D, Stokes, P. The dopamine theory of addiction: 40 years of highs and lows. Nature Reviews Neuroscience 2015; 16: 305-312. DOI: https://doi.org/10.1038/nrn3939

[40] Diana M. The dopamine hypothesis of drug addiction and its potential therapeutic value. Front Psychiatry. 2011;2:64. DOI: 10.3389/fpsyt.2011.00064.

[41] Li P, Snyder GL, Vanover KE. Dopamine Targeting Drugs for the Treatment of Schizophrenia: Past, Present and Future. Curr Top Med Chem. 2016;16(29):3385-3403. DOI: 10.2174/1568026616666160608084834.